Translational Medicine Research

Translational medicine converts promising laboratory discoveries into clinical applications and elucidates clinical questions with the use of bench work, aiming to facilitate the prediction, prevention, diagnosis and treatment of diseases. The development of translational medicine will accelerate disease control and the process of finding solutions to key health problems. It is a multidisciplinary endeavor that integrates research from the medical sciences, basic sciences and social sciences, with the aim of optimizing patient care and preventive measures that may extend beyond health care services. Therefore, close and international collaboration between all parties involved is essential to the advancement of translational medicine.

To enhance the aforementioned international collaboration as well as to provide a forum for communication and cross-pollenation between basic, translational and clinical research practitioners from all relevant established and emerging disciplines, the book series "Translational Medicine Research" features original and observational investigations in the broad fields of laboratory, clinical and public health research, aiming to provide practical and up-to-date information on significant research from all subspecialties of medicine and to broaden readers' vision horizons, from bench to bed and bed to bench.

Produced in close collaboration with National Infrastructures for Translational Medicine (Shanghai), the largest translational medicine research center in China, the book series offers a state-of-the-art resource for physicians and researchers alike who are interested in the rapidly evolving field of translational medicine. Prof. Zhu Chen, the Editor-in-Chief of the series, is a hematologist at Shanghai Jiao Tong University, China's former Minister of Health, and chairman of the center's scientific advisory board.

Allan I. Pack • Qing Yun Li
Editors

Sleep and its Disorders

Translational Medicine

Springer

上海交通大學出版社
SHANGHAI JIAO TONG UNIVERSITY PRESS

Editors
Allan I. Pack
John Miclot Professor, Division of Sleep Medicine
University of Pennsylvania
Philadelphia, PA, USA

Qing Yun Li
Department of Pulmonary and Critical Care Medicine
Ruijin Hospital, Shanghai Jiaotong University School of Medicine
Shanghai, China

ISSN 2451-991X ISSN 2451-9928 (electronic)
Translational Medicine Research
ISBN 978-94-024-2166-8 ISBN 978-94-024-2168-2 (eBook)
https://doi.org/10.1007/978-94-024-2168-2

Jointly published with Shanghai Jiao Tong University Press

This Springer imprint is published by the registered company Springer Nature B.V.
The registered company address is: Van Godewijckstraat 30, 3311 GX Dordrecht, The Netherlands

Contents

Part I Basic Sleep Mechanisms

1 Evolving Approaches to Identifying Genetic Risk Variants for Sleep Disorders 3
Allan I. Pack

2 Neurobiology of Sleep–Wake Control 21
Leszek Kubin

3 Prostaglandins, Adenosine, and Histaminergic System in the Regulation of Sleep and Wakefulness 49
Zhi-Li Huang, Ze Zhang, and Wei-Min Qu

4 Sleep and Neuronal Plasticity 71
Marcos G. Frank

Part II Insufficient Sleep and Its Consequences

5 Epidemiology of Insufficient Sleep 95
Michael A. Grandner

6 Social Factors in Insufficient Sleep 115
Mathias Basner

7 Sleep Loss and the Unfolded Protein Response 127
Nirinjini Naidoo

Part III Sleep Apnea

8 Biological and Genetic Mechanisms of Sleepiness in Obstructive Sleep Apnea and Cardiovascular Disease 151
Victoria M. Pak

9 Diaphragm EMG Recording and Its Application in Sleep Medicine 163
Ying-Mei Luo and Yuan-Ming Luo

10 Chronic Intermittent Hypoxia in Patients with OSA 177
Qing Yun Li, Chen Juan Gu, Ying Ni Lin, and Qiong Wang

11 Neural Injury in Models of Intermittent Hypoxia 209
Sigrid C. Veasey

Part IV Narcolepsy

12 Narcolepsy and Orexin/Hypocretin 229
Fu Long Xiao, Jun Zhang, and Fang Han

Part V Circadian Rhythm Disorders

13 Circadian Rhythm Sleep–Wake Disorders: Mechanisms and Treatment 265
Sabra M. Abbott and Phyllis C. Zee

Part I
Basic Sleep Mechanisms

Chapter 1
Evolving Approaches to Identifying Genetic Risk Variants for Sleep Disorders

Allan I. Pack

Abstract There has been recent substantial progress in elucidating gene variants that confer risk for common sleep disorders, and also for those associated with different quantitative aspects of the sleep/circadian phenotype. The major strategy employed has been genome-wide association studies (GWAS). Initially, the approach was to recruit and phenotype large numbers of cases with specific sleep disorders and controls. This was used to identify gene variants conferring risk for Restless Legs Syndrome (RLS) and narcolepsy. This approach is, however, time-consuming and expensive. Newer approaches have involved establishing biobanks with large numbers of subjects with a variety of disorders and controls, all of whom are genotyped. One of the most successful such efforts has been the UK Biobank. Studies using data from the UK Biobank have led to successful GWAS for sleep duration, chronotype, excessive sleepiness, and insomnia. The challenge is that the phenotype data are quite limited. Moreover, the UK Biobank has large numbers of relatively healthy subjects so the prevalence of any specific disorder is low. This approach has been complemented by development of large biobanks based on specific health systems in which patients have given blood samples for genotyping. These biobanks have a much larger prevalence of disorders, including sleep disorders. The use of these biobanks for a specific disorder requires development of algorithms to identify individuals with a specific disorder using data in the electronic health record (EHR). This approach is starting to be used for the study of variants conferring risk for specific sleep disorders. Results from GWAS are being used to develop polygenic risk scores (PRS) for specific disorders. This, when combined with other information, can be used to predict who will develop specific disorders, opening the opportunity for prevention.

Keywords Genetics · GWAS · PheWAS · UK Biobank · FinnGen · Big data · Sleep duration · Insomnia · Obstructive sleep apnea · Chronotype

---

A. I. Pack (✉)
Translational Research Laboratories, Division of Sleep Medicine, Department of Medicine, Perelman School of Medicine, University of Pennsylvania, Philadelphia, PA, USA
e-mail: pack@pennmedicine.upenn.edu

A. I. Pack, Q. Y. Li (eds.), *Sleep and its Disorders*, Translational Medicine Research,
https://doi.org/10.1007/978-94-024-2168-2_1

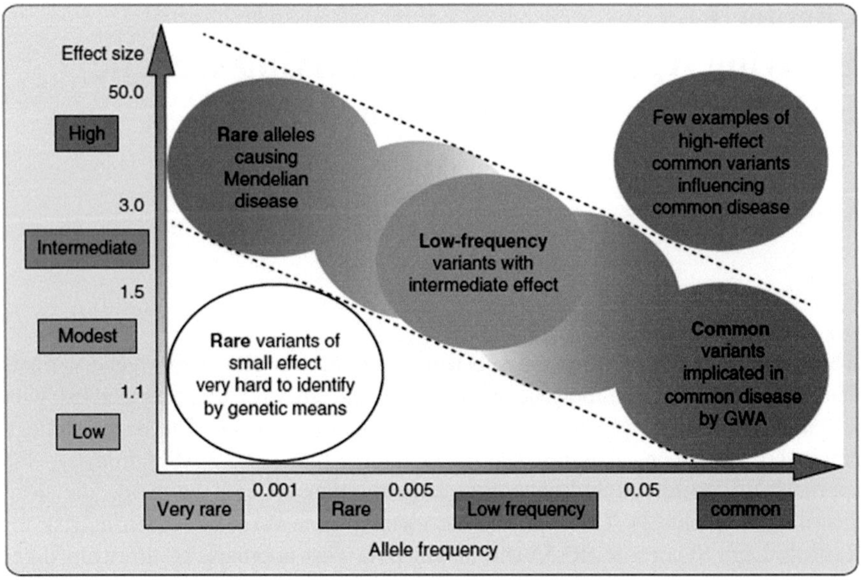

Fig. 1.1 Diagram illustrating the concept of common and rare variants. The plot shows the frequency of the allele (x-axis) and effect size for the allele on the phenotype of interest. Common alleles (bottom right) have, in general, a low effect size. There are examples including narcolepsy where common variants have large effect sizes since it makes the individual susceptible to a particular environmental challenge. Rare variants (left side) typically have large effects on the phenotype [From Manolio et al. (2009) with permission]

There are rapidly evolving approaches and resources to identify genetic variants that provide risk for, or protection against, common sleep disorders. Moreover, since almost all aspects of sleep are heritable (Pack et al. 2021), there are efforts to understand the genetic regulation of sleep in humans. In considering genetic approaches, it is helpful to think about common variants with small effects and rare variants with large effects (Manolio et al. 2009) (see Fig. 1.1). Common variants occur in >5% of the population. A single common variant has a small effect with an odds ratio typically in the range of 1.1–1.4. There are examples where common variants have a large effect size. This typically occurs when the variant makes the individual susceptible to an environmental challenge. Many individuals can have this variant but not have the disorder, since they have not been exposed to the relevant challenge. Rare variants occur typically in <1% of the population. Each rare variant has a large effect on the relevant phenotype. While each variant is rare, there are a lot of them. Different variants can occur in the same gene and there are statistical approaches to allow analysis of all such variants combined. Common and rare variants conferring risk for a particular disorder can occur in the same genes, i.e., there are mutation hot spots. The variants being discussed here are single nucleotide polymorphisms (SNPs). Common variants typically occur in introns or in the regulatory region of the gene. Rare variants with large effects are typically in exons, i.e., in protein coding regions of the gene. Exon sequencing that is now routine assesses the presence of these variants across the whole genome. In addition to SNPs, copy number variants (CNVs) including insertions and deletions of genomic regions (Conrad et al. 2010; Redon et al. 2006) provide additional mechanisms for genetic underpinnings of disease.

Currently, the major approach to identifying variants of genes conferring risk for, or protection to, sleep disorders, and that associate with various aspects of the sleep phenotype is using a genome-wide association study (GWAS). The first GWAS was published in 2005 for macular degeneration (Klein et al. 2005). There has been an explosion of GWAS with the availability of online resources that catalog results of previous GWAS (Welter et al. 2014; Visscher et al. 2012; MacArthur et al. 2017).

The first major GWAS for a sleep disorder was in 2007 for Restless Legs Syndrome (Winkelmann et al. 2007; Stefansson et al. 2007). There were in that year publications from Germany/Canada (Winkelmann et al. 2007) and from Iceland (Stefansson et al. 2007). The German study was based on a detailed questionnaire (Allen et al. 2003), while in Iceland use was made of leg actigrams to evaluate periodic limb movements during sleep (Allen et al. 2003). The latter allowed identification of risk variants associated with the motor component of RLS rather than the sensory component. The two studies identified the same risk variants in BTDP9 and MEIS1. The prevailing strategy for GWAS at the time was to assemble large numbers of well-studied cases and controls. This had the advantage that the phenotype was rigorously defined and in-depth phenotyping of subjects was possible. However, it was time-consuming and expensive to recruit and study the large sample of participants that is required to protect against false-positive associations. The findings from these GWAS in RLS have been replicated in many subsequent studies (Kemlink et al. 2009; Yang et al. 2011; Moore et al. 2014).

GWAS has also been used to study the genetics of narcolepsy. It has long been known that a particular HLA antigen has been implicated as conferring risk for narcolepsy, i.e., DQB1*0602 (Juji et al. 1984). Recent data from the European Narcolepsy Network showed a very robust association with narcolepsy cases with cataplexy and DQB1*0602 in multiple European countries (see Table 1.1) (Tafti et al. 2014). The odds ratio averaged across countries is 251. But the genetic variant is common occurring in 6.93–24.32% of controls without narcolepsy in different European countries (Tafti et al. 2014). The average occurrence in controls is 17.68%. Thus, this is an example of a common variant with a large effect. It makes individuals susceptible to an environmental challenge such as a particular infection or particular type of influenza vaccine.

DQB1*0602 is, however, not the only genetic risk factor. Given how robust this effect is makes it difficult to identify other genetic risk factors. Hallmayer et al. (2009) did an innovative GWAS (see Fig. 1.2) to address this challenge. They recruited cases with narcolepsy and cataplexy and controls but all had the DQB1*0602 variant, i.e., in both cases and controls. They did so in multiple ethnic groups (see Fig. 1.2). They then applied a GWAS analysis and identified variants in the T cell receptor alpha locus as conferring risk for narcolepsy with cataplexy. The finding was replicated in most groups but did not replicate in African Americans; this

Table 1.1 Association in European countries with DQB1*0602 in cases with narcolepsy and cataplexy

Country (case, control)	Case-DQB1+N (%)	Control-DQBI+N (%)	OR	*p*
DE (232, 296)	227 (97.84)	72 (24.3.2)	141.24	9.71E-26
CH (66, 473)	65 (98.48)	102 (21.56)	236.42	7.01E-8
NL (323, 469)	318 (98.45)	114 (24.31)	198.05	3.62E-30
PL (63, 197)	63 (100)	44 (22.33)	438.08	2.65E-09
SP (127, 1174)	126 (99.21)	170 (14.48)	744.14	5.25E-11
FR (341, 499)	335 (98.24)	94 (18.84)	240.56	1.18R-37
IT (66, 433)	64 (96.97)	30 (6.93)	429.87	3.21E-16
Mantel-Haenszel (meta-analysis)	1198 (98.36)	626 (17.68)	251.12	1.04E-120

DE Germany, *CH* Switzerland, *NL* Netherlands, *PL*, Poland, *SP* Spain, *FR* France, *IT* Italy, *OR* odds ratio

The frequency of DQB1*0602 in cases and controls with OR for increased risk and the *p*-value for the association are shown [From Tafti et al. (2014) with permission]

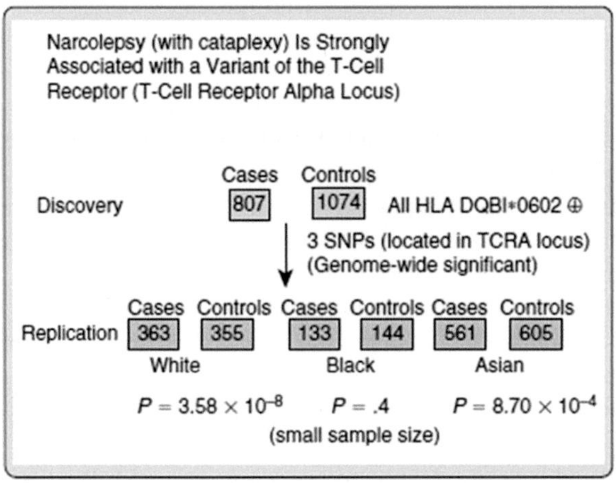

Fig. 1.2 Design of a genome-wide association study to identify variants other than HLA DQB1*0602 that confer risk for narcolepsy. To do so, all cases and controls were positive for this variant. There was an initial discovery phase with 807 cases and 1074 controls that identified 3 SNPs in the T cell alpha locus that had a genome-wide significant association. This finding was replicated in separate samples of White subjects and Asians but not in African Americans. The latter had the smallest sample size [From Hallmayer et al. (2009) with permission]

may be the result of the much smaller sample size in this group. This result adds further evidence that narcolepsy is an autoimmune disorder with a specific antigen-presenting HLA and a specific subtype of a T cell receptor.

Thus, this initial approach to GWAS led to a significant new understanding of genetic risk for RLS and narcolepsy/cataplexy. The expense and time-consuming nature of the subject recruitment has led to development of new approaches but still using GWAS, as will now be described.

1.1 UK Biobank

An initial large-scale GWAS examined in one study genetic risks for seven common diseases using 14,000 cases and 3000 controls (Wellcome Trust Case Control Consortium 2007). This study was supported by the Wellcome Trust in the United Kingdom. Subsequently, the Wellcome Trust funded the UK Biobank. The study recruited approximately 500,000 individuals in the United Kingdom. Participants provided samples for extraction of DNA, as well as other blood samples, filled out questionnaires, and their medical records were available in their electronic health records. Initially, genotyping was done using arrays to assess common SNP variants. More recently, exome sequencing data are becoming available. Whole-genome sequencing data will be available in the future. The remarkable aspect of this program is that all of these data (genetic, phenotypes) are shared with the international research community who can apply for access. The UK Biobank provides the data in a download. They have realized that this requires large-scale computing resources at institutions receiving the data. They are working to provide mechanisms for investigators at institutions without such computer resources to do analyses on the computers provided by the UK Biobank.

The questionnaires used to phenotype individuals are broad and lack depth in any particular area. There are, however, more in-depth phenotyping in a subset of subjects. Approximately 100,000 individuals were studied with an accelerometer. While not originally intended to provide estimates of sleep duration, this can be obtained from the data obtained (van Hees et al. 2018). Approximately the same number of subjects have had extensive imaging studies, e.g., brain MRIs, and these data can also be obtained by interested investigators. Currently, there are no data on objectively studied sleep, an area of opportunity.

There is a similar program now being developed in the United States. This was initially called the Precision Medicine Initiative, now the All of US Program. The vision is to evaluate multiple chronic diseases and to use wearables to phenotype the 1.0 million subjects who are to be recruited (Collins and Varmus 2015). Given the rapid advances in wearables to study sleep (Chinoy et al. 2021), including continuous remote assessment of EEG, sleep is ideally positioned to be assessed in these developing efforts.

Despite the current lack of in-depth information on participants in the UK Biobank, this resource has contributed greatly to elucidating the genetic basis of sleep and circadian rhythm. There have been successful GWAS for the following: chronotype (Jones et al. 2019a; Lane et al. 2016; Hu et al. 2016; Kalmbach et al. 2017), sleep duration based on self-report (Jones et al. 2016; Lane et al. 2017; Dashti et al. 2019; Doherty et al. 2018), sleep duration assessed objectively from data obtained by accelerometers (Dashti et al. 2019; Doherty et al. 2018; Jones et al.

2019b), excessive sleepiness (Wang et al. 2019), and insomnia (Lane et al. 2017, 2019; Jansen et al. 2019).

There have been three separate GWAS to assess variants associated with chronotype (Jones et al. 2019a; Lane et al. 2016; Hu et al. 2016) [for review, see Kalmbach et al. (2017)]. The studies that have been conducted involved data from the UK Biobank and 23andMe. The latter is a commercial program that provides for fee information on an individual's genotype. For this program, questionnaires have been used for participants who had provided samples and who agree to be part of research studies. These GWAS were based on questionnaires. They were not full chronotype questionnaires such as the Horne and Ostberg (1976) but rather individuals were questioned as to whether they believed they were a morning person, night person, or neither. All three GWAS reported associations for chronotype for SNPs in PER2, RGS1E, FBXL13, and AK5 (Jones et al. 2019a; Lane et al. 2016; Hu et al. 2016; Kalmbach et al. 2017). Both PER2 and RGS17 are known to play a role in the molecular clock.

GWAS assessing self-report sleep duration has consistently shown an association with PAX8 (Jones et al. 2016; Lane et al. 2017; Dashti et al. 2019). This is a transcription factor. The genes whose expression is altered by PAX8 that could be involved in the regulation of sleep are currently unknown. The other variant that has been consistently identified is VRK2. It is a kinase. Variants of this gene have been shown to be associated with schizophrenia, major depressive Illness, and genetic generalized epilepsy (Li and Yue 2018).

Studies with sleep duration determined by accelerometry have not surprisingly been more fruitful. Heritability estimates of objectively measured sleep (19% [95% CI: 18.2–19.8%]) are larger than self-report sleep duration (8.8% [95%CI: 8.5–9.0%]) (Jones et al. 2019b). GWAS of objectively measured sleep identified variants in both studies of this type in DPYD, MEIS1, PAX8, and LOC IO1928419 (Doherty et al. 2018; Jones et al. 2019b). Other variants were identified in one of the studies (Doherty et al. 2018; Jones et al. 2019b), including BTBD9 and ANK1. As described earlier, both MEIS1 and BTBD9 variants have been shown to be associated with RLS (Winkelmann et al. 2007; Stefansson et al. 2007). This raises the question as to whether there is a large number of individuals in the UK Biobank with unrecognized RLS.

Another GWAS was conducted on excessive sleepiness (Collins and Varmus 2015). It was based on a single question—how likely are you to doze off or fall asleep during the daytime when you do not mean to (e.g., when working or driving)? Forty-two variants were identified to be associated with this response. (It is remarkable how much can be learned from just one question!) Since little is known about actual sleep disorders in the UK Biobank, some of these variants may be associated with specific sleep disorders such as obstructive sleep apnea.

To study insomnia a different question was asked. The largest GWAS to date included 1,331,010 subjects! This was based on 386,539 from the UK Biobank and 944,471 from 23andMe (Jansen et al. 2019). Two hundred two loci were identified to be associated with an insomnia phenotype. Both variants in MEIS1 and BTBD9 were among these variants. This may be the result of unrecognized RLS in this population. Investigators in this study studied where the genes they identified were expressed and using databases for gene expression in different brain regions, they found that these genes were overrepresented among expressed genes in the frontal cortex, and the anterior cingulate cortex.

Thus, much has been learned from this resource and we can anticipate more contributions in the future. There are currently large biobanks in China, e.g., the Kadoorie Biobank of 0.5 million subjects (Chen et al. 2011). It is unclear if they have information about sleep/chronotype or sleep/circadian disorders. Given the scale of this biobank, there is great potential for sleep/circadian research in China using this resource.

1.2 The Emerge Network/Health System Biobanks

An alternative to these population-based approaches is biobanks in large health systems. Large institutions have introduced programs to have individual patients provide consent for research and give samples of blood for DNA extraction. Some biobanks also obtain samples to allow proteomics, metabolomics, etc. to be employed. These biobanks are in institutions with well-developed electronic health records and informatics infrastructure.

The concept that underlies these health system biobanks is to achieve a broad representation of individuals with different disorders, including sleep disorders. Different institutions have used different approaches. Resources to establish these biobanks typically came from the institutions. One of the first such biobanks was at Vanderbilt University Medical Center. They used a process whereby the individual did not have to give consent but could opt out. This allowed them to utilize blood leftover from laboratory tests for extraction of DNA. While this simplifies the process, it has the distinct disadvantage of limiting the ability to recontact the individual for research studies since individual consent was not obtained. Other biobanks, including those at the University of Pennsylvania (Penn) and Geisinger Clinic, obtained blood samples not only for DNA extraction but also samples to allow different OMIC approaches. NIH provided funds to several such institutions that are part of the eMERGE Network to obtain genotype data (Gottesman et al. 2013).

Funds were provided either by NIH or by interested pharma companies to genotype the samples. Genotyping is done broadly for individuals in the biobank. The challenge is now for investigators to identify in the biobank the specific subjects that the investigator is interested in. This requires using an algorithm to identify specific subjects using diagnostic codes and other information in the EHR. We have developed and validated a specific algorithm for obstructive sleep apnea (OSA) (Keenan et al. 2020). This was based on individuals having a diagnostic code (there are multiple such CPT codes) for OSA in two or more occasions in the EHR. Individuals with only one code may have had the diagnosis suspected but a subsequent sleep study was negative. This algorithm was validated by randomly selecting

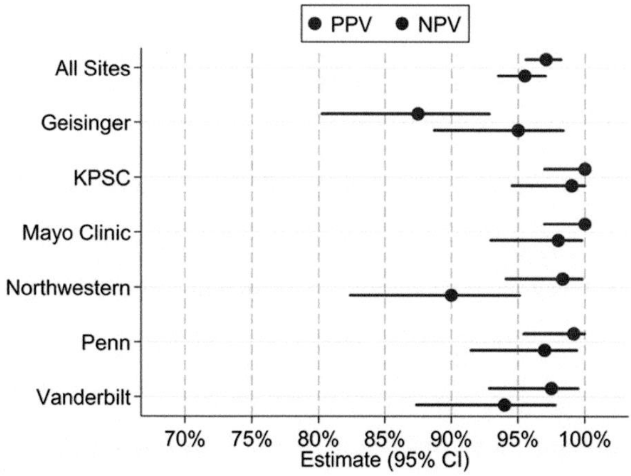

Fig. 1.3 Positive (PPV) and negative (NPV) predictive values for algorithm to identify OSA from data in the EHR. The data shown are estimates and 95% confidence intervals (CI). Data are shown by aggregating across all sites and for individual sites—Geisinger Clinic, Kaiser Permanente Southern California (KPSC), Mayo Clinic, Northwestern University, University of Pennsylvania (Penn), and Vanderbilt University [From Keenan et al. (2020) with permission]

a sample of individuals who met this criteria (cases) and a random sample of controls who had no diagnostic codes for OSA. We did this validation using random samples from multiple institutions (see Fig. 1.3). The clinical records of these samples were examined by trained staff to see whether they were indeed cases or controls. The majority of cases (72.2%) had sleep study reports that confirmed the diagnosis, or had evidence of treatment of OSA (22.3%). Only in a minority of cases did we have to rely on clinical-based notes (5.5%). The validation showed that we had in all institutions a high positive and negative predictive value using this algorithm. Averaged across all institutions in our network, the positive and negative predictive value was over 90%. At Geisinger Clinic the positive predictive value was <90%. We, therefore, evaluated an algorithm that used ≥3 occasions with a diagnostic code for OSA as being a case. This improved the positive predictive value but at the expense of losing cases, i.e., some cases with a diagnosis on at least two occasions did not have a third such encounter. The loss was not major at Geisinger Clinic but was much greater at Penn. This likely reflects that Penn is very much a tertiary care health system. Thus, investigators using this approach should seek to validate the algorithm they plan to use in their biobank.

There has currently been active development of these algorithms for multiple disorders. Fifty three such algorithms that use a combination of clinical variables to define a particular phenotype are in a public repository—Phenotype Knowledge Base (PheKB) (Kirby et al. 2016).

While many of these algorithms use CPT codes, as we have done for OSA (Keenan et al. 2020), these codes are intended primarily for billing purposes. They are, therefore suboptimal to define a specific disease (Hripcsak and Albers 2013). Thus, information from CPT codes can be amplified with other clinical information such as results of laboratory tests. This will add specificity. The example described for OSA could use, in addition to CPT codes, information from clinical sleep studies.

While using CPT codes has worked well for OSA (Keenan et al. 2020), algorithms based solely on diagnostic codes may not work for all diagnoses. We have worked with our colleagues at Geisinger Clinic to develop a similar algorithm for Alzheimer's disease (AD) (unpublished observations). We found that for those individuals evaluated in specialized clinics an algorithm worked well. They had extensive testing including brain imaging, neurocognitive tests, and studies of biomarkers. However, there are a large number of individuals where the diagnosis of AD was made by primary care physicians without such tests. It is, therefore, unclear if these individuals have AD. Thus, for AD, an algorithm that is based not only on CPT codes but also on data from other tests is required.

Recently, as described in an excellent review (Li et al. 2020), use is now being made of machine learning approaches to derive specific phenotypes based on multiple sources of data in the EHR (Banda et al. 2018). A machine learning approach has been used to define an algorithm to identify type 2 diabetes mellitus using EHR data (Zheng et al. 2017).

These approaches need to be replicated in EHR data from multiple institutions. This requires efforts at standardization of data. EHR data can be mapped to common data models, e.g., the Observational Medical Outcomes Partnership (OMOP) standardized vocabulary (Stang et al. 2010). A recent review has developed the argument that there needs to be systematic adoption of standardized terminologies in all areas of sleep medicine, with development of an integrated infrastructure (Mazzotti 2021).

The approach to identifying OSA in EHR data has allowed us to identify more than 20,000 cases with OSA who have genotype data. This permits us to do a very large GWAS. It permits us not only to do case/control analysis, but we can also obtain quantitative data relevant to OSA from sleep study reports and actual raw sleep study data for additional analyses. Thus, large-scale quantitative trait analyses can also be conducted.

A similar approach to case/control analyses has already been published from the large FinnGen program in Finland (Strausz et al. 2021). They identified OSA from inpatient records in Finland and from death registry data. Thus, it is a somewhat biased sample since most OSA are determined in outpatient studies. Moreover, as pointed out in an editorial (Wang et al. 2021) that accompanied this report, there was no ability to do quantitative analyses.

This important study in Finland identified several obesity-related genes that conferred risk for OSA (see Fig. 1.4). By doing analyses when controlling for BMI or not, it can be shown that some variants such as in FTO (fat mass obesity gene) are in the obesity pathway to OSA, other variants that were identified are in the non-obesity pathway (see Fig. 1.4) (Strausz et al. 2021). Patel et al. had previously proposed that the way to think about genetics of OSA was in terms of obesity- and non-obesity-related pathways (Patel 2005).

The Finnish group has developed a polygenic risk score for OSA (Strausz et al. 2021). A polygenic risk score for insomnia has also been developed based on findings from the large GWAS described above. This is one of the goals of

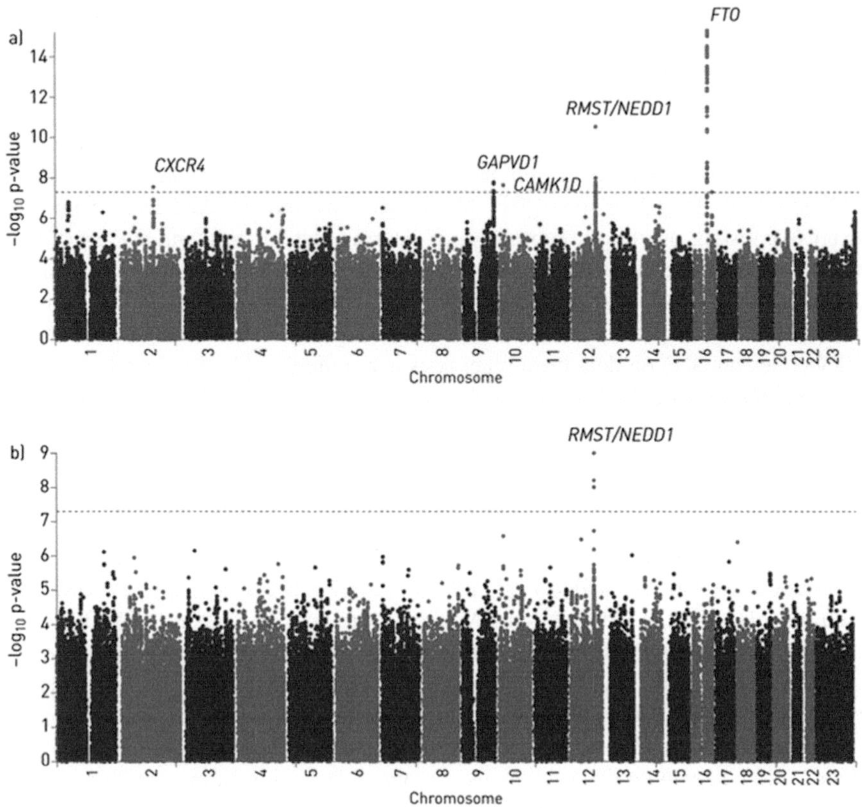

Fig. 1.4 Manhattan plots for GWAS of OSA with 16,761 cases and 201,194 controls. The x-axis shows the position of each variant across all the chromosomes and the y-axis the $-\log_{10} p$-value for association. The dashed line on each plot indicates the $-\log p$-value for genome-wide significance, i.e., after correcting for multiple comparisons. The top panel (**a**) shows the results for uncorrected analyses while the bottom panel (**b**) shows the results after controlling for BMI. The latter analysis had fewer subjects (12,759 cases and 146,972 controls). Most of the genome-wide significant associations, including FTO (fat mass and obesity-associated protein), are no longer significant after controlling for BMI (see panel **b**). One variant, i.e., RMST/NEDD1 (rhabdomyosarcoma 2 associated transcript/NEDD1 γ tubulin ring complex targeting factor), continues to be significant after correcting for BMI [From Strausz et al. (2021) with permission]

GWAS and related genetic studies, i.e., to identify individuals with high genetic risk for the disorder (PREDICT) and allow clinicians to move from treatment of the disorder to PREVENTION. For OSA, prevention may involve the future use of mandibular advancement devices in such individuals to prevent the slow progression of the disorder (Newman et al. 2005).

But PRS are only one source of data for prediction of risk. Prediction can be improved by using additional sources of data such as family history and relevant environmental exposures (Li et al. 2020). The iCARE package jointly models data from multiple sources to define relative and absolute risk and risk factor distributions

(Pal Choudhury et al. 2020). Currently, disease risk predictions using PRS are starting to be applied clinically, in particular, for psychiatric disorders (Kember et al. 2021). For example, PRS have been shown to be significantly associated with risk for schizophrenia (Zheutlin et al. 2019).

Currently, however, these polygenic risk scores both for OSA and for insomnia only explain a small proportion of the genetic variance. There is missing heritability. This is related to several issues. First, GWAS does not necessarily identify the causative variant. There are other gene variants that are correlated. Current approaches also do not address the interactive effects of different gene variants, i.e., epistasis. There are also other sources of genetic variations. This includes rare variants (there are as described earlier many of these) and copy number variants (CNVs) (Conrad et al. 2010; Redon et al. 2006). There are also epigenetic modifications that alter gene transcription (Murphy and Mill 2014). For many disorders there are ongoing efforts to address all of these issues thereby improving prediction.

Another approach that EHR data can be used for is PheWAS (Verma et al. 2019; Bush et al. 2016). This is based on seeking an association with a specific gene variant and all diagnoses in the EHR. This can serve to replicate previously described associations and potentially identify pathophysiological mechanisms. For example, a variant associated with OSA might also be associated with nasal septal deviation indicating why this variant is a risk variant for OSA. We have conducted a PheWAS on variants shown to be associated with OSA (Veatch et al. 2020). We did not replicate an association with OSA for the majority of previously described associations. SNPs in LEPR, MMP-9, and GABBR1 validated for an association with a diagnosis of OSA in European Americans from two different clinic-based biobanks at Geisinger Clinic and Vanderbilt. LEPR encodes for a receptor for the adipocyte-specific leptin hormone. This SNP is not associated, however, with obesity (Gozal et al. 2016; Olza et al. 2017; Rojano-Rodriguez et al. 2016; Chavarria-Avila et al. 2015). GABBR1 encodes for a receptor for GABA, an inhibitory neurotransmitter.

For many existing biobanks, there is increasing information on other sources of genetic variation, in particular exome sequence data. Eventually, these biobanks will have whole-genome sequence data. Extensive exome sequence data are available in the UK Biobank, and in the biobanks at Geisinger Clinic and the University of Pennsylvania. One of the first biobanks to assess exome sequence data was at the Geisinger Clinic. This clinic provides care to over 3.0 million individuals in a rural areas of Pennsylvania. Individuals obtaining care from this clinic seldom move. Thus, there is less than 1% loss of individuals from this system. Individuals who use this system for their care do so from birth to death. Thus, it allows long-term follow-up of individuals. One can examine longitudinal change in laboratory values and in key measures such as blood pressure. This is part of what has been described as a learning health system (Williams et al. 2018). In the first description of exome sequence data from this biobank (Dewey et al. 2016), it was shown that 92% of genes have a rare variant and 7% of sequenced genes are predicted to have a homozygous loss of function variant of that gene. Although the variants are rare, the average human carries 21 predicted loss of function rare variants. Using exome sequencing, data can be particularly valuable to identify relevant genes when there are extreme phenotypes. Extreme phenotypes of OSA have been described, e.g., severe OSA in individuals with a low likelihood of OSA based on age, gender, and BMI (Rizzatti et al. 2020).

Availability of exome sequence data also allows a new strategy, i.e., callbacks. With this approach, one can identify individuals in the biobank with a predicted loss of function variants of genes of interest and then determine their phenotype. This may be done using data already available from clinical studies, e.g., laboratory values, such as sleep studies and images. They can also be recontacted for in-depth phenotyping for specific areas of focus. For example, if a gene is thought to be involved in sleep regulation, individuals with a predicted loss of function of this gene could have their sleep assessed. This general approach has been used in subjects in the Human Knock Out Project (Saleheen et al. 2017), i.e., to determine differences in phenotype in individuals with loss of function of specific genes. This resource is based on studies in Pakistan where there is a high level of consanguineous marriage such that many individuals have homozygous loss of function variants (Saleheen et al. 2017).

PheWAS can also be done with exome sequence data as was described above for common variants (Verma et al. 2019; Bush et al. 2016). A recent major publication did a genome-wide study looking at association with all rare variants and all diagnoses in the EHR (Park et al. 2021). The study replicated known associations such as rare variants of BRAC and breast cancer as well as new associations (Park et al. 2021) (see Fig. 1.5).

Since each individual variant is rare, loss of function variants in a single gene or targeted set of genes were aggregated, i.e., they conducted a gene burden PheWAS. They identified 97 gene burdens with association with specific phenotypes at $p < 10^{-6}$. The initial analysis was using data from the biobank at Penn. They sought to replicate the findings in other clinical biobanks, e.g., at Geisinger, and in the UK Biobank. They found more replication with data from other health system biobanks than with data from the UK Biobank. The UK Biobank is recognized to have a healthy volunteer selection bias (Fry et al. 2017). There is, therefore, a lower prevalence of specific disorders in the UK Biobank compared to biobanks developed by health systems. For sleep disorders, there is the added complication that participants in the UK Biobank may have undiagnosed sleep disorders such as RLS and OSA. The prevalence of OSA in the UK Biobank is much less than the estimated prevalence based on age, gender, and BMI (Peppard et al. 2013) (unpublished observations).

1.3 Trans-omics for Precision Medicine (TOPMed)

Another key resource that has been developed is the Trans-Omics for Precision Medicine (TOPMed) (Burgess 2021) that is supported by the National Heart, Lung and Blood Institute. This is an innovative grant mechanism that has allowed a major resource for genetic studies to be developed. Applicants for this program apply for

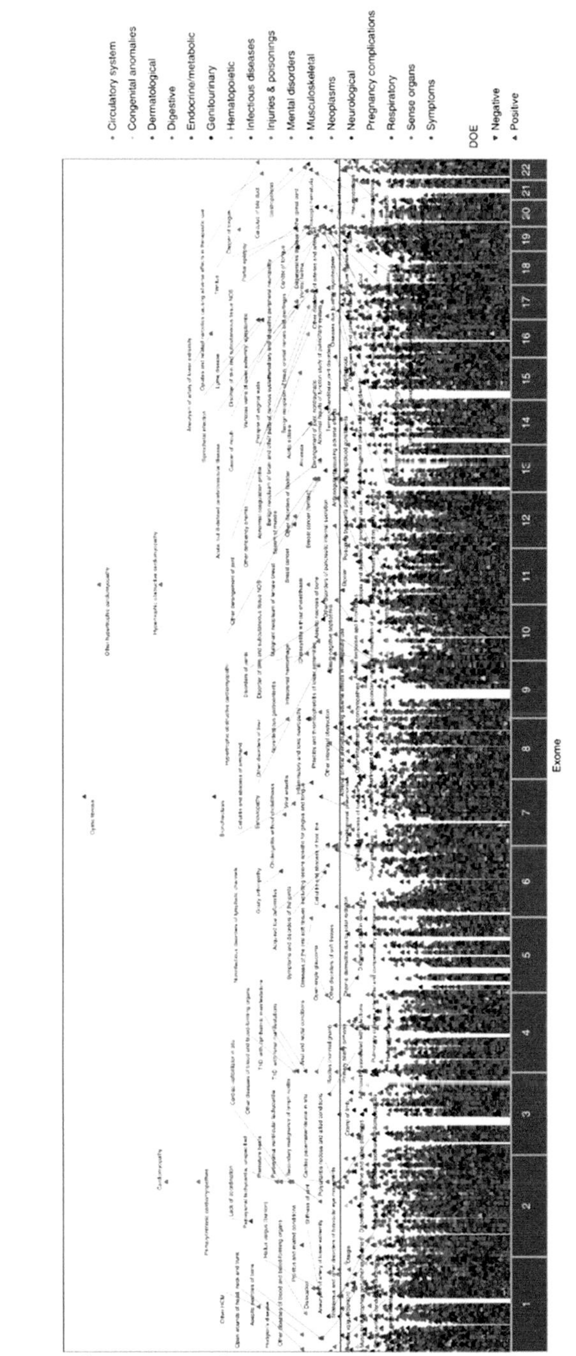

Fig. 1.5 The plot shows the landscape of gene–phenotype associations across the exome and phenotype data from the Penn Medicine Biobank. The *x*-axis represents the location across the genome. The $-\log_{10}$ of the *p*-value is shown for the association in the *y*-axis. The association for each of the 97 genome burdens with 1000 phecodes is shown. Colors are used to represent different phecode groups [From Park et al. (2021) with permission]

grants that do not provide support for the efforts of the applicant, but rather provide resources to do analyses of samples provided by the investigators who apply. These analyses include whole-genome sequencing (WGS), whole-genome DNA methylation, and metabolomics. Much of the effort has gone into whole-genome sequencing. The initial results from analysis of WGS in 53,831 individuals have recently been reported (Taliun et al. 2021). More than 400 million variants were detected. A large number of rare variants that occur in $<1\%$ of individuals were found. Given the scale of this effort, data from TOPMed will likely be used as the reference genome for future genetic studies.

Currently, in TOPMed there are somewhat limited data from individuals with sleep disorders. These largely come from sleep studies that have been performed on individuals in population-based cohort studies (Zhang et al. 2018). Many of these cohorts were developed to assess variables, including genetic variants that are associated with cardiovascular risk. But some have argued that sleep apnea identified in population-based studies is different from that found in patients who present clinically (Arnardottir et al. 2016). The data from sleep studies obtained in these cohorts is available from the National Sleep Research Resource (Zhang et al. 2018). This contains data on 26,808 subjects and there are 31,166 files of sleep studies available in the European Data Format (EDF). These data can be obtained by interested investigators. Genetic analysis using these data with WGS generated in TOPMed has shown that six coding and 51 noncoding variants in the gene for GTPase-activating proteins (DLC1) are associated with average oxygen saturation during sleep (Liang et al. 2019). Recently, new data are being added to TOPMed from a sample of 3000 clinical patients with OSA.

1.4 Conclusion

The identification of gene variants conferring risk for specific sleep disorders is accelerating. The approach is moving from the laborious recruitment of large numbers of cases and controls to use of resources that have been developed in different countries to make investigation of genetic variants more efficient. Extensive use is being made of data from electronic health records as part of the phenotyping strategy. Ultimately, however, we need to prove that the variants identified are indeed casual. This will require functional studies not only using assays in specific cells but also use of model systems such as zebrafish and mice. The efforts currently underway in Europe and the USA could be duplicated in China, thereby further accelerating progress in this area.

References

Allen RP, Picchietti D, Hening WA, Trenkwalder C, Walters AS, Montplaisi J, et al. Restless legs syndrome: diagnostic criteria, special considerations, and epidemiology. A report from the restless legs syndrome diagnosis and epidemiology workshop at the National Institutes of Health. Sleep Med. 2003;4(2):101–19.

Arnardottir ES, Bjornsdottir E, Olafsdottir KA, Benediktsdottir B, Gislason T. Obstructive sleep apnoea in the general population: highly prevalent but minimal symptoms. Eur Respir J. 2016;47(1):194–202.

Banda JM, Seneviratne M, Hernandez-Boussard T, Shah NH. Advances in electronic phenotyping: from rule-based definitions to machine learning models. Annu Rev Biomed Data Sci. 2018;1: 53–68.

Burgess DJ. The TOPMed genomic resource for human health. Nat Rev Genet. 2021;22(4):200.

Bush WS, Oetjens MT, Crawford DC. Unravelling the human genome-phenome relationship using phenome-wide association studies. Nat Rev Genet. 2016;17(3):129–45.

Chavarria-Avila E, Vazquez-Del Mercado M, Gomez-Banuelos E, Ruiz-Quezada SL, Castro-Albarran J, Sanchez-Lopez L, et al. The impact of LEP G-2548A and LEPR Gln223Arg polymorphisms on adiposity, leptin, and leptin-receptor serum levels in a Mexican Mestizo population. Biomed Res Int. 2015;2015:539408.

Chen Z, Chen J, Collins R, Guo Y, Peto R, Wu F, et al. China Kadoorie Biobank of 0.5 million people: survey methods, baseline characteristics and long-term follow-up. Int J Epidemiol. 2011;40(6):1652–66.

Chinoy ED, Cuellar JA, Huwa KE, Jameson JT, Watson CH, Bessman SC, et al. Performance of seven consumer sleep-tracking devices compared with polysomnography. Sleep. 2021;44(5): zsaa291.

Collins FS, Varmus H. A new initiative on precision medicine. N Engl J Med. 2015;372(9):793–5.

Conrad DF, Pinto D, Redon R, Feuk L, Gokcumen O, Zhang Y, et al. Origins and functional impact of copy number variation in the human genome. Nature. 2010;464(7289):704–12.

Dashti HS, Jones SE, Wood AR, Lane JM, van Hees VT, Wang H, et al. Genome-wide association study identifies genetic loci for self-reported habitual sleep duration supported by accelerometer-derived estimates. Nat Commun. 2019;10(1):1100.

Dewey FE, Murray MF, Overton JD, Habegger L, Leader JB, Fetterolf SN, et al. Distribution and clinical impact of functional variants in 50,726 whole-exome sequences from the DiscovEHR study. Science. 2016;354(6319):aaf6814.

Doherty A, Smith-Byrne K, Ferreira T, Holmes MV, Holmes C, Pulit SL, et al. GWAS identifies 14 loci for device-measured physical activity and sleep duration. Nat Commun. 2018;9(1):5257.

Fry A, Littlejohns TJ, Sudlow C, Doherty N, Adamska L, Sprosen T, et al. Comparison of sociodemographic and health-related characteristics of UK Biobank participants with those of the general population. Am J Epidemiol. 2017;186(9):1026–34.

Gottesman O, Kuivaniemi H, Tromp G, Faucett WA, Li R, Manolio TA, et al. The electronic medical records and genomics (eMERGE) network: past, present, and future. Genet Med. 2013;15(10):761–71.

Gozal D, Ham SA, Mokhlesi B. Sleep apnea and cancer: analysis of a nationwide population sample. Sleep. 2016;39(8):1493–500.

Hallmayer J, Faraco J, Lin L, Hesselson S, Winkelmann J, Kawashima M, et al. Narcolepsy is strongly associated with the T-cell receptor alpha locus. Nat Genet. 2009;41(6):708–11.

Horne JA, Ostberg O. A self-assessment questionnaire to determine morningness-eveningness in human circadian rhythms. Int J Chronobiol. 1976;4(2):97–110.

Hripcsak G, Albers DJ. Next-generation phenotyping of electronic health records. J Am Med Inform Assoc. 2013;20(1):117–21.

Hu Y, Shmygelska A, Tran D, Eriksson N, Tung JY, Hinds DA. GWAS of 89,283 individuals identifies genetic variants associated with self-reporting of being a morning person. Nat Commun. 2016;7:10448.

Jansen PR, Watanabe K, Stringer S, Skene N, Bryois J, Hammerschlag AR, et al. Genome-wide analysis of insomnia in 1,331,010 individuals identifies new risk loci and functional pathways. Nat Genet. 2019;51(3):394–403.

Jones SE, Tyrrell J, Wood AR, Beaumont RN, Ruth KS, Tuke MA, et al. Genome-wide association analyses in 128,266 individuals identifies new morningness and sleep duration loci. PLoS Genet. 2016;12(8):e1006125.

Jones SE, Lane JM, Wood AR, van Hees VT, Tyrrell J, Beaumont RN, et al. Genome-wide association analyses of chronotype in 697,828 individuals provides insights into circadian rhythms. Nat Commun. 2019a;10(1):343.

Jones SE, van Hees VT, Mazzotti DR, Marques-Vidal P, Sabia S, van der Spek A, et al. Genetic studies of accelerometer-based sleep measures yield new insights into human sleep behaviour. Nat Commun. 2019b;10(1):1585.

Juji T, Satake M, Honda Y, Doi Y. HLA antigens in Japanese patients with narcolepsy. All the patients were DR2 positive. Tissue Antigens. 1984;24(5):316–9.

Kalmbach DA, Schneider LD, Cheung J, Bertrand SJ, Kariharan T, Pack AI, et al. Genetic basis of chronotype in humans: insights from three landmark GWAS. Sleep. 2017;40(2):zsw048.

Keenan BT, Kirchner HL, Veatch OJ, Borthwick KM, Davenport VA, Feemster JC, et al. Multisite validation of a simple electronic health record algorithm for identifying diagnosed obstructive sleep apnea. J Clin Sleep Med. 2020;16(2):175–83.

Kember RL, Merikangas AK, Verma SS, Verma A, Judy R, Regeneron Genetics C, et al. Polygenic Risk of Psychiatric Disorders Exhibits Cross-trait Associations in Electronic Health Record Data From European Ancestry Individuals. Biol Psychiatry. 2021;89(3):236–45.

Kemlink D, Polo O, Frauscher B, Gschliesser V, Hogl B, Poewe W, et al. Replication of restless legs syndrome loci in three European populations. J Med Genet. 2009;46(5):315–8.

Kirby JC, Speltz P, Rasmussen LV, Basford M, Gottesman O, Peissig PL, et al. PheKB: a catalog and workflow for creating electronic phenotype algorithms for transportability. J Am Med Inform Assoc. 2016;23(6):1046–52.

Klein RJ, Zeiss C, Chew EY, Tsai JY, Sackler RS, Haynes C, et al. Complement factor H polymorphism in age-related macular degeneration. Science. 2005;308(5720):385–9.

Lane JM, Vlasac I, Anderson SG, Kyle SD, Dixon WG, Bechtold DA, et al. Genome-wide association analysis identifies novel loci for chronotype in 100,420 individuals from the UK Biobank. Nat Commun. 2016;7:10889.

Lane JM, Liang J, Vlasac I, Anderson SG, Bechtold DA, Bowden J, et al. Genome-wide association analyses of sleep disturbance traits identify new loci and highlight shared genetics with neuropsychiatric and metabolic traits. Nat Genet. 2017;49(2):274–81.

Lane JM, Jones SE, Dashti HS, Wood AR, Aragam KG, van Hees VT, et al. Biological and clinical insights from genetics of insomnia symptoms. Nat Genet. 2019;51(3):387–93.

Li M, Yue W. VRK2, a candidate gene for psychiatric and neurological disorders. Mol Neuropsychiatry. 2018;4(3):119–33.

Li R, Chen Y, Ritchie MD, Moore JH. Electronic health records and polygenic risk scores for predicting disease risk. Nat Rev Genet. 2020;21(8):493–502.

Liang J, Cade BE, He KY, Wang H, Lee J, Sofer T, et al. Sequencing analysis at 8p23 identifies multiple rare variants in DLC1 associated with sleep-related oxyhemoglobin saturation level. Am J Hum Genet. 2019;105(5):1057–68.

MacArthur J, Bowler E, Cerezo M, Gil L, Hall P, Hastings E, et al. The new NHGRI-EBI Catalog of published genome-wide association studies (GWAS Catalog). Nucleic Acids Res. 2017;45(D1): D896–901.

Manolio TA, Collins FS, Cox NJ, Goldstein DB, Hindorff LA, Hunter DJ, et al. Finding the missing heritability of complex diseases. Nature. 2009;461(7265):747–53.

Mazzotti DR. Landscape of biomedical informatics standards and terminologies for clinical sleep medicine research: a systematic review. Sleep Med Rev. 2021;60:101529.

Moore H, Winkelmann J, Lin L, Finn L, Peppard P, Mignot E. Periodic leg movements during sleep are associated with polymorphisms in BTBD9, TOX3/BC034767, MEIS1, MAP2K5/SKOR1, and PTPRD. Sleep. 2014;37(9):1535–42.

Murphy TM, Mill J. Epigenetics in health and disease: heralding the EWAS era. Lancet. 2014;383 (9933):1952–4.

Newman AB, Foster G, Givelber R, Nieto FJ, Redline S, Young T. Progression and regression of sleep-disordered breathing with changes in weight: the Sleep Heart Health Study. Arch Intern Med. 2005;165(20):2408–13.

Olza J, Ruperez AI, Gil-Campos M, Leis R, Canete R, Tojo R, et al. Leptin receptor gene variant rs11804091 is associated with BMI and insulin resistance in Spanish female obese children: a case-control study. Int J Mol Sci. 2017;18(8):1690.

Pack AI, Keenan BT, Gehrman PR, Justice AE. Genetics and genomic basis of sleep disorders in humans. In: Kryger M, editor. Principles and practices of sleep medicine. Philadelphia, PA: Elsevier; 2021.

Pal Choudhury P, Maas P, Wilcox A, Wheeler W, Brook M, Check D, et al. iCARE: an R package to build, validate and apply absolute risk models. PLoS One. 2020;15(2):e0228198.

Park J, Lucas AM, Zhang X, Chaudhary K, Cho JH, Nadkarni G, et al. Exome-wide evaluation of rare coding variants using electronic health records identifies new gene-phenotype associations. Nat Med. 2021;27(1):66–72.

Patel SR. Shared genetic risk factors for obstructive sleep apnea and obesity. J Appl Physiol. 2005;99(4):1600–6.

Peppard PE, Young T, Barnet JH, Palta M, Hagen EW, Hla KM. Increased prevalence of sleep-disordered breathing in adults. Am J Epidemiol. 2013;177(9):1006–14.

Redon R, Ishikawa S, Fitch KR, Feuk L, Perry GH, Andrews TD, et al. Global variation in copy number in the human genome. Nature. 2006;444(7118):444–54.

Rizzatti FG, Mazzotti DR, Mindel J, Maislin G, Keenan BT, Bittencourt L, et al. Defining extreme phenotypes of OSA across international sleep centers. Chest. 2020;158(3):1187–97.

Rojano-Rodriguez ME, Beristain-Hernandez JL, Zavaleta-Villa B, Maravilla P, Romero-Valdovinos M, Olivo-Diaz A. Leptin receptor gene polymorphisms and morbid obesity in Mexican patients. Hereditas. 2016;153:2.

Saleheen D, Natarajan P, Armean IM, Zhao W, Rasheed A, Khetarpal SA, et al. Human knockouts and phenotypic analysis in a cohort with a high rate of consanguinity. Nature. 2017;544(7649): 235–9.

Stang PE, Ryan PB, Racoosin JA, Overhage JM, Hartzema AG, Reich C, et al. Advancing the science for active surveillance: rationale and design for the Observational Medical Outcomes Partnership. Ann Intern Med. 2010;153(9):600–6.

Stefansson H, Rye DB, Hicks A, Petursson H, Ingason A, Thorgeirsson TE, et al. A genetic risk factor for periodic limb movements in sleep. N Engl J Med. 2007;357(7):639–47.

Strausz S, Ruotsalainen S, Ollila HM, Karjalainen J, Kiiskinen T, Reeve M, et al. Genetic analysis of obstructive sleep apnoea discovers a strong association with cardiometabolic health. Eur Respir J. 2021;57:2003091.

Tafti M, Hor H, Dauvilliers Y, Lammers GJ, Overeem S, Mayer G, et al. DQB1 locus alone explains most of the risk and protection in narcolepsy with cataplexy in Europe. Sleep. 2014;37 (1):19–25.

Taliun D, Harris DN, Kessler MD, Carlson J, Szpiech ZA, Torres R, et al. Sequencing of 53,831 diverse genomes from the NHLBI TOPMed Program. Nature. 2021;590(7845):290–9.

van Hees VT, Sabia S, Jones SE, Wood AR, Anderson KN, Kivimaki M, et al. Estimating sleep parameters using an accelerometer without sleep diary. Sci Rep. 2018;8(1):12975.

Veatch OJ, Bauer CR, Keenan BT, Josyula NS, Mazzotti DR, Bagai K, et al. Characterization of genetic and phenotypic heterogeneity of obstructive sleep apnea using electronic health records. BMC Med Genet. 2020;13(1):105.

Verma A, Bang L, Miller JE, Zhang Y, Lee MTM, Zhang Y, et al. Human-disease phenotype map derived from PheWAS across 38,682 individuals. Am J Hum Genet. 2019;104(1):55–64.

Visscher PM, Brown MA, McCarthy MI, Yang J. Five years of GWAS discovery. Am J Hum Genet. 2012;90(1):7–24.

Wang H, Lane JM, Jones SE, Dashti HS, Ollila HM, Wood AR, et al. Genome-wide association analysis of self-reported daytime sleepiness identifies 42 loci that suggest biological subtypes. Nat Commun. 2019;10(1):3503.

Wang H, Goodman MO, Sofer T, Redline S. Cutting the fat: advances and challenges in sleep apnoea genetics. Eur Respir J. 2021;57(5):2004644.

Wellcome Trust Case Control Consortium. Genome-wide association study of 14,000 cases of seven common diseases and 3,000 shared controls. Nature. 2007;447(7145):661–78.

Welter D, MacArthur J, Morales J, Burdett T, Hall P, Junkins H, et al. The NHGRI GWAS Catalog, a curated resource of SNP-trait associations. Nucleic Acids Res. 2014;42(Database issue): D1001–6.

Williams MS, Buchanan AH, Davis FD, Faucett WA, Hallquist MLG, Leader JB, et al. Patient-centered precision health in a learning health care system: Geisinger's Genomic Medicine Experience. Health Aff (Millwood). 2018;37(5):757–64.

Winkelmann J, Schormair B, Lichtner P, Ripke S, Xiong L, Jalilzadeh S, et al. Genome-wide association study of restless legs syndrome identifies common variants in three genomic regions. Nat Genet. 2007;39(8):1000–6.

Yang Q, Li L, Chen Q, Foldvary-Schaefer N, Ondo WG, Wang QK. Association studies of variants in MEIS1, BTBD9, and MAP2K5/SKOR1 with restless legs syndrome in a US population. Sleep Med. 2011;12(8):800–4.

Zhang GQ, Cui L, Mueller R, Tao S, Kim M, Rueschman M, et al. The National Sleep Research Resource: towards a sleep data commons. J Am Med Inform Assoc. 2018;25(10):1351–8.

Zheng T, Xie W, Xu L, He X, Zhang Y, You M, et al. A machine learning-based framework to identify type 2 diabetes through electronic health records. Int J Med Inform. 2017;97:120–7.

Zheutlin AB, Dennis J, Karlsson Linner R, Moscati A, Restrepo N, Straub P, et al. Penetrance and pleiotropy of polygenic risk scores for schizophrenia in 106,160 patients across four health care systems. Am J Psychiatry. 2019;176(10):846–55.

Chapter 2
Neurobiology of Sleep–Wake Control

Leszek Kubin

Abstract The chapter provides an introduction to the mechanism underlying the generation and regulation of sleep under physiologic conditions. Sleep–wake behavior is gated by circadian rhythm and paced by the ultradian rhythm called the basic rest–activity cycle (BRAC). Within the framework of these two rhythms, three distinct behavioral states—wakefulness, non-rapid eye movement (NREM) sleep, and REM sleep—are generated by neuronal groups that differ based on their neurotransmitter phenotypes, anatomic locations, and relationship of their activity to the phases of the sleep–wake cycle. Gamma-aminobutyric acid (GABA) plays a major role in this network, with different groups of GABAergic cells contributing to the generation of each of the three behavioral states. Different groups of cholinergic cells support wakefulness or REM sleep. Norepinephrine-, serotonin-, histamine-, and orexin-containing neurons subserve different aspects of wakefulness. The entire network possesses multiple mechanisms that support the homeostatic regulation of sleep. These include the use-dependent control of neurotransmitter synthesis, neurotransmitter receptor trafficking, cellular effects of metabolites (e.g., adenosine), response to depletion of energy stores (e.g., glycogen), as well as actions of sleep-promoting cytokines and growth factors responsive to inflammation and external environment (e.g., synaptic plasticity supporting memory).

Keywords Adenosine · Circadian rhythm · GABA · Sleep homeostasis · Hypothalamus · Pons · Ultradian rhythm

2.1 Introduction

Three major discoveries and the associated fundamental concepts have shaped our current understanding of the basic neurobiology of sleep–wake states. Chronologically, they were: (a) the recognition that sleep is actively generated within a

L. Kubin (✉)
Department of Biomedical Sciences 209E/VET, School of Veterinary Medicine, University of Pennsylvania, Philadelphia, PA, USA
e-mail: lkubin@vet.upenn.edu

A. I. Pack, Q. Y. Li (eds.), *Sleep and its Disorders*, Translational Medicine Research,
https://doi.org/10.1007/978-94-024-2168-2_2

delimited part of the forebrain (von Economo 1930); (b) the determination that what has been earlier seen as a single state of sleep, comprises two distinct entities, the non-Rapid Eye Movement (NREM) sleep and REM sleep (Aserinsky and Kleitman 1953); and (c) introduction of a model of the relationship between the circadian and homeostatic regulations of sleep, commonly referred to as the two-process model (Borbély 1982).

Prior to the groundbreaking observations of von Economo (1930), sleep was commonly regarded as a passive state resulting from a temporal suspension of the active processes that maintain wakefulness and everything it entails, including the ability to perceive and process external stimuli, respond to them emotionally and physically, and create a memory of past events. Indeed, equating sleep with death was not uncommon in pre-twentieth-century literature in both Europe and Asia (e.g., Dante's *Divine Comedy*). The passive nature of sleep did not mean, however, that the "refreshing" and "strength-restoring" qualities of sleep were not recognized. For example, to account for the common observation that a sumptuous meal promotes sleepiness, Aristotle considered a causal relationship between the occurrence of sleep and accumulation of nutrients. Along similar lines, in ancient China, sleep was attributed to alterations in the composition of circulating blood (Inoue et al. 1995). Hence, the modern concepts of sleep as a restorative process evolved from ancient science and philosophy.

Analogously to the identification of the anterior and posterior parts of the hypothalamus as the key sites for the generation of sleep and wakefulness, respectively, the formal recognition of REM sleep as a distinct behavioral state (Aserinsky and Kleitman 1953) was followed by the finding that the neuroanatomical origin of the state is in the pontomedullary reticular formation, with the dorsomedial pontine tegmentum being the key site (Jouvet 1962). This, and the finding that mesopontine acetylcholine and amines (serotonin and norepinephrine) exert opposing effects on REM sleep, has led to the formulation of the "reciprocal interaction model," which emphasized the mutually inhibitory interaction between pontine aminergic neurons (especially those containing serotonin and noradrenergic neurons of the locus coeruleus, a.k.a. the catecholaminergic A6 group) and those containing acetylcholine (specifically, the Ch5 and Ch6 groups) (McCarley and Hobson 1975). Since its original publication, the model has been modified and expanded, with some of its core assumptions being questioned (Lu et al. 2006; Luppi et al. 2012; Reiner 1995). In addition, following the discovery of the excitatory peptides, orexins (a.k.a. hypocretins), for which the posterior hypothalamus is the only source in the brain (de Lecea et al. 1998) and whose absence results in narcolepsy-cataplexy, a disorder of REM sleep (Chemelli et al. 1999), attention has considerably shifted from the brainstem to the hypothalamus and its role in the control of REM sleep. Nevertheless, the reciprocal interaction model, as originally proposed, stimulated studies of cellular behaviors in relation to the stages of sleep and wakefulness that continue to this day and yield novel findings [for reviews, see Hassani et al. (2009a) and Hobson et al. (1986)].

The basic principle of the interaction between the circadian and homeostatic regulations of sleep illustrated in Fig. 2.1 was widely adapted in sleep medicine

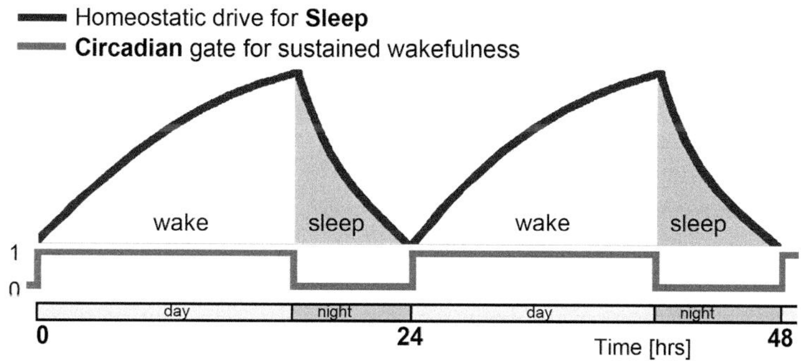

Fig. 2.1 In its simplest form, the interaction between the drive for sleep and the central circadian clock can be visualized as a circadian gate that prevents entry into sleep (promotes wakefulness) over a pre-set portion of the 24 h circadian cycle. In diurnal species, the circadian system actively supports wakefulness during the day, thereby effectively disallowing sleep despite the progressive accumulation of sleep drive with time spent awake. During the night, when sleep can actually occur, the homeostatic drive for sleep is gradually dissipated

thanks to the concurrent refinements of the techniques for electroencephalographic (EEG) recording and application of the fast Fourier transform to decompose complex brain signals into sine waves of different frequencies. In particular, the delta power (EEG signal energy carried by delta frequencies, i.e., those lower than 4 Hz) became recognized as a convenient and reliable measure of sleep propensity [process S, for sleep, in the originally proposed model (Borbély 1982)]. Thus, although changes in electrical activity of the cortex reflect, rather than initiate, the generation of sleep–wake states, measurement of delta power is commonly used as a tool with which to study the biochemical, cellular, genetic, and systemic mechanisms of the regulation of sleep (Franken et al. 2001; Qiu et al. 2015; Rector et al. 2009; Vyazovskiy et al. 2011).

The formalization of the concept of sleep as a homeostatically regulated behavioral response that inevitably follows a period of wakefulness in order to fulfill the restorative function of sleep required a definition of sleep that would distinguish it from other states characterized by the absence of conscious awareness of the external environment, such as coma or anesthesia. As discussed elsewhere, reversibility (ability to instantly terminate sleep and elicit wakefulness) and the homeostatic response to deprivation distinguish sleep from other states characterized by a disconnection from external environment (Brown et al. 2010; Lydic and Baghdoyan 2005). This definition appears to exclude at least some pharmacologically altered states of vigilance even though certain endogenous neurochemical structures and targets are shared between anesthesia and natural sleep (Sukhotinsky et al. 2007; Vanini et al. 2014; Zecharia et al. 2009). Notably, the ability of caffeine to reduce rest in flies has been used as a supportive argument for expanding the definition of sleep to non-vertebrate species (Hendricks et al. 2000).

2.2 Circadian Control of Sleep–Wake Behavior

When compared to circadian regulation that is under a relatively stringent control exerted by molecular pacemakers and physical environment (light, temperature, availability of food), the regulation of sleep is relatively subtle which may offer certain adaptive benefits. Indeed, in all likelihood, the genetic, biochemical, neurobiological, and structural features important for the generation and regulation of sleep evolved superimposed onto the circadian system. This, in turn, suggests that the emergence of sleep–wake behavior was an important step in support of the development of advanced brain functions, such as learning, memory, abstract thinking, and advanced forms of communication.

The hierarchical organization of the circadian and sleep regulations gives the circadian system a powerful control over the regulation of sleep and wakefulness. In mammals, the occurrence of sleep is gated by the central rhythm generated in the suprachiasmatic nucleus (SCN) of the ventromedial anterior hypothalamus (Bass and Takahashi 2010; Kalsbeek et al. 2010; Mistlberger 2005; Silver and Lesauter 2008) (Fig. 2.1). Furthermore, the same molecular machinery that sets the basic circadian rhythm within the SCN, is also present in other regions and cells in the brain, as well as in peripheral organs (Albrecht 2012; Tong and Yin 2013). Under the baseline conditions, these additional pacemakers are being synchronized through both humoral and neural pathways with the master pacemaker in the SCN. However, when the normal circadian rhythm of daily activity is disrupted (e.g., shift work or jet lag), or physiologic synchronizers (zeitgebers) are absent or desynchronized (e.g., no light–dark cycle, chronic disruption of the normal rest–activity cycle), dissociated rhythms may occur and this may lead to pathologies (Kim et al. 2007; Paul et al. 2009; Reid and Abbott 2015).

The most important effector hormones of the circadian clock as far as sleep effects are concerned are melatonin (produced in the pineal gland, causes drowsiness and lowers body temperature) and cortisol (produced in the adrenal gland, mobilizes glucose and enables anti-stress, and anti-inflammatory functions). In diurnal mammals, the period of rest/sleep coincides with decreasing core body temperature and increased melatonin concentration, with both peaking toward the end of the sleep period (Emens and Burgess 2015).

While the detailed mechanisms underlying the generation of circadian rhythm and its interaction with the sleep–wake cycle are outside of the scope of this chapter, circadian regulation needs to be recognized as a major "confounder" in research on the mechanisms of sleep. Typically, all experimental manipulations whose goal is to isolate genuine sleep-dependent processes need to control for any concurrent circadian effects. For example, the circadian phase at which measurements are collected must be kept constant when putative sleep-dependent effects are investigated. The model shown in Fig. 2.1 can be used as the basic tool with which to achieve this goal. Additionally, one needs to take into account any potential effects of sleep manipulations on the circadian pacemakers. This is important because, despite the principally top-down organization of the circadian and sleep controls, there is evidence that various cellular circadian pacemakers can be adversely affected by disruptions of sleep–wake behavior (Buckley and Schatzberg 2005; Rolls et al. 2015).

2.3 Basic Rest–Activity Cycle (BRAC) and the Sleep–Wake Cycle

Evidence that a distinct ultradian rhythm can be detected in various behavioral measures taken during both wakefulness and sleep was explored by Nathaniel Kleitman (1949, 1963, 1982) who also provided the first thorough characterization of REM sleep as a distinct behavioral state (Aserinsky and Kleitman 1953). He named the underlying ultradian rhythm the Basic Rest-Activity Cycle (BRAC). One expression of BRAC during the active phase of the circadian cycle is that EEG activity shows a periodic variation. Associated with this is a rhythmic waxing and waning of alertness and attention (Fig. 2.2). The ultradian clock of BRAC is separate from the circadian rhythm generator. While numerous behavioral studies explored different properties and manifestations of BRAC (D'Olimpio and Renzi 1998), its biochemical and neuronal basis have not been established.

The relevance of BRAC for the generation of sleep–wake behavior is that the semi-rhythmic sequential transitions from wakefulness to NREM and then to REM sleep that may include a transient awakening occur with the frequency characteristic of BRAC. In humans, BRAC has a period of 90–110 min; in rodents, it is about 12–20 min (Kleitman 1982). Therefore, the mechanisms associated with BRAC may

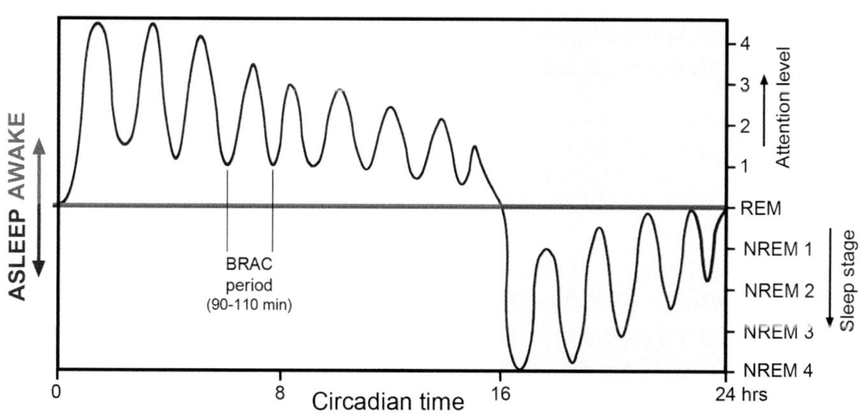

Fig. 2.2 The basic rest–activity cycle (BRAC) (Kleitman 1963, 1982) is, after circadian rhythm, the second major endogenous rhythm that determines the timing and pattern of sleep during the night and waxing and waning of attention during the day. While the neurobiological basis of this ultradian rhythm remains to be identified, its presence is strongly manifest across the entire circadian cycle. During the active phase of the circadian cycle, BRAC determines the periodic variation in attention; during the rest/sleep phase, BRAC is responsible for rhythmic cycling between successive substages of NREM sleep (NREM 1–4) and REM sleep

influence the timing of transitions from NREM sleep to REM sleep and also the durations and "intensities" of individual episodes of wakefulness, NREM and REM sleep (Lavie 1991; McPartland and Kupfer 1978). If BRAC is the clock for the wake-NREM-REM sleep cycle, it is plausible that the sleep–wake cycle is generated by a three-, rather than two-, phase oscillator. If so, this would be analogous to the central pattern generator for breathing. As with the sleep–wake rhythm, the respiratory generator was originally seen as a bistable oscillator that alternated between inspiration and expiration. However, it then became recognized that the original expiratory phase consisted of two functionally distinct sub-phases, the post-inspiratory phase, and active expiratory phase [for reviews, see Feldman et al. (2003) and Richter and Spyer (2001)]. Accordingly, it may be productive to see the sleep–wake cycle as a three-phase cycle (wake–NREM sleep–REM sleep), rather than a process resulting from an interaction between two relatively independent bistable and reciprocally organized oscillators, one for NREM sleep and wakefulness, and the other for REM sleep and wakefulness (or REM and NREM sleep). Although recent models include connections between such two bistable oscillators (Saper et al. 2010) (see also Sect. 2.4.2), a fully integrated three-phase model of the sleep–wake cycle remains to be developed. It is also of note that, in humans, four phases of NREM sleep are often distinguished and referred to as NREM 1 through NREM 4, of these NREM 3–4 can be also collectively named slow–wake sleep (SWS); in animals, the entire period of NREM sleep is referred to as SWS.

Thus, the baseline sleep–wake behavior is shaped by two rhythmic processes, one derived from the endogenous circadian clocks and the other from BRAC. Figure 2.3 shows one nearly full circadian cycle of natural sleep–wake behavior in the rat which, together with mice, is the most commonly used vertebrate model for studies on the regulation of sleep. Both the day–night difference in the amounts of sleep and wake and the recurrent sequential occurrence of wake, SWS and REM sleep are well expressed in this typical record.

2.4 Neuroanatomy and Neurochemistry of Wakefulness and Sleep

2.4.1 Locations and Neurochemical Phenotypes of State-Dependent Neurons

Identification of the hypothalamus as a major center for the maintenance of sleep and vigilance and the pons as the site for the generation of REM sleep by means of brain lesion and transection experiments enabled and focused the search for specific groups and types of neurons responsible for the generation of sleep–wake behavior. These studies, conducted mainly by means of electrophysiological recordings from single cells and to some extent using c-Fos immunohistochemistry as indirect means of assessing cell activity (Basheer et al. 1997; Boissard et al. 2002; Dentico et al.

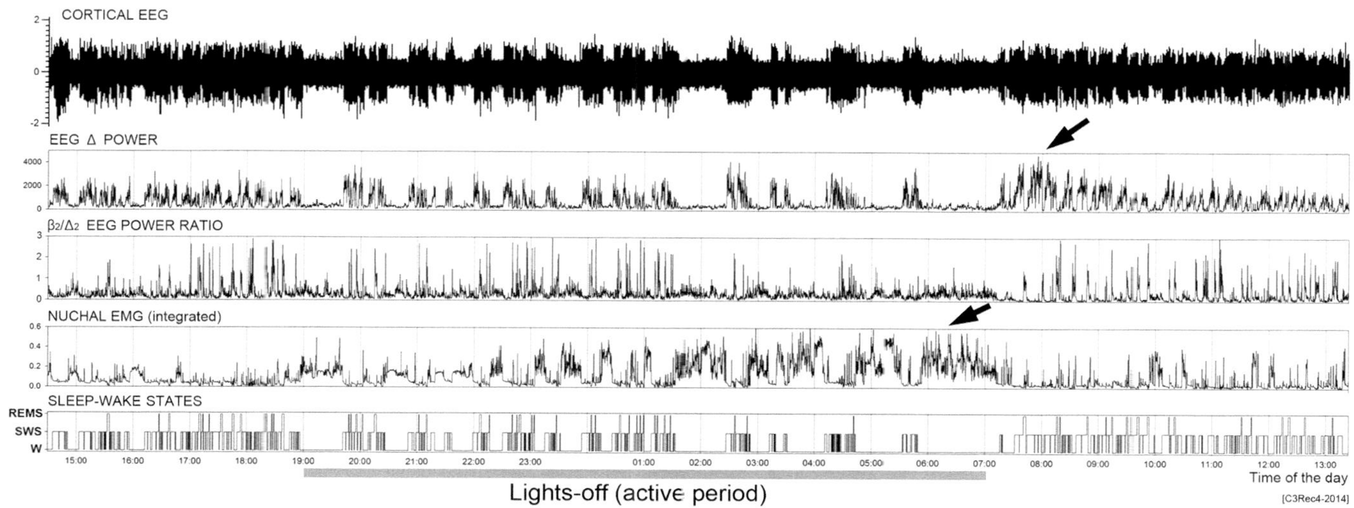

Fig. 2.3 Polygraphic record of natural sleep–wake behavior during a period of 23 h in a freely behaving rat. The example illustrates how the circadian, ultradian, and homeostatic processes converge and collectively control the rest–activity and sleep–wake rhythms. Successive bouts of slow-wave sleep (SWS) are marked by periods of high-amplitude signal in cortical electroencephalogram (EEG) (top trace). The second trace from the top shows EEG power in delta (Δ) range (<4 Hz), which characteristically dominates during SWS. The third trace shows the ratio of EEG powers in β2 range (12–14 Hz) and Δ2 range (0.5–2 Hz), which in rodents greatly increases during each transition from SWS to rapid eye movement sleep (REMS). The fourth trace shows integrated electromyogram (EMG) of dorsal neck muscles. It is high during wakefulness (W) and lowest during REMS. The bottom trace shows the hypnogram for this recording session. The following characteristic features are noteworthy: (1) the circadian difference in the amount of SWS between the rest period and active period (marked by the bar below the record); (2) the semi-rhythmic occurrence of the SWS-REMS-W cycle, reflecting the modulation of the sleep–wake behavior by BRAC; (3) diminished probability of sleep and an extended period of W with motor activity near the end of the active period (arrow above the nuchal EMG trace) which reflects the circadian reinforcement of W against the accumulating drive for sleep; and (4) increased delta power during the initial sleep episodes after the end of the lights-off/active period (arrow above the delta power trace), reflecting the increased pressure for sleep that accumulated during the active period. (Unpublished data from L. Kubin, K. Herr & G.L. Mann at the University of Pennsylvania, Philadelphia, PA)

2009; Gvilia et al. 2006; Leger et al. 2009; Maloney et al. 2000; Modirrousta et al. 2005; Sherin et al. 1996) indicated that groups of cells exhibiting different activity patterns relative to the distinct states of sleep and wake aggregate together and belong to different neurochemical phenotypes (Figs. 2.4 and 2.5). At the very basic level, cells located in the anterior hypothalamic median and ventrolateral preoptic nuclei (MnPO and VLPO) were identified as containing gamma-amino butyric acid (GABA), an inhibitory transmitter, and the peptide galanin and have increased discharge in association with NREM sleep. These cells have widespread axonal projections to the forebrain, midbrain, and hindbrain where they target different cell groups whose activity is associated with wakefulness (Uschakov et al. 2007). More recently, another group of SWS-active and GABAergic cells was localized in the reticular formation near the pontomedullary junction medial to the fibers of the facial nerve (Anaclet et al. 2012, 2014). Thus, the main executive units responsible for the generation of SWS are located in two brain regions and all appear to be GABAergic. Notably, the magnitude of their activation during SWS increases with the increasing need for sleep (Gvilia et al. 2006, 2011; Alam et al. 2014). As such, the anterior hypothalamic sleep-active neurons may accumulate and then discharge the drive for sleep, thereby mediating a component of the signal responsible for the homeostatic regulation of sleep.

Whereas the occurrence of SWS appears to be achieved by activation of two groups of GABAergic neurons, wake-active neurons are distributed more broadly and belong to at least six different neurochemical phenotypes. The main distinct groups contain the following neuromodulators, neurotransmitters, and peptides: norepinephrine (NE), serotonin (5HT), histamine (HI), acetylcholine (ACh), dopamine (DA), and orexins (ORX). These neurons are located in the posterior hypothalamus (HI and ORX), the basal forebrain or rostral pons/caudal midbrain (ACh), and in the midbrain, pons, and medulla (NE, 5HT, DA). Like the sleep-active neurons, the wake-active groups have widespread axonal projections throughout the brain (including the cortex and thalamus), as well as the spinal cord. Through their direct and indirect connections, when active, they suppress activity of NREM-active neurons. Hence, there is a mutually reciprocal inhibitory interaction between sleep- and wake-active neurons. Common to all wake-active neuronal groups is that activation of any one of them alone is sufficient to terminate sleep and elicit wakefulness, which may be taken to suggest a high degree of redundancy within the wake-active network. However, studies also indicate specialization and complementary roles of different groups in the generation of various aspects of wakefulness. For example, basal forebrain ACh neurons and NE neurons of the locus coeruleus (LC) are distinctly activated in association with cortical activation and support attention to, and processing of, external stimuli. DA, medullary 5HT, and pontomedullary NE neurons other than LC are particularly activated in connection with motor activation. ORX cells appear to reinforce wake-related activation of other wake-active groups. Furthermore, activation of NE, 5HT, and ORX neurons actively opposes the occurrence of REM sleep and, as such, they are important components of most models explaining the generation of this state (next section).

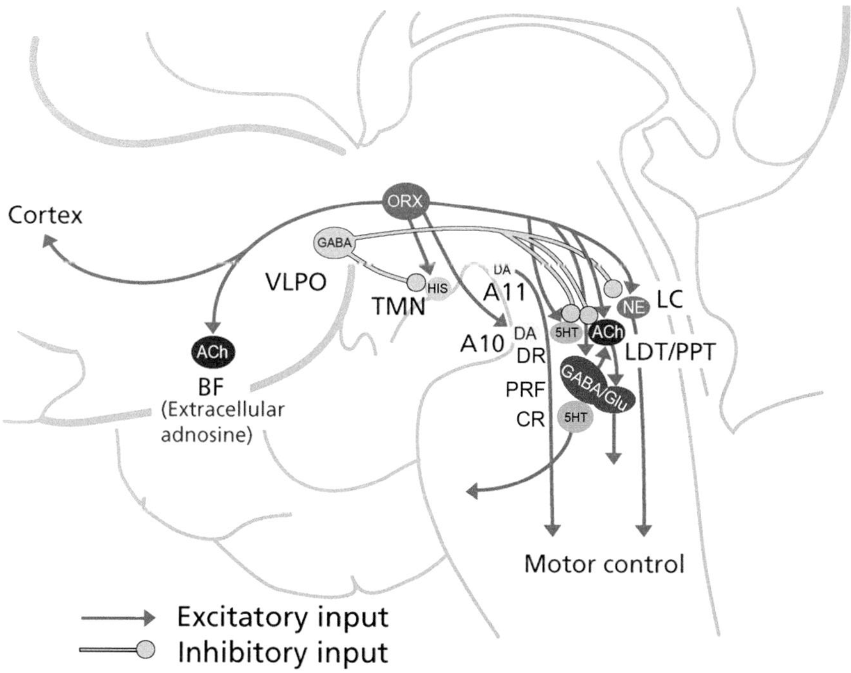

Fig. 2.4 Network of key connections among sleep active neurons of the anterior hypothalamus and wake-active neurons of the forebrain and hindbrain responsible for the generation of sleep–wake states. The anterior hypothalamic cells of the ventrolateral preoptic nucleus (VLPO) synthesize the inhibitory gamma-aminobutyric acid (GABA) and the inhibitory neuropeptide, galanin (blue). They are maximally active during NREM sleep and have extensive descending projections that primarily target different groups of wake-active neurons. As such, they represent the key component of the sleep-promoting and maintaining part of the network. The wake-active counterpart of the network includes cholinergic (ACh) neurons of the basal forebrain (BF), histaminergic (HIS) neurons of the tuberomammillary region (TMN), orexin (ORX, a.k.a. hypocretin)-containing neurons of the posterior lateral hypothalamus, pontine noradrenergic (NE) neurons symbolized here by the largest member of this group, the locus coeruleus (LC), dopaminergic (DA) neurons of the A10 and A11 groups which contribute to motor activation during wakefulness, and serotonin (5HT)-containing neurons of the dorsal and caudal raphé nuclei (DR and CR). Included in the scheme is adenosine which is one of the established metabolites that accumulate in extracellular space during periods of sustained cellular activation (e.g., during wakefulness) and provide negative feedback that limit further activation. As such, adenosine is one of the biochemical substrates of the drive for sleep (Sect. 2.5). Also, embedded within the network of NE, 5HT, and ACh neuronal groups of the caudal midbrain and rostral pons is a sub-network of GABA- and glutamate (Glu)-containing neurons that are responsible for the generation and maintenance of REM sleep. The scheme is adapted with permission from Fig. 1B in Mignot et al. (2002). Additional contributors to the generation of sleep–wake states have been discovered and characterized, including distinct subpopulations of hypothalamic and brainstem GABAergic neurons that play important roles in switching between NREM and REM sleep (Luppi et al. 2017)

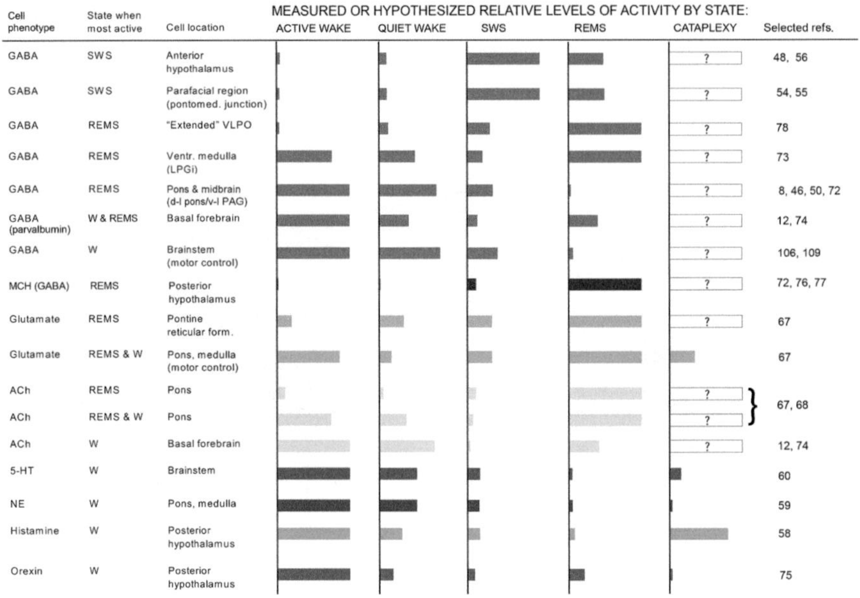

Fig. 2.5 At least 17 groups of neurons important for the generation and maintenance of sleep–wake states can be distinguished based on the combination of three criteria: anatomical location, main transmitter, or peptide that they use for communication with other neurons, and pattern of their activity across sleep–wake states. The data set included here distinguishes between active and quiet wakefulness and, where available, provides information about cell activity during cataplexy. Cataplexy is a dissociated state that occurs in the disorder of REM sleep called narcolepsy-cataplexy. During cataplectic attacks, patients experience muscle weakness, or a fully developed postural atonia like that during REM sleep, but are awake and aware of the external environment. Information about differences, or lack thereof, in cell firing between active and quiet wakefulness, on the one hand, and between REM sleep and cataplexy, on the other hand, helps define the specific roles of different groups of cells in different aspects of behavioral state control. For example, the histaminergic wake-active cells of the posterior hypothalamus maintain a high level of activity during cataplectic episodes when subjects are awake but have no postural muscle tone, whereas noradrenergic and serotonergic wake-active cells are silent or profoundly depressed during cataplexy. This distinction suggests a major role for histaminergic cells in the maintenance of wake-related cortical activation and an important contribution of noradrenergic and serotonergic neurons to the wake-related maintenance of muscle tone. Abbreviations unique for the Figure: *d-l* dorsolateral, *LPGi* lateral paragigantoccellular region, *PAG* periaqueductal gray, *v-l* ventrolateral

In contrast to NE, 5HT, and ORX neurons, activation of HI cells is important for the maintenance of consciousness (and cortical activation) but appears to have a weak relationship to motor activation or the absence thereof. Supporting this distinction are single-cell recordings obtained during cataplectic episodes from dogs selectively bred as genetic models of narcolepsy-cataplexy. Cataplectic attacks are dissociated states in which motor activity is suppressed through activation of a subset of the same neural mechanisms that are being activated during natural REM sleep but, in contrast to REM sleep, awareness of the external environment is preserved. Under these conditions, HI cells maintain high levels of activity whereas

NE and 5HT cell activity is abolished, or at least profoundly suppressed, like during natural REM sleep (John et al. 2004; Wu et al. 1999, 2004). Recordings from different sleep- and wake-active neurons during dissociated states such as cataplexy can provide more information about specific roles of different state-dependent neuronal groups in the generation of different external characteristics of distinct states of sleep and vigilance. To date, only a limited number of different neuronal groups have been investigated (Fig. 2.5). The availability of genetic mouse models of narcolepsy-cataplexy (Chemelli et al. 1999; Zhang et al. 2007) may help to expand such studies (Thankachan et al. 2009).

The scheme in Fig. 2.4 is an example of the basic network responsible for the generation of sleep–wake states [adapted from Mignot et al. (2002)]. It emphasizes a major role of the anterior hypothalamic GABAergic and NREM sleep-active neurons in the generation of sleep and a major role of posterior hypothalamic orexin neurons in the generation and maintenance of wakefulness. The scheme includes selected brainstem components of the sleep–wake network but they are given a relatively subordinate role, and the local mesopontine elements and connections responsible for the generation and maintenance of REM sleep are not detailed. Other published variants of the basic sleep–wake network include the components shown in Fig. 2.4 but differ in the level of detail and relative importance ascribed to neurochemically different cell groups and their interconnections (Saper et al. 2010; Fort et al. 2009; Jones 2005; Siegel 2009).

A notable development in the studies of the neuronal network responsible for the generation of sleep–wake states is the growing evidence for only a limited correspondence between neurochemically different cell groups and different states of vigilance that they support. Such a diversity occurs in the case of pontine cholinergic neurons, of which some are distinctly active during all states associated with cortical activation (during both wakefulness and REM sleep), some have relatively selective activity increases during REM sleep, and still some are distinctly activated during eye movements and/or other phasic events occurring during this state (Boucetta et al. 2014; el Mansari et al. 1989; Steriade et al. 1990). A similar functional diversity involves GABAergic neurons (Maloney et al. 2000). In particular, data indicate that the caudal midbrain and rostral pons contain different populations of GABAergic neurons of which some are wake-active and some are REM sleep-active. These neurons locally interact with excitatory glutamatergic neurons, and probably also with a separate population of ventromedial medullary REM sleep-active GABAergic neurons, to generate REM sleep, as well as to terminate this state (Boucetta et al. 2014; Lai et al. 1993, 1999; Luppi et al. 2017; Weber et al. 2015). Furthermore, a subpopulation of GABAergic neurons that are intermixed among cholinergic neurons within the basal forebrain is wake active (Xu et al. 2015), whereas another population of posterior hypothalamic GABAergic neurons intermixed among wake-active orexin-containing neurons are SWS active (Hassani et al. 2010). Additionally, the melanin-concentrating hormone (MCH) containing posterior hypothalamic neurons are preferentially activated during REM sleep and are also GABAergic (Hassani et al. 2009b; Peyron et al. 2009). Finally, there is a population of GABA- and galanin-containing neurons in the region of "extended" VLPO that is preferentially activated during REM sleep (Lu et al. 2000). Thus, GABAergic transmission is important, if not essential, for the generation and maintenance of all three major behavioral states.

Figure 2.5 provides a summary of activity patterns among neurochemically different cell groups that support the generation of sleep–wake states. This landscape, albeit still evolving, provides the basis for the design of different network models of the generation and maintenance of the states of NREM sleep, REM sleep and wake, as discussed in the next section.

2.4.2 Network Models of Generation of Sleep–Wake States

The original aminergic-cholinergic reciprocal interaction model of the generation of REM sleep (McCarley and Hobson 1975) proposed specific network interactions and neuronal properties and stimulated the search for supportive experimental evidence. The findings against the original model included the evidence that cholinergic activation, albeit sufficient, is not a necessary prerequisite for the occurrence of REM sleep (Reiner 1995; Jones 1991; Shouse and Siegel 1992) and that the interactions between aminergic and cholinergic neurons are either not direct or not mutually inhibitory. Encouraging for the design of alternate models were also the findings that antagonism of endogenous inhibition mediated by $GABA_A$ receptors directed toward the dorsomedial pontine network was very effective in triggering REM sleep-like episodes (Boissard et al. 2002; Fenik and Kubin 2009; Pollock and Mistlberger 2003; Sanford et al. 2003; Xi et al. 1999) [for review, see Kubin (2001)]. The discovery of the powerful role of orexins in protecting against random entries into REM sleep shifted the attention to a distributed network in which inputs descending from the hypothalamus converged onto local networks of the dorsal pontine tegmentum. Within the latter, different types of GABAergic neurons were identified and their interaction with local glutamatergic neurons has been proposed to be key for the generation of REM sleep (Luppi et al. 2017).

With the discovery that a single genetic mutation that disrupts synthesis of orexins or their receptors results in cataplectic attacks (Chemelli et al. 1999; Lin et al. 1999; Liu et al. 2008; Willie et al. 2003) came the appreciation for the need to maintain state stability and protect the network from random transitions among different behavioral states. The so-called “flip-flop” models have been designed in response to this need, first to model the transitions between wakefulness and NREM sleep and incorporate the proposed state-stabilizing role of hypothalamic orexin-containing neurons (Fig. 2.6a) (Saper et al. 2001), and then to incorporate the role of local and remote GABAergic inhibition in the generation of REM sleep within the mesopontine reticular formation (Fig. 2.6b) (Lu et al. 2006). The two models were ultimately combined and attempts were made to define their properties in mathematical terms [reviewed in Saper et al. (2010)].

The current “flip-flop” models of state switching (Saper et al. 2010) assign specific roles to most of the neurochemically and neuroanatomically different

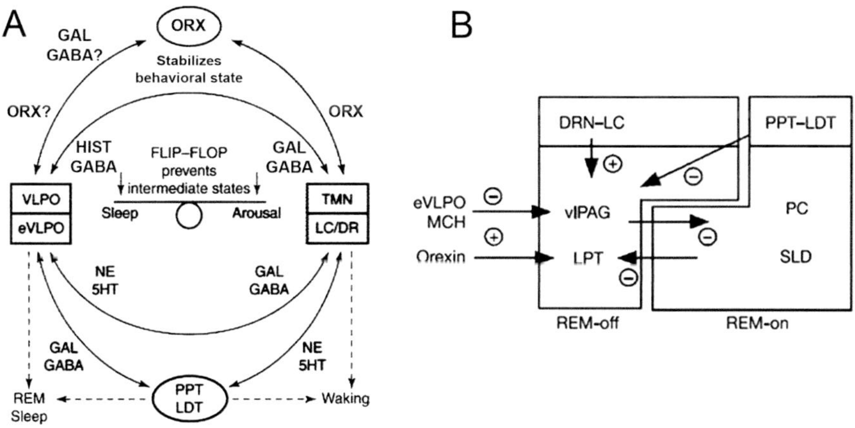

Fig. 2.6 Models of the interactions among neurochemically and neuroanatomically distinct groups of neurons that contribute to the generation of sleep–wake states. (**a**): A model designed to generate stable states of wakefulness and sleep in which GABA- and galanin (GAL)-containing cells located in the ventrolateral preoptic nucleus (VLPO) and the extended (e) VLPO of the anterior hypothalamus play an active role generating NREM sleep and enabling the emergence of REM sleep from the former. These cells have extensive efferent connections through which they inhibit multiple cell groups responsible for the maintenance of wakefulness, such as histaminergic (HIST) cells of the posterior hypothalamic tuberomammillary region (TMN), noradrenergic (NE) cells of the pontine locus coeruleus (LC), midbrain serotonergic (5HT) cells of the dorsal raphé nucleus (DR), and mesopontine acetylcholine-containing cells of the pedunculopontine and laterodorsal tegmental nuclei (PPT and LDT). The latter are shown in a position to promote both wakefulness and REM sleep. When active, all wake-related cell groups inhibit sleep-promoting neurons of the VLPO. In this model, a special role in stabilization of behavioral states is proposed for the wake-related cells of the posterior lateral hypothalamus that contain the excitatory peptides orexins (ORX). These cells, when active, reinforce activation of all other wake-active groups. They are themselves inhibited by sleep-active neurons of the VLPO. The model emphasizes the reciprocal interactions between sleep- and wake-promoting brain regions in a manner that results in alternative generation of distinct and stable states and secures rapid and reliable state switching. To emphasize the latter aspect, the model is referred to as a "flip-flop" switch model. Reproduced with permission from Saper et al. (2001). (**b**): A model of interactions among neurochemically different groups of dorsal pontomesencephalic neurons important for the generation and maintenance of REM sleep. Similar to the original reciprocal interaction model (McCarley and Hobson 1975), this model also includes a reciprocal arrangement between serotonergic and noradrenergic neurons (DRN-LC), on the one hand, and mesopontine cholinergic neurons (PPT-LDT), on the other hand. However, in contrast to the original model, the interaction is indirect, whereas a key role is ascribed to mutually inhibitory interaction between inhibitory (GABAergic) REM sleep-active (REM-on) neurons of the pontine sublaterodorsal region (SLD) and another group of inhibitory neurons located in the ventrolateral periaqueductal gray region (vlPAG) and in the lateral pontine tegmentum (LPT) that are silent during REM sleep (REM-off). Additionally, the REM-on part of the circuit includes excitatory neurons of the caudal pontine (PC) reticular formation whose proposed function is to generate external manifestations of REM sleep, such as cortical activation and postural atonia. This core reciprocally organized oscillator is externally enabled by inhibitory REM sleep-related inputs that descend onto its REM-off component from the melanin-concentrating hormone (MCH) cells of the posterior lateral hypothalamus and eVLPO cells of the anterior hypothalamus (both GABAergic). Conversely, external activation of the REM-off component is mediated by excitatory projections from hypothalamic ORX neurons. This model of flip-flop switching between REM sleep and the other two major states of vigilance (W and SWS) accounts for two distinct roles of inhibition mediated by GABA, one to prevent, and the other to promote, REM sleep. Reproduced with permission from Lu et al. (2006)

neuronal groups that have state-dependent activity patterns (see Fig. 2.5) and propose specific connections among these groups. As such, they offer an attractive framework on which to build specific experiments testing different aspects of these models. One obstacle toward this goal is the increasing recognition that sleep–wake circuits are often physically intertwined with networks controlling other vital functions, such as mood or metabolism, in a way that makes neuroanatomical and neurochemical signatures of studied cells of limited use for their unique identification as neurons specifically involved in the generation of one or another state of sleep or wakefulness (e.g., GABAergic cells in the posterior hypothalamus, or GABAergic cells of the dorsal mesopontine tegmentum). Genetic models and the selectivity offered by optogenetic activation or inhibition of genetically unique cell groups should help overcome the methodical problems with unique identification of different members of the network generating sleep–wake states. Once the basic models that can generate a tri-phasic sleep–wake rhythm are validated, there will be a need to better define and model their efferent pathways responsible for the production and shaping of different external manifestations of behavioral states, such as electrocortical changes, sleep effects on motor activity, or distinct regulations of memory and cognitive functions during sleep and wake. Also, while the current "flip-flop" models emphasize the need for stable maintenance of distinct behavioral states, the cellular and subcellular mechanisms that allow, trigger, and shape the process of transitions among different states (actual state switching) have not been well elaborated. This needs further study.

2.4.3 Atonia of REM Sleep

Different sleep–wake states are recognized based on different external manifestations (signs) that alone, or in combination, indicate the status of the state-controlling neuronal network. For NREM sleep, in addition to the absence of consciousness, such key signs include high delta power in cortical EEG, relaxed muscles with no phasic activity, regular breathing and heart rate. For REM sleep, cortical activation, and theta rhythm generated in the ponto-septo-hippocampal circuits are similar to active wakefulness but combined with the absence of consciousness, irregular breathing and heart rate, REMs, and muscle twitches superimposed on the absence of background tonic muscle activity (atonia) are some of the cardinal signs.

The mechanisms responsible for the suppression of motor activity during REM sleep have received extensive attention. The postural atonia of REM sleep is an important phenomenon that prevents motor enactment of the contents of dreams that predominantly occur during this stage of sleep (Uguccioni et al. 2013). Interestingly, motor suppression does not uniformly affect all muscles. Oculomotor muscles and muscles of the inner ear and the tongue maintain high levels of phasic activity during REM sleep, with patterns characteristic of this behavioral state (e.g., eye movements and muscle twitches). Activity of the main respiratory pump muscle, the diaphragm, also maintains rhythmic activity that, albeit highly variable from breath to breath, adequately supports ventilation (Orem 1980; Orem and Kubin 2005). On the other hand, activity of many accessory respiratory muscles that in some individuals need to be active in order to keep the upper airway open for breathing is profoundly diminished during REM sleep (or both NREM and REM sleep) which enables the disorder known as the obstructive sleep apnea syndrome (White and Younes 2012). Moreover, among the different trunk, proximal limb, and distant limb muscles, motor suppression is least prominent in the latter, which explains the occurrence of twitches in the foot and hand muscles. Data also indicate that a gradual deterioration of motor suppression during REM sleep precedes the occurrence of overt clinical signs of aging-related degenerative disorders (Howell and Schenck 2015; Iranzo et al. 2013; Postuma et al. 2009). Hence, there are substantial quantitative differences in the REM sleep-related control of different pools of motor neurons, both cranial and spinal, and monitoring of the magnitude and pattern of motor activation, or the absence thereof, during REM sleep may be of diagnostic value.

There is now evidence that three neuroanatomically and neurochemically distinct mechanisms may contribute to the suppression of motor activity during REM sleep. They may utilize the following processes: (a) REM sleep-related withdrawal of motoneuronal activation that is exerted in other states by norepinephrine, serotonin, and associated neuropeptides (thyrotropin-releasing hormone, substance P, orexins); (b) active inhibition of motoneurons by cholinergic pathways that are activated during REM sleep; and (c) active, postsynaptic inhibition of motoneurons by REM sleep-specific pathways that terminate on motoneurons and release inhibitory amino acids, such as glycine or GABA. The last of the three potential mechanisms have been by far most widely considered because intracellular recordings from lumbar motoneurons during REM sleep revealed the presence of inhibitory postsynaptic potentials (IPSPs) of which some had uniquely large amplitudes (Glenn and Dement 1981; Morales and Chase 1982; Morales et al. 1987). Similar potentials were also detected in trigeminal and hypoglossal motoneurons (Chandler et al. 1980; Fung and Chase 2015; Pedroarena et al. 1994; Yamuy et al. 1999). Furthermore, in lumbar motoneurons, these IPSPs were abolished by strychnine, an antagonist of chloride-dependent inhibition mediated by glycine, when the drug was administered onto individual motoneurons (Chase et al. 1989).

Collectively, the presence of strychnine-sensitive IPSPs in motoneurons supports the concept that the atonia of REM sleep is caused by an active, postsynaptic inhibition of motoneurons (Chase and Morales 1990). However, all studies attempting to block the REM sleep-related suppression of activity in trigeminal or hypoglossal motoneurons (or their target muscles) by local delivery of antagonists of the inhibitory glycine or GABA receptors indicated that active inhibition does not cause the atonia because these well-established antagonists could not abolish, or even substantially diminish, the atonia (Brooks and Peever 2008; Fenik et al. 2005a; Kubin et al. 1993; Morrison et al. 2003; Soja et al. 1987). Indeed, all these studies pointed to a small, if any, role of glycine or GABA in causing the REM sleep-related suppression of motoneuronal activity. Consequently, one had to conclude that, at least in hypoglossal and trigeminal motoneurons, REM sleep-specific IPSPs occur but they are not the main cause of depression of motoneuronal activity during this state (Kubin 2008). It must, however, be noted that experiments designed similar to those with hypoglossal and trigeminal motoneurons are yet to be conducted with postural motoneurons of the spinal cord. Until then, one has to be open to the possibility that REM sleep-specific active inhibition has a more prominent role in the spinal motor circuits than in cranial motoneurons that innervate orofacial muscles.

Withdrawal of aminergic activation of motoneurons (disfacilitation) that must occur during REM sleep when noradrenergic and serotonergic neurons cease firing (Fig. 2.5) has been tested in hypoglossal and trigeminal motoneurons as a mechanism of the atonia of REM sleep alternative to the concept of active amino acid-mediated inhibition. Consistent with the disfacilitation hypothesis, studies revealed that pharmacological antagonism of appropriate serotonin and/or norepinephrine receptors located within the regions of the trigeminal or hypoglossal motor nuclei resulted in decrements of motoneuronal activity comparable in magnitude to those observed during REM sleep (Chan et al. 2006; Fenik et al. 2005b; Kubin et al. 1992; Veasey et al. 1996). As the next step in the exploration of this concept, experiments were designed to test whether a combined withdrawal from motoneurons of excitations mediated by norepinephrine and serotonin causes a depression of motoneuronal activity that is functionally equivalent to the depression of motoneuronal activity during REM sleep (Fenik et al. 2004, 2005a, b). These experiments, conducted in a rat pharmacological model of REM sleep, used combined antagonism of appropriate serotonergic and adrenergic receptors to reduce hypoglossal nerve activity. Importantly, when episodes of REM sleep-like state were elicited while the endogenous aminergic effects were fully blocked, there was no further reduction of XII nerve activity. This indicated that, in hypoglossal motoneurons, a combined withdrawal from motoneurons of the activations mediated by just two modulators, norepinephrine and serotonin, were functionally equivalent to the endogenous neurochemical processes causing the atonia of REM sleep (Fenik et al. 2005b).

The third mechanism that is proposed to be a potentially important contributor to the atonia of REM sleep is based on active inhibition mediated by cholinergic pathways to motoneurons that are specifically activated during REM sleep. The concept is based on data indicating that there is a subset of brainstem cholinergic neurons that have axonal projections within the brainstem and to the spinal cord (Rukhadze and Kubin 2007; Weng et al. 2014), and are selectively activated during REM sleep (see Fig. 2.5). In support of the cholinergic mechanism, tongue muscle activity was significantly increased when a broad spectrum muscarinic cholinergic receptor antagonist, scopolamine, was delivered to the hypoglossal nucleus region by means of reverse microdialysis during REM sleep (Grace et al. 2013, 2014). Although activity was also increased during wakefulness and NREM sleep, the prominent increases obtained during REM sleep were quite remarkable when compared to weak effects reported in earlier studies with antagonists of inhibitory glycine or GABA receptors. Thus, while the state-specificity of the cholinergic effect remains to be further investigated, the data show that it is possible to pharmacologically overcome the depression of activity of hypoglossal motoneurons during REM sleep.

Thus, the current landscape of the field of studies on the mechanisms of motor depression during REM sleep shows that a combination of several distinct neurotransmitters and pathways may be involved and that their relative contributions may vary among different pools of motoneurons [for reviews, see Kubin (2008), Arrigoni et al. (2016), and Kubin (2016)].

2.5 Mechanisms of Sleep–Wake Homeostasis

Superimposed on the basic ability of the sleep–wake network to generate different behavioral states is the need for homeostatic regulation of the daily amounts of sleep and wake. According to the two-process model described in the Introduction, sleep need increases with the duration of wakefulness, and an extension of vigilance beyond its normal range is followed by sleep rebound expressed in the form of "deeper" sleep (increased delta power and reduced arousability) and increased sleep duration. There is some uncertainty whether REM sleep counts as wakefulness or sleep in the balance of sleep–wake homeostasis (Franken et al. 2001; Benington and Heller 1994; Horne 2000; Nykamp et al. 1998). Regardless of this, however, there is evidence that REM sleep amounts are homeostatically regulated because selective REM sleep deprivation is followed by a REM sleep rebound (Leger et al. 2009; Ocampo-Garces and Vivaldi 2002).

Sleep homeostasis is achieved through multiple mechanisms that operate at different levels of the sleep–wake network. These mechanisms may be divided into distinct categories based on their mechanistic principles and putative functions. One category represents a specialized case of a general principle of homeostatic plasticity that likely operates within most neuronal networks and whose role is to maintain a balance between excitation and inhibition in order to maintain long-term network stability and support its adaptation to varying levels of use (Nelson et al. 2002; Turrigiano 2008). This category includes the mechanisms that increase and decrease the production of transmitters and regulate neurotransmitter receptor expression, utilization, and trafficking in a homeostatic (negative feedback-driven and use-dependent) manner. A generic example of such a mechanism would be an increased synthesis of functional inhibitory receptors in a neuron subjected to intense excitatory inputs, with or without a concurrent degradation and reduction of synthesis of the postsynaptic receptors that receive the excitation. Collectively, the purpose of this regulation is to protect the excited neuron from excessive excitation.

Neurochemical processes that ensure network stability can support generation and maintenance of sleep and wake provided that their time constant is compatible with the rhythms regulating sleep and wake, such as the circadian rhythm and BRAC. With this condition fulfilled, it is easy to imagine how prolonged wakefulness and the associated activation of certain wake-active neurons may lead to increased synthesis of inhibitory receptors on these neurons which, in turn, make them more sensitive and receptive to inhibition imparted on them by sleep-related neurons.

There is now considerable evidence that homeostatic regulation of receptor expression and trafficking indeed occurs in brain regions and cells important for the regulation of sleep, as well as in the networks controlling cortical activation/ deactivation with sleep–wake states. Relevant adaptive changes occur on the time scale of hours, rather than days or weeks, and can be detected following sleep deprivation of moderate duration (e.g., 2–6 h). Examples of such a regulation revealed to date include robust downregulation of mRNA levels for multiple subunits of $GABA_A$ receptors and GABA synthesizing enzyme (GAD-65) elicited in brain slices in vitro obtained from the wake-active regions of the posterior hypothalamus when endogenous GABA levels are increased by inhibition of GABA reuptake for periods as short as 1.5 h. Conversely, in the same in vitro setting, increased stimulation of $GABA_A$ receptors reduces GAD-65 mRNA levels (Volgin and Kubin 2007). Importantly, similar mRNA changes also occur in the same brain region in vivo following 6 h of gentle sleep deprivation, and proteins for selected $GABA_A$ receptor subunits and GAD exhibit homeostatic changes (Volgin et al. 2014). Increased expression of α_1 subunit of $GABA_A$ receptor has been detected in wake-active orexin neurons following 6 h of sleep deprivation (Matsuki et al. 2015). On the other hand, a pool of inhibitory α_2-adrenergic receptors on orexin neurons was inactive under the baseline conditions but became activated (or made available) after 2 h of sleep deprivation (Uschakov et al. 2011). Collectively, these studies indicated that homeostatic changes involving $GABA_A$ and adrenergic inhibitory receptors located in the posterior hypothalamus respond to sleep loss in a manner suggesting that they contribute to the homeostatic regulation of sleep. Increased expression of proteins for the $\beta2/\beta3$ subunits of $GABA_A$ receptor located on cholinergic neurons also occurs following sleep deprivation in the basal forebrain where such changes probably reinforce sleep-related suppression of activity of these wake-active neurons (Modirrousta et al. 2007).

Another major category of mechanism by which the amounts of sleep and wake are regulated in a homeostatic manner is related to the concept of sleep as an obligatory period of rest and recovery that follows a period of wakefulness during which certain vital organismal resources are depleted and certain potentially toxic by-products accumulate. Among the sleep-promoting factors that belong to this category are adenosine (Benington et al. 1995; Landolt 2008; Radulovacki 1985) which is produced from adenosine triphosphate (ATP) when cells are metabolically active, various by-products of glycogen utilization (Petit et al. 2015), uridine-5-′-triphosphate (UTP) which contributes to both restoration of energy stores and synthesis of new RNA, and glutathione, an endogenous antioxidant (Inoue et al. 1995; Ikeda et al. 2005). Studies of the role and mode of action of adenosine indicate that it has sleep-inducing effects in multiple brain regions important for the regulation of sleep, most prominently in the basal forebrain (Dworak et al. 2010; Mackiewicz et al. 2003; Rai et al. 2010; Blanco-Centurion et al. 2006), and that it accumulates in response to sleep deprivation (Porkka-Heiskanen et al. 2000; Thakkar et al. 2003; Yanik and Radulovacki 1987). Data also indicate that astroglia and its interaction with neurons represent the main source and control local accumulation and removal of adenosine (Bjorness et al. 2016; Frank 2013; Halassa et al. 2009).

A number of endogenous compounds associated with fever and inflammation have NREM sleep-promoting properties but data indicate that their role is not limited to the modulation of sleep during infection and other challenges. Several cytokines typically generated as a part of immune response facilitate sleep. This includes interleukin-1β (IL-1β) and tumor necrosis factor α (TNFα) (Krueger 2008; Krueger et al. 2011). The effects of IL-1β are mediated by the growth hormone-releasing hormone (GHRH) (Obal and Krueger 2004, Obal et al. 1995), and IL-1β effects depend on adenosine generated by both neurons and glia (Ingiosi et al. 2015; Nadjar et al. 2013; Opp and Krueger 2015).

Local cell activation and the use-/activity-dependent generation of ATP and nitric oxide synthase (NOS) contribute to local modulation of cellular excitability in a homeostatic manner (Krueger et al. 2013). These and other local cellular and molecular processes promote local rest/sleep in cortical networks following a period of intense activation (Krueger et al. 2013; Krueger and Tononi 2011; Vyazovskiy et al. 2009). Together with a host of other activity-dependent biochemical and molecular changes, they act as intermediaries for the use-dependent structural plasticity, such as synaptic scaling and generation or retraction of dendritic spines, that are necessary for processing and consolidation of memory (Havekes et al. 2016; Huber et al. 2004; Naidoo et al. 2012; Nelson et al. 2004).

Thus, the different mechanisms put in motion during alternating periods of increased use and disuse of selected networks and neuronal connections interact and complement each other in a manner that ensures long-term homeostasis at both local and organismal levels and supports adaptation to the changing environment.

2.6 Conclusion

A major goal of sleep research and sleep medicine is to identify the mechanisms responsible for the generation and regulation of natural sleep–wake states and develop remedies for sleep disorders in humans. To achieve this, a major research effort is directed toward the exploration of animal models. The underlying premise is that most fundamental mechanisms are common to all mammals and may even have their origin in simpler vertebrate and non-vertebrate species. Accordingly, the state of knowledge discussed in this chapter is extensively informed by experimental findings derived from animals. Over the last 20 years, rodents, in particular, have become models of choice for sleep research due to their suitable size, good availability across a broad and ever-increasing range of genetic modifications, and sophisticated infrastructure of research tools, such as gene and protein data bases, well-characterized drugs and antibodies, brain atlases, and data collection equipment. Information derived from this research effort has repeatedly proven to be applicable to sleep–wake control in humans. Still, beyond fundamental principles, major species differences exist and need to be considered in translational medicine.

Most rodents, for example, are nocturnal and tend to have more robust circadian regulation than humans. The metabolic rate of rodents is faster than humans' which is probably the reason for the relatively high frequency of most of their rhythmic processes, including sleep–wake cycling, respiratory rate, and heart rate (Lo et al. 2004). These interspecies differences, albeit important for the practice of medicine, are beyond consideration in this overview of fundamental principles of sleep–wake regulation that are common across many species.

Under normal, physiologic conditions, sleep and wake rhythmically alternate as a result of external gating and pacing imposed on a distributed network of neurons responsible for the generation and maintenance of each of the three distinct behavioral states, wakefulness, NREM sleep, and REM sleep. The system is robust but also vulnerable to external and internal perturbations. Major sleep fragmentation, such as the obstructive sleep apnea syndrome, neuropsychiatric disorders, such as anxiety disorders or post-traumatic stress disorder (PTSD), shift work, metabolic derangements, degenerative disorders of aging, and pain are among the factors and conditions associated with severe sleep disruptions. They occur and exert their detrimental effects on the development, health status, and quality of life of individuals by altering the properties and functions of the neural networks and cellular processes discussed in this chapter. The pathophysiology of these changes and various established and emerging therapies are discussed in other sections of this volume.

Acknowledgments Our research discussed in this review has been supported by the following grants from the National Institutes of Health (USA): HL042236, HL047600, HL060287, HL071097, and HL074385.

References

Alam MA, Kumar S, McGinty D, Alam MN, Szymusiak R. Neuronal activity in the preoptic hypothalamus during sleep deprivation and recovery sleep. J Neurophysiol. 2014;111(2): 287–99.

Albrecht U. Timing to perfection: the biology of central and peripheral circadian clocks. Neuron. 2012;74(2):246–60.

Anaclet C, Lin JS, Vetrivelan R, Krenzer M, Vong L, Fuller PM, et al. Identification and characterization of a sleep-active cell group in the rostral medullary brainstem. J Neurosci. 2012;32(50):17970–6.

Anaclet C, Ferrari L, Arrigoni E, Bass CE, Saper CB, Lu J, et al. The GABAergic parafacial zone is a medullary slow wave sleep-promoting center. Nat Neurosci. 2014;17(9):1217–24.

Arrigoni E, Chen MC, Fuller PM. The anatomical, cellular and synaptic basis of motor atonia during rapid eye movement sleep. J Physiol. 2016;594(19):5391–414.

Aserinsky E, Kleitman N. Regularly occurring periods of eye motility, and concomitant phenomena, during sleep. Science. 1953;118(3062):273–4.

Basheer R, Sherin JE, Saper CB, Morgan JI, McCarley RW, Shiromani PJ. Effects of sleep on wake-induced c-fos expression. J Neurosci. 1997;17(24):9746–50.

Bass J, Takahashi JS. Circadian integration of metabolism and energetics. Science. 2010;330 (6009):1349–54.

Benington JH, Heller HC. Does the function of REM sleep concern non-REM sleep or waking? Prog Neurobiol. 1994;44(5):433–49.

Benington JH, Kodali SK, Heller HC. Stimulation of A1 adenosine receptors mimics the electroencephalographic effects of sleep deprivation. Brain Res. 1995;692(1–2):79–85.

Bjorness TE, Dale N, Mettlach G, Sonneborn A, Sahin B, Fienberg AA, et al. An adenosine-mediated glial-neuronal circuit for homeostatic sleep. J Neurosci. 2016;36(13):3709–21.

Blanco-Centurion C, Xu M, Murillo-Rodriguez E, Gerashchenko D, Shiromani AM, Salin-Pascual RJ, et al. Adenosine and sleep homeostasis in the Basal forebrain. J Neurosci. 2006;26(31): 8092–100.

Boissard R, Gervasoni D, Schmidt MH, Barbagli B, Fort P, Luppi PH. The rat ponto-medullary network responsible for paradoxical sleep onset and maintenance: a combined microinjection and functional neuroanatomical study. Eur J Neurosci. 2002;16(10):1959–73.

Borbély AA. A two process model of sleep regulation. Hum Neurobiol. 1982;1(3):195–204.

Boucetta S, Cisse Y, Mainville L, Morales M, Jones BE. Discharge profiles across the sleep-waking cycle of identified cholinergic, GABAergic, and glutamatergic neurons in the pontomesencephalic tegmentum of the rat. J Neurosci. 2014;34(13):4708–27.

Brooks PL, Peever JH. Glycinergic and $GABA_A$-mediated inhibition of somatic motoneurons does not mediate rapid eye movement sleep motor atonia. J Neurosci. 2008;28(14):3535–45.

Brown EN, Lydic R, Schiff ND. General anesthesia, sleep, and coma. N Engl J Med. 2010;363(27): 2638–50.

Buckley TM, Schatzberg AF. On the interactions of the hypothalamic-pituitary-adrenal (HPA) axis and sleep: normal HPA axis activity and circadian rhythm, exemplary sleep disorders. J Clin Endocrinol Metab. 2005;90(5):3106–14.

Chan E, Steenland HW, Liu H, Horner RL. Endogenous excitatory drive modulating respiratory muscle activity across sleep-wake states. Am J Respir Crit Care Med. 2006;174(11):1264–73.

Chandler SH, Chase MH, Nakamura Y. Intracellular analysis of synaptic mechanisms controlling trigeminal motoneuron activity during sleep and wakefulness. J Neurophysiol. 1980;44(2): 359–71.

Chase MH, Morales FR. The atonia and myoclonia of active (REM) sleep. Annu Rev Psychol. 1990;41:557–84.

Chase MH, Soja PJ, Morales FR. Evidence that glycine mediates the postsynaptic potentials that inhibit lumbar motoneurons during the atonia of active sleep. J Neurosci. 1989;9(3):743–51.

Chemelli RM, Willie JT, Sinton CM, Elmquist JK, Scammell T, Lee C, et al. Narcolepsy in orexin knockout mice: molecular genetics of sleep regulation. Cell. 1999;98(4):437–51.

D'Olimpio F, Renzi P. Ultradian rhythms in young and adult mice: further support for the basic rest-activity cycle. Physiol Behav. 1998;64(5):697–701.

de Lecea L, Kilduff TS, Peyron C, Gao X, Foye PE, Danielson PE, et al. The hypocretins: hypothalamus-specific peptides with neuroexcitatory activity. Proc Natl Acad Sci U S A. 1998;95(1):322–7.

Dentico D, Amici R, Baracchi F, Cerri M, Del Sindaco E, Luppi M, et al. c-Fos expression in preoptic nuclei as a marker of sleep rebound in the rat. Eur J Neurosci. 2009;30(4):651–61.

Dworak M, McCarley RW, Kim T, Kalinchuk AV, Basheer R. Sleep and brain energy levels: ATP changes during sleep. J Neurosci. 2010;30(26):9007–16.

el Mansari M, Sakai K, Jouvet M. Unitary characteristics of presumptive cholinergic tegmental neurons during the sleep-waking cycle in freely moving cats. Exp Brain Res. 1989;76(3): 519–29.

Emens JS, Burgess HJ. Effect of light and melatonin and other melatonin receptor agonists on human circadian physiology. Sleep Med Clin. 2015;10(4):435–53.

Feldman JL, Mitchell GS, Nattie EE. Breathing: rhythmicity, plasticity, chemosensitivity. Annu Rev Neurosci. 2003;26:239–66.

Fenik VB, Kubin L. Differential localization of carbachol- and bicuculline-sensitive pontine sites for eliciting REM sleep-like effects in anesthetized rats. J Sleep Res. 2009;18(1):99–112.

Fenik V, Davies RO, Kubin L. Combined antagonism of aminergic excitatory and amino acid inhibitory receptors in the XII nucleus abolishes REM sleep-like depression of hypoglossal motoneuronal activity. Arch Ital Biol. 2004;142(3):237–49.

Fenik VB, Davies RO, Kubin L. Noradrenergic, serotonergic and GABAergic antagonists injected together into the XII nucleus abolish the REM sleep-like depression of hypoglossal motoneuronal activity. J Sleep Res. 2005a;14(4):419–29.

Fenik VB, Davies RO, Kubin L. REM sleep-like atonia of hypoglossal (XII) motoneurons is caused by loss of noradrenergic and serotonergic inputs. Am J Respir Crit Care Med. 2005b;172(10): 1322–30.

Fort P, Bassetti CL, Luppi PH. Alternating vigilance states: new insights regarding neuronal networks and mechanisms. Eur J Neurosci. 2009;29(9):1741–53.

Frank MG. Astroglial regulation of sleep homeostasis. Curr Opin Neurobiol. 2013;23(5):812–8.

Franken P, Chollet D, Tafti M. The homeostatic regulation of sleep need is under genetic control. J Neurosci. 2001;21(8):2610–21.

Fung SJ, Chase MH. Postsynaptic inhibition of hypoglossal motoneurons produces atonia of the genioglossal muscle during rapid eye movement sleep. Sleep. 2015;38(1):139–46.

Glenn LL, Dement WC. Membrane potential, synaptic activity, and excitability of hindlimb motoneurons during wakefulness and sleep. J Neurophysiol. 1981;46(4):839–54.

Grace KP, Hughes SW, Horner RL. Identification of the mechanism mediating genioglossus muscle suppression in REM sleep. Am J Respir Crit Care Med. 2013;187(3):311–9.

Grace KP, Hughes SW, Horner RL. Identification of a pharmacological target for genioglossus reactivation throughout sleep. Sleep. 2014;37(1):41–50.

Gvilia I, Xu F, McGinty D, Szymusiak R. Homeostatic regulation of sleep: a role for preoptic area neurons. J Neurosci. 2006;26(37):9426–33.

Gvilia I, Suntsova N, Angara B, McGinty D, Szymusiak R. Maturation of sleep homeostasis in developing rats: a role for preoptic area neurons. Am J Physiol Regul Integr Comp Physiol. 2011;300(4):R885–94.

Halassa MM, Florian C, Fellin T, Munoz JR, Lee SY, Abel T, et al. Astrocytic modulation of sleep homeostasis and cognitive consequences of sleep loss. Neuron. 2009;61(2):213–9.

Hassani OK, Lee MG, Henny P, Jones BE. Discharge profiles of identified GABAergic in comparison to cholinergic and putative glutamatergic basal forebrain neurons across the sleep-wake cycle. J Neurosci. 2009a;29(38):11828–40.

Hassani OK, Lee MG, Jones BE. Melanin-concentrating hormone neurons discharge in a reciprocal manner to orexin neurons across the sleep-wake cycle. Proc Natl Acad Sci U S A. 2009b;106(7): 2418–22.

Hassani OK, Henny P, Lee MG, Jones BE. GABAergic neurons intermingled with orexin and MCH neurons in the lateral hypothalamus discharge maximally during sleep. Eur J Neurosci. 2010;32 (3):448–57.

Havekes R, Park AJ, Tudor JC, Luczak VG, Hansen RT, Ferri SL, et al. Sleep deprivation causes memory deficits by negatively impacting neuronal connectivity in hippocampal area CA1. eLife. 2016;5:e13424.

Hendricks JC, Finn SM, Panckeri KA, Chavkin J, Williams JA, Sehgal A, et al. Rest in Drosophila is a sleep-like state. Neuron. 2000;25(1):129–38.

Hobson JA, Lydic R, Baghdoyan HA. Evolving concepts of sleep cycle generation: from brain centers to neuronal populations. Behav Brain Sci. 1986;9:371–448.

Horne JA. REM sleep—by default? Neurosci Biobehav Rev. 2000;24(8):777–97.

Howell MJ, Schenck CH. Rapid eye movement sleep behavior disorder and neurodegenerative disease. JAMA Neurol. 2015;72(6):707–12.

Huber R, Ghilardi MF, Massimini M, Tononi G. Local sleep and learning. Nature. 2004;430(6995): 78–81.

Ikeda M, Ikeda-Sagara M, Okada T, Clement P, Urade Y, Nagai T, et al. Brain oxidation is an initial process in sleep induction. Neuroscience. 2005;130(4):1029–40.

Ingiosi AM, Raymond RM Jr, Pavlova MN, Opp MR. Selective contributions of neuronal and astroglial interleukin-1 receptor 1 to the regulation of sleep. Brain Behav Immun. 2015;48:244–57.
Inoue S, Honda K, Komoda Y. Sleep as neuronal detoxification and restitution. Behav Brain Res. 1995;69(1–2):91–6.
Iranzo A, Tolosa E, Gelpi E, Molinuevo JL, Valldeoriola F, Serradell M, et al. Neurodegenerative disease status and post-mortem pathology in idiopathic rapid-eye-movement sleep behaviour disorder: an observational cohort study. Lancet Neurol. 2013;12(5):443–53.
John J, Wu MF, Boehmer LN, Siegel JM. Cataplexy-active neurons in the hypothalamus: implications for the role of histamine in sleep and waking behavior. Neuron. 2004;42(4):619–34.
Jones BE. Paradoxical sleep and its chemical/structural substrates in the brain. Neuroscience. 1991;40(3):637–56.
Jones BE. From waking to sleeping: neuronal and chemical substrates. Trends Pharmacol Sci. 2005;26(11):578–86.
Jouvet M. [Research on the neural structures and responsible mechanisms in different phases of physiological sleep]. Arch Ital Biol 1962;100(2):125–206.
Kalsbeek A, Yi CX, la Fleur SE, Buijs RM, Fliers E. Suprachiasmatic nucleus and autonomic nervous system influences on awakening from sleep. Int Rev Neurobiol. 2010;93:91–107.
Kim Y, Laposky AD, Bergmann BM, Turek FW. Repeated sleep restriction in rats leads to homeostatic and allostatic responses during recovery sleep. Proc Natl Acad Sci U S A. 2007;104(25):10697–702.
Kleitman N. Biological rhythms and cycles. Physiol Rev. 1949;29(1):1–30.
Kleitman N. Sleep and wakefulness. Chicago: University of Chicago Press; 1963.
Kleitman N. Basic rest-activity cycle—22 years later. Sleep. 1982;5(4):311–7.
Krueger JM. The role of cytokines in sleep regulation. Curr Pharm Des. 2008;14(32):3408–16.
Krueger JM, Tononi G. Local use-dependent sleep; synthesis of the new paradigm. Curr Top Med Chem. 2011;11(19):2490–2.
Krueger JM, Clinton JM, Winters BD, Zielinski MR, Taishi P, Jewett KA, et al. Involvement of cytokines in slow wave sleep. Prog Brain Res. 2011;193:39–47.
Krueger JM, Huang YH, Rector DM, Buysse DJ. Sleep: a synchrony of cell activity-driven small network states. Eur J Neurosci. 2013;38(2):2199–209.
Kubin L. Carbachol models of REM sleep: recent developments and new directions. Arch Ital Biol. 2001;139(1–2):147–68.
Kubin L. Adventures and tribulations in the search for the mechanisms of the atonia of REM sleep. Sleep. 2008;31(11):1473–6.
Kubin L. Neural control of the upper airway: respiratory and state-dependent mechanisms. Compr Physiol. 2016;6(4):1801–50.
Kubin L, Tojima H, Davies RO, Pack AI. Serotonergic excitatory drive to hypoglossal motoneurons in the decerebrate cat. Neurosci Lett. 1992;139(2):243–8.
Kubin L, Kimura H, Tojima H, Davies RO, Pack AI. Suppression of hypoglossal motoneurons during the carbachol-induced atonia of REM sleep is not caused by fast synaptic inhibition. Brain Res. 1993;611(2):300–12.
Lai YY, Clements JR, Siegel JM. Glutamatergic and cholinergic projections to the pontine inhibitory area identified with horseradish peroxidase retrograde transport and immunohistochemistry. J Comp Neurol. 1993;336(3):321–30.
Lai YY, Clements JR, Wu XY, Shalita T, Wu JP, Kuo JS, et al. Brainstem projections to the ventromedial medulla in cat: retrograde transport horseradish peroxidase and immunohistochemical studies. J Comp Neurol. 1999;408(3):419–36.
Landolt HP. Sleep homeostasis: a role for adenosine in humans? Biochem Pharmacol. 2008;75(11): 2070–9.
Lavie P. REM periodicity under ultrashort sleep/wake cycle in narcoleptic patients. Can J Psychol. 1991;45(2):185–93.

Leger L, Goutagny R, Sapin E, Salvert D, Fort P, Luppi PH. Noradrenergic neurons expressing Fos during waking and paradoxical sleep deprivation in the rat. J Chem Neuroanat. 2009;37(3): 149–57.

Lin L, Faraco J, Li R, Kadotani H, Rogers W, Lin X, et al. The sleep disorder canine narcolepsy is caused by a mutation in the hypocretin (orexin) receptor 2 gene. Cell. 1999;98(3):365–76.

Liu M, Thankachan S, Kaur S, Begum S, Blanco-Centurion C, Sakurai T, et al. Orexin (hypocretin) gene transfer diminishes narcoleptic sleep behavior in mice. Eur J Neurosci. 2008;28(7): 1382–93.

Lo CC, Chou T, Penzel T, Scammell TE, Strecker RE, Stanley HE, et al. Common scale-invariant patterns of sleep-wake transitions across mammalian species. Proc Natl Acad Sci U S A. 2004;101(50):17545–8.

Lu J, Greco MA, Shiromani P, Saper CB. Effect of lesions of the ventrolateral preoptic nucleus on NREM and REM sleep. J Neurosci. 2000;20(10):3830–42.

Lu J, Sherman D, Devor M, Saper CB. A putative flip-flop switch for control of REM sleep. Nature. 2006;441(7093):589–94.

Luppi PH, Clement O, Sapin E, Peyron C, Gervasoni D, Leger L, et al. Brainstem mechanisms of paradoxical (REM) sleep generation. Pflugers Arch. 2012;463(1):43–52.

Luppi PH, Peyron C, Fort P. Not a single but multiple populations of GABAergic neurons control sleep. Sleep Med Rev. 2017;32:85–94.

Lydic R, Baghdoyan HA. Sleep, anesthesiology, and the neurobiology of arousal state control. Anesthesiology. 2005;103(6):1268–95.

Mackiewicz M, Nikonova EV, Zimmerman JE, Galante RJ, Zhang L, Cater JR, et al. Enzymes of adenosine metabolism in the brain: diurnal rhythm and the effect of sleep deprivation. J Neurochem. 2003;85(2):348–57.

Maloney KJ, Mainville L, Jones BE. c-Fos expression in GABAergic, serotonergic, and other neurons of the pontomedullary reticular formation and raphe after paradoxical sleep deprivation and recovery. J Neurosci. 2000;20(12):4669–79.

Matsuki T, Takasu M, Hirose Y, Murakoshi N, Sinton CM, Motoike T, et al. $GABA_A$ receptor-mediated input change on orexin neurons following sleep deprivation in mice. Neuroscience. 2015;284:217–24.

McCarley RW, Hobson JA. Neuronal excitability modulation over the sleep cycle: a structural and mathematical model. Science. 1975;189(4196):58–60.

McPartland RJ, Kupfer DJ. Rapid eye movement sleep cycle, clock time and sleep onset. Electroencephalogr Clin Neurophysiol. 1978;45(2):178–85.

Mignot E, Taheri S, Nishino S. Sleeping with the hypothalamus: emerging therapeutic targets for sleep disorders. Nat Neurosci. 2002;5(Suppl):1071–5.

Mistlberger RE. Circadian regulation of sleep in mammals: role of the suprachiasmatic nucleus. Brain Res Brain Res Rev. 2005;49(3):429–54.

Modirrousta M, Mainville L, Jones BE. Orexin and MCH neurons express c-Fos differently after sleep deprivation vs. recovery and bear different adrenergic receptors. Eur J Neurosci. 2005;21 (10):2807–16.

Modirrousta M, Mainville L, Jones BE. Dynamic changes in $GABA_A$ receptors on basal forebrain cholinergic neurons following sleep deprivation and recovery. BMC Neurosci. 2007;8:15.

Morales FR, Chase MH. Repetitive synaptic potentials responsible for inhibition of spinal cord motoneurons during active sleep. Exp Neurol. 1982;78(2):471–6.

Morales FR, Boxer P, Chase MH. Behavioral state-specific inhibitory postsynaptic potentials impinge on cat lumbar motoneurons during active sleep. Exp Neurol. 1987;98(2):418–35.

Morrison JL, Sood S, Liu H, Park E, Liu X, Nolan P, et al. Role of inhibitory amino acids in control of hypoglossal motor outflow to genioglossus muscle in naturally sleeping rats. J Physiol. 2003;552(Pt 3):975–91.

Nadjar A, Blutstein T, Aubert A, Laye S, Haydon PG. Astrocyte-derived adenosine modulates increased sleep pressure during inflammatory response. Glia. 2013;61(5):724–31.

Naidoo N, Ferber M, Galante RJ, McShane B, Hu JH, Zimmerman J, et al. Role of Homer proteins in the maintenance of sleep-wake states. PLoS One. 2012;7(4):e35174.
Nelson SB, Sjostrom PJ, Turrigiano GG. Rate and timing in cortical synaptic plasticity. Philos Trans R Soc Lond Ser B Biol Sci. 2002;357(1428):1851–7.
Nelson SE, Duricka DL, Campbell K, Churchill L, Krueger JM. Homer1a and 1bc levels in the rat somatosensory cortex vary with the time of day and sleep loss. Neurosci Lett. 2004;367(1): 105–8.
Nykamp K, Rosenthal L, Folkerts M, Roehrs T, Guido P, Roth T. The effects of REM sleep deprivation on the level of sleepiness/alertness. Sleep. 1998;21(6):609–14.
Obal F Jr, Krueger JM. GHRH and sleep. Sleep Med Rev. 2004;8(5):367–77.
Obal F Jr, Fang J, Payne LC, Krueger JM. Growth-hormone-releasing hormone mediates the sleep-promoting activity of interleukin-1 in rats. Neuroendocrinology. 1995;61(5):559–65.
Ocampo-Garces A, Vivaldi EA. Short-term homeostasis of REM sleep assessed in an intermittent REM sleep deprivation protocol in the rat. J Sleep Res. 2002;11(1):81–9.
Opp MR, Krueger JM. Sleep and immunity: a growing field with clinical impact. Brain Behav Immun. 2015;47:1–3.
Orem J. Neuronal mechanisms of respiration in REM sleep. Sleep. 1980;3(3–4):251–67.
Orem J, Kubin L. Respiratory physiology: central neural control. In: Kryger MH, Roth T, Dement WC, editors. Principles and practice of sleep medicine. 4th ed. Philadelphia, PA: Elsevier-Saunders; 2005. p. 213–23.
Paul KN, Losee-Olson S, Pinckney L, Turek FW. The ability of stress to alter sleep in mice is sensitive to reproductive hormones. Brain Res. 2009;1305:74–85.
Pedroarena C, Castillo P, Chase MH, Morales FR. The control of jaw-opener motoneurons during active sleep. Brain Res. 1994;653(1–2):31–8.
Petit JM, Burlet-Godinot S, Magistretti PJ, Allaman I. Glycogen metabolism and the homeostatic regulation of sleep. Metab Brain Dis. 2015;30(1):263–79.
Peyron C, Sapin E, Leger L, Luppi PH, Fort P. Role of the melanin-concentrating hormone neuropeptide in sleep regulation. Peptides. 2009;30(11):2052–9.
Pollock MS, Mistlberger RE. Rapid eye movement sleep induction by microinjection of the GABA-A antagonist bicuculline into the dorsal subcoeruleus area of the rat. Brain Res. 2003;962(1–2): 68–77.
Porkka-Heiskanen T, Strecker RE, McCarley RW. Brain site-specificity of extracellular adenosine concentration changes during sleep deprivation and spontaneous sleep: an in vivo microdialysis study. Neuroscience. 2000;99(3):507–17.
Postuma RB, Gagnon JF, Vendette M, Montplaisir JY. Markers of neurodegeneration in idiopathic rapid eye movement sleep behaviour disorder and Parkinson's disease. Brain. 2009;132(Pt 12): 3298–307.
Qiu MH, Chen MC, Lu J. Cortical neuronal activity does not regulate sleep homeostasis. Neuroscience. 2015;297:211–8.
Radulovacki M. Role of adenosine in sleep in rats. Rev Clin Basic Pharm. 1985;5(3–4):327–39.
Rai S, Kumar S, Alam MA, Szymusiak R, McGinty D, Alam MN. A1 receptor mediated adenosinergic regulation of perifornical-lateral hypothalamic area neurons in freely behaving rats. Neuroscience. 2010;167(1):40–8.
Rector DM, Schei JL, Van Dongen HP, Belenky G, Krueger JM. Physiological markers of local sleep. Eur J Neurosci. 2009;29(9):1771–8.
Reid KJ, Abbott SM. Jet lag and shift work disorder. Sleep Med Clin. 2015;10(4):523–35.
Reiner PB. Are mesopontine cholinergic neurons either necessary or sufficient components of the ascending reticular activating system? Semin Neurosci. 1995;7(5):355–9.
Richter DW, Spyer KM. Studying rhythmogenesis of breathing: comparison of in vivo and in vitro models. Trends Neurosci. 2001;24(8):464–72.
Rolls A, Pang WW, Ibarra I, Colas D, Bonnavion P, Korin B, et al. Sleep disruption impairs haematopoietic stem cell transplantation in mice. Nat Commun. 2015;6:8516.

Rukhadze I, Kubin L. Mesopontine cholinergic projections to the hypoglossal motor nucleus. Neurosci Lett. 2007;413(2):121–5.

Sanford LD, Tang X, Xiao J, Ross RJ, Morrison AR. GABAergic regulation of REM sleep in reticularis pontis oralis and caudalis in rats. J Neurophysiol. 2003;90(2):938–45.

Saper CB, Chou TC, Scammell TE. The sleep switch: hypothalamic control of sleep and wakefulness. Trends Neurosci. 2001;24(12):726–31.

Saper CB, Fuller PM, Pedersen NP, Lu J, Scammell TE. Sleep state switching. Neuron. 2010;68(6): 1023–42.

Sherin JE, Shiromani PJ, McCarley RW, Saper CB. Activation of ventrolateral preoptic neurons during sleep. Science. 1996;271(5246):216–9.

Shouse MN, Siegel JM. Pontine regulation of REM sleep components in cats: integrity of the pedunculopontine tegmentum (PPT) is important for phasic events but unnecessary for atonia during REM sleep. Brain Res. 1992;571(1):50–63.

Siegel JM. The neurobiology of sleep. Semin Neurol. 2009;29(4):277–96.

Silver R, Lesauter J. Circadian and homeostatic factors in arousal. Ann N Y Acad Sci. 2008;1129: 263–74.

Soja PJ, Finch DM, Chase MH. Effect of inhibitory amino acid antagonists on masseteric reflex suppression during active sleep. Exp Neurol. 1987;96(1):178–93.

Steriade M, Datta S, Pare D, Oakson G, Curro Dossi RC. Neuronal activities in brain-stem cholinergic nuclei related to tonic activation processes in thalamocortical systems. J Neurosci. 1990;10(8):2541–59.

Sukhotinsky I, Zalkind V, Lu J, Hopkins DA, Saper CB, Devor M. Neural pathways associated with loss of consciousness caused by intracerebral microinjection of GABA A-active anesthetics. Eur J Neurosci. 2007;25(5):1417–36.

Thakkar MM, Winston S, McCarley RW. A1 receptor and adenosinergic homeostatic regulation of sleep-wakefulness: effects of antisense to the A1 receptor in the cholinergic basal forebrain. J Neurosci. 2003;23(10):4278–87.

Thankachan S, Kaur S, Shiromani PJ. Activity of pontine neurons during sleep and cataplexy in hypocretin knock-out mice. J Neurosci. 2009;29(5):1580–5.

Tong X, Yin L. Circadian rhythms in liver physiology and liver diseases. Compr Physiol. 2013;3 (2):917–40.

Turrigiano GG. The self-tuning neuron: synaptic scaling of excitatory synapses. Cell. 2008;135(3): 422–35.

Uguccioni G, Golmard JL, de Fontreaux AN, Leu-Semenescu S, Brion A, Arnulf I. Fight or flight? Dream content during sleepwalking/sleep terrors vs. rapid eye movement sleep behavior disorder. Sleep Med. 2013;14(5):391–8.

Uschakov A, Gong H, McGinty D, Szymusiak R. Efferent projections from the median preoptic nucleus to sleep- and arousal-regulatory nuclei in the rat brain. Neuroscience. 2007;150(1): 104–20.

Uschakov A, Grivel J, Cvetkovic-Lopes V, Bayer L, Bernheim L, Jones BE, et al. Sleep-deprivation regulates alpha-2 adrenergic responses of rat hypocretin/orexin neurons. PLoS One. 2011;6(2): e16672.

Vanini G, Nemanis K, Baghdoyan HA, Lydic R. GABAergic transmission in rat pontine reticular formation regulates the induction phase of anesthesia and modulates hyperalgesia caused by sleep deprivation. Eur J Neurosci. 2014;40(1):2264–73.

Veasey SC, Panckeri KA, Hoffman EA, Pack AI, Hendricks JC. The effects of serotonin antagonists in an animal model of sleep-disordered breathing. Am J Respir Crit Care Med. 1996;153 (2):776–86.

Volgin DV, Kubin L. Regionally selective effects of GABA on hypothalamic $GABA_A$ receptor mRNA in vitro. Biochem Biophys Res Commun. 2007;353(3):726–32.

Volgin DV, Lu JW, Stettner GM, Mann GL, Ross RJ, Morrison AR, et al. Time- and behavioral state-dependent changes in posterior hypothalamic $GABA_A$ receptors contribute to the regulation of sleep. PLoS One. 2014;9(1):e86545.

von Economo C. Sleep as a problem of localization. J Nerv Ment Dis. 1930;71:249–59.

Vyazovskiy VV, Olcese U, Lazimy YM, Faraguna U, Esser SK, Williams JC, et al. Cortical firing and sleep homeostasis. Neuron. 2009;63(6):865–78.

Vyazovskiy VV, Cirelli C, Tononi G. Electrophysiological correlates of sleep homeostasis in freely behaving rats. Prog Brain Res. 2011;193:17–38.

Weber F, Chung S, Beier KT, Xu M, Luo L, Dan Y. Control of REM sleep by ventral medulla GABAergic neurons. Nature. 2015;526(7573):435–8.

Weng FJ, Williams RH, Hawryluk JM, Lu J, Scammell TE, Saper CB, et al. Carbachol excites sublaterodorsal nucleus neurons projecting to the spinal cord. J Physiol. 2014;592(7):1601–17.

White DP, Younes MK. Obstructive sleep apnea. Compr Physiol. 2012;2(4):2541–94.

Willie JT, Chemelli RM, Sinton CM, Tokita S, Williams SC, Kisanuki YY, et al. Distinct narcolepsy syndromes in Orexin receptor-2 and Orexin null mice: molecular genetic dissection of Non-REM and REM sleep regulatory processes. Neuron. 2003;38(5):715–30.

Wu MF, Gulyani SA, Yau E, Mignot E, Phan B, Siegel JM. Locus coeruleus neurons: cessation of activity during cataplexy. Neuroscience. 1999;91(4):1389–99.

Wu MF, John J, Boehmer LN, Yau D, Nguyen GB, Siegel JM. Activity of dorsal raphe cells across the sleep-waking cycle and during cataplexy in narcoleptic dogs. J Physiol. 2004;554(Pt 1): 202–15.

Xi MC, Morales FR, Chase MH. Evidence that wakefulness and REM sleep are controlled by a GABAergic pontine mechanism. J Neurophysiol. 1999;82(4):2015–9.

Xu M, Chung S, Zhang S, Zhong P, Ma C, Chang WC, et al. Basal forebrain circuit for sleep-wake control. Nat Neurosci. 2015;18(11):1641–7.

Yamuy J, Fung SJ, Xi M, Morales FR, Chase MH. Hypoglossal motoneurons are postsynaptically inhibited during carbachol-induced rapid eye movement sleep. Neuroscience. 1999;94(1):11–5.

Yanik G, Radulovacki M. REM sleep deprivation up-regulates adenosine A1 receptors. Brain Res. 1987;402(2):362–4.

Zecharia AY, Nelson LE, Gent TC, Schumacher M, Jurd R, Rudolph U, et al. The involvement of hypothalamic sleep pathways in general anesthesia: testing the hypothesis using the $GABA_A$ receptor beta3N265M knock-in mouse. J Neurosci. 2009;29(7):2177–87.

Zhang S, Lin L, Kaur S, Thankachan S, Blanco-Centurion C, Yanagisawa M, et al. The development of hypocretin (orexin) deficiency in hypocretin/ataxin-3 transgenic rats. Neuroscience. 2007;148(1):34–43.

Additional Web Resources Offering a Complementary Overview of the Subject

McCarley RW, Sinton CM. Neurobiology of sleep and wakefulness. Scholarpedia. 2008;3:3313. http://www.scholarpedia.org/article/Neurobiology_of_sleep_and_wakefulness. Accessed Nov 2021.

National Institute of Neurological Disorders and Stroke. Brain basics: understanding sleep. https://www.ninds.nih.gov/Disorders/Patient-Caregiver-Education/Understanding-Sleep. Accessed Nov 2021.

Wikipedia. Neuroscience of sleep. https://en.wikipedia.org/wiki/Neuroscience_of_sleep. Accessed Nov 2021.

Chapter 3
Prostaglandins, Adenosine, and Histaminergic System in the Regulation of Sleep and Wakefulness

Zhi-Li Huang, Ze Zhang, and Wei-Min Qu

Abstract This chapter provides an overview of the current knowledge about the roles of prostaglandins, adenosine, and the histaminergic system in sleep–wake regulation, focusing on prostaglandins, adenosine, and histamine in the central nervous system, their level regulation, their receptors, and pharmacological and molecular biological manipulations of the adenosine and histaminergic systems. Prostaglandin (PG) D_2 is an endogenous somnogen that can increase the extracellular adenosine under the subarachnoid space of the basal forebrain, thereby induce physiological sleep. Adenosine is found neither stored nor released as a classical neurotransmitter, which is formed inside cells or on their surface and derived from adenine nucleotide breakdown. Prolonged wakefulness increases extracellular adenosine concentration in the cortex and basal forebrain and the concentration will go back during the sleep recovery period. Therefore, adenosine has been thought of as a homeostatic regulator of sleep and a link between the humoral and neural mechanisms of sleep–wake regulation. Both the adenosine A_1 receptor (A_1R) and the $A_{2A}R$ are involved in sleep induction. The somnogenic effects of PGD_2 are predominantly dependent on $A_{2A}R$. In addition, it is proved that the $A_{2A}R$ is necessary for the arousal effect of caffeine by using gene-manipulated mice. In contrast, the role of the A_1R is more complicated. Although stimulation of A_1R in wake-promoting brain areas increases sleep, activation of A_1R in the lateral preoptic area induces wakefulness, indicating that the A_1R acts in a site-dependent manner in sleep–wake regulation. The histaminergic system also plays an essential role in sleep–wake regulation and is indispensable for the sleep/wakefulness-promoting effects induced by the A_1R and $A_{2A}R$. A brief discussion about the potential therapeutic applications of agonists and antagonists of these receptors in sleep disorders is also included at the end of this chapter.

Z.-L. Huang (✉) · Z. Zhang · W.-M. Qu
Department of Pharmacology, School of Basic Medical Sciences, State Key Laboratory of Medical Neurobiology, Institutes of Brain Science and Collaborative Innovation Center for Brain Science, Shanghai Medical College, Fudan University, Shanghai, China
e-mail: huangzl@fudan.edu.cn

A. I. Pack, Q. Y. Li (eds.), *Sleep and its Disorders*, Translational Medicine Research,
https://doi.org/10.1007/978-94-024-2168-2_3

Keywords Adenosine · Prostaglandin D_2 · Histamine · Receptor · Sleep · Wakefulness

Abbreviations

ADA	Adenosine deaminase
AK	Adenosine kinase
ATP	Adenosine triphosphate
cAMP	Cyclic adenosine 3′, 5′-monophosphate
cN	Cytosolic nucleotidase
CPA	N6-cyclopentyladenosine
CSF	Cerebrospinal fluid
dnSNARE	The SNARE domain of the protein synaptobrevin II
DP_1R	PGD_2 receptor
GPCR	G protein-coupled receptors
H_1R	Histamine H_1 receptor
H-PGDS	Hematopoietic PGDS
KO	Knockout
L-PGDS	Lipocalin-type PGDS
NBTI	S-(4-nitrobenzyl)-6-thioinosine
NREM	Non-rapid eye movement
PLC	Phospholipase C
PG	Prostaglandin
PGDS	PGD synthase
R	Receptor
REM	Rapid eye movement
SAHH	*S*-adenosyl-homocysteine hydrolase
Se^{4+}	Tetravalent selenium
$SeCl_4$	Selenium tetrachloride
SWA	Slow wave activity
TMN	Tuberomammillary nucleus
VLPO	Ventrolateral preoptic area
WT	Wild type

3.1 Introduction

Sleep propensity rises with the prolonged wakefulness time and dissipates with the progression of sleep. The waxing and waning of the sleep drive are presumed to be regulated by endogenous sleep factors acting on specific neurons in the brain (Porkka-Heiskanen et al. 1999). One of these sleep factors is adenosine, a purine nucleoside naturally occurring in all cells (Fredholm 2007), the other one is prostaglandin (PG) D_2, an eicosanoid acting as tissue or local hormone (Huang et al. 2007). Both adenosine and PGD_2 are released as neuromodulators in the brain. Here, we are discussing some aspects of high general complexity: (a) adenosine is a key signaling molecule for PGD_2-induced sleep; (b) the metabolism of adenosine, which is ubiquitously present in all cells; (c) key roles of the A_{2A} receptor ($A_{2A}R$) in sleep induction; (d) adenosine A_1R plays a role in sleep–wake regulation in a site-dependent manner.

3.2 Adenosine Is a Key Signaling Molecule for PGD_2-Induced Sleep

The discovery that adenosine acts as a mediator of PGD_2-induced sleep led to the identification of the mechanism by which endogenous PGD_2 promotes sleep (Fig. 3.1) (Satoh et al. 1996). PGD_2 was found to be one of the most potent somnogens and also the most abundant prostaglandin in the brains of rats (Narumiya et al. 1982) and other mammals including humans (Ogorochi et al. 1984) involved in physiological sleep (Urade and Hayaishi 2010) The PGD_2 concentration in the cerebrospinal fluid (CSF) of rats fluctuates along with the sleep–wake rhythms (Pandey et al. 1995) and elevates with an increase of sleep propensity during sleep deprivation (Ram et al. 1997), implying that PGD_2 may have some important role in the CNS. The sleep-inducing activity of PGD_2 was discovered while the scientists were trying to investigate its neural function (Ueno et al. 1982). Both non-rapid eye

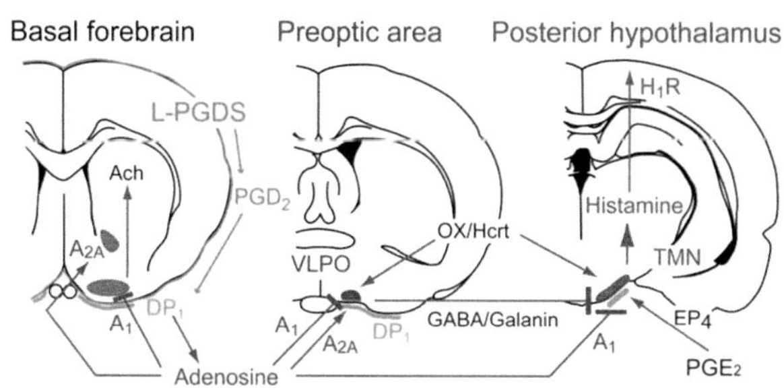

Fig. 3.1 Molecular mechanism of sleep–wake regulation. The endogenous somnogen PGD_2 (green), produced by L-PGDS, circulates within the CSF, stimulates DP_1R (light blue) on the ventral surface from the basal forebrain to the hypothalamus, and increases the level of extracellular adenosine. Adenosine (purple) diffuses into the brain parenchyma as the secondary somnogen, inhibits arousal neurons in the basal forebrain (orange area) and TMN (red area) via A_1R (blue lines), and activates sleep–active VLPO neurons (blue area) via $A_{2A}R$ (red arrows) to induce sleep. The flip-flop switch of sleep–wakefulness regulation between the VLPO and TMN is stabilized by their OX/Hcrt-mediated activation and adenosine A_1R-mediated suppression. *Ach* Acetylcholine, *EP_4* Prostaglandin E_2 receptor, subtype EP_4, *H_1R* Histamine H1 receptor, *Hcrt* Hypocretin, *L-PGDS* Lipocalin-type prostaglandin D synthase, *OX* Orexin, *TMN* Tuberomammillary nucleus, *VLPO* Ventrolateral preoptic area. Adapted and modified from Urade and Hayaishi (2010) with permission

movement (non-REM, NREM) and REM sleep increased in the rat brain just by microinjection of nanomolar quantities of PGD_2 (Ueno et al. 1983). The same sleep-inducing effect was found in the rhesus monkey by an i.c.v. infusion of PGD_2 (Onoe et al. 1988). The PGD_2 can significantly induce sleep with as small as picomolar quantities per minute, which is almost identical to physiological sleep as judged by several electrophysiological and behavioral criteria.

PGD_2 can be produced by two distinct types of PGD synthase (PGDS) in the CNS: one is lipocalin-type PGDS (L-PGDS), substantially locates in the arachnoid membrane, choroid plexus, and oligodendrocytes (Mizoguchi et al. 2001; Urade et al. 1993); and the other, hematopoietic PGDS (H-PGDS), expresses in microglia (Mohri et al. 2003). PGD_2 that are produced by either of these two enzymes will be secreted into the CSF, and the level of PGD_2 there shows a circadian change in freely moving rats (Pandey et al. 1995). L-PGDS is the same as β-trace, a major protein in human CSF. Also, the serum L-PGDS/β-trace concentration exhibits a circadian alteration with a nocturnal increase, which is suppressed by total sleep deprivation but not influenced during REM sleep deprivation in humans (Jordan et al. 2004). In patients with narcolepsy and idiopathic hypersomnia, L-PGDS levels were reported to be increased (Wang et al. 2021).

Furthermore, sleep is inhibited in a time- and dose-dependent fashion and is reversible when rats are administered the specific and reversible inhibitors of PGDS, inorganic tetravalent selenium (Se^{4+}) compounds such as selenium tetrachloride ($SeCl_4$) (Islam et al. 1991; Matsumura et al. 1991; Takahata et al. 1993). These results suggest that PGD_2/PGDS plays a key role in sleep induction.

To investigate the mechanism of PGD_2 in regulating physiological sleep, we tested the effect of inhibition of PGD_2 synthesis by $SeCl_4$ on the sleep in wild-type (WT) mice as well as PGDS and PGD_2 receptor (DP_1R) knockout (KO) mice, and the effect of a DP_1R antagonist, ONO-4127Na, on sleep in rats. The PGD_2 concentration in the brain of WT mice decreased by the i.p. injection of $SeCl_4$ without affecting the amounts of PGE_2 and $PGF_{2\alpha}$. The injection dose-dependently suppressed sleep and induced almost complete insomnia after the administration during the light phase when mice normally sleep. The $SeCl_4$-induced insomnia was observed in H-PGDS KO mice but not in L-PGDS KO, H- and L-PGDS double KO, or DP_1R KO mice. Furthermore, the amount of sleep decreased when the DP_1R antagonist ONO-4127Na was infused into the subarachnoid space under the rostral basal forebrain in rats (Qu et al. 2006). These findings indicate that the L-PGDS/PGD_2/DP_1R system is critical for physiological sleep regulation.

The extracellular adenosine concentration was increased dose dependently while PGD_2 was infused into the subarachnoid space of the basal forebrain of WT mice (Mizoguchi et al. 2001), in which DP_1Rs are remarkably abundant, whereas the mechanism linking PGD_2 and adenosine accumulation is still unclear. The increase of extracellular adenosine induced by PGD_2 was only observed in WT mice, but not in DP_1R KO mice (Fig. 3.2) (Mizoguchi et al. 2001). Moreover, the sleep-promoting effect of PGD_2 can be eliminated by i.p. injection of the $A_{2A}R$-selective antagonist KF 17837. These results suggest that the adenosine increase was dependent on the activation of DP_1R and that endogenous adenosine acting at $A_{2A}Rs$ may mediate the

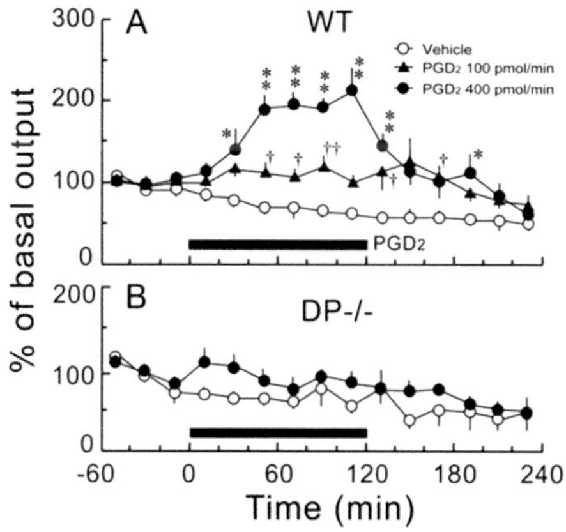

Fig. 3.2 Effect of PGD_2 perfusion on the extracellular adenosine level in the subarachnoid space below the rostral basal forebrain of WT and $DP^{-/-}$ mice. Vehicle or PGD_2 was perfused for 2 h (black bar) into the subarachnoid space below the rostral basal forebrain of WT (**a**) and $DP^{-/-}$ (**b**) mice under anesthesia. The basal level of adenosine for 1 h before the PGD_2 perfusion was 0.46 ± 0.04 pmol/20 μl in WT mice and 0.24 ± 0.04 pmol/20 μl in $DP^{-/-}$ mice. The data are expressed as a percentage of the baseline value (mean ± SEM, $n = 5–8$). $^{*,\dagger}P < 0.05$; $^{**,\dagger\dagger}P < 0.01$, compared with the vehicle group. Adapted from Mizoguchi et al. (2001) with modification and permission

PGD_2-induced sleep (Fig. 3.1). In addition, it was found that PGD_2-induced sleep attenuated in animals with adenosine $A_{2A}R$ deficiency (Oishi et al. 2017), suggesting that adenosine $A_{2A}R$ is necessary for this process.

3.3 Formation, Metabolism, and Transport of Adenosine in the CNS

As shown in Fig. 3.3, adenosine is a nucleoside that consists of one molecule of adenine attached to a ribose sugar molecule (ribofuranose) via a β-N9-glycosidic bond for its chemical structure. It is produced inside or on the surface of the cell and is majorly produced by the breakdown of intra- or extracellular adenine nucleotides (Zimmermann 2000). Inside the cell, adenosine is produced from adenosine triphosphate (ATP) by intracellular 5′-nucleotidase and then transported outside the cell by bidirectional nucleoside transporters. It also can be generated outside the cell by the metabolism of released nucleotides by ectonucleotidases. Two intracellular 5-′-nucleotidase enzymes have been cloned, with cytosolic nucleotidase (cN)-I breaking down AMP to adenosine, and (cN)-II breaking down inosine 5′-monophosphate and guanosine monophosphate to inosine and guanosine, respectively (Sala-Newby et al. 1999). There is a family of ectonucleotidases that can generate adenosine from ATP, but in physiological conditions the major enzyme that is responsible for this is ecto-5′-nucleotidase (Zimmermann et al. 1998). Adenosine can also arise from

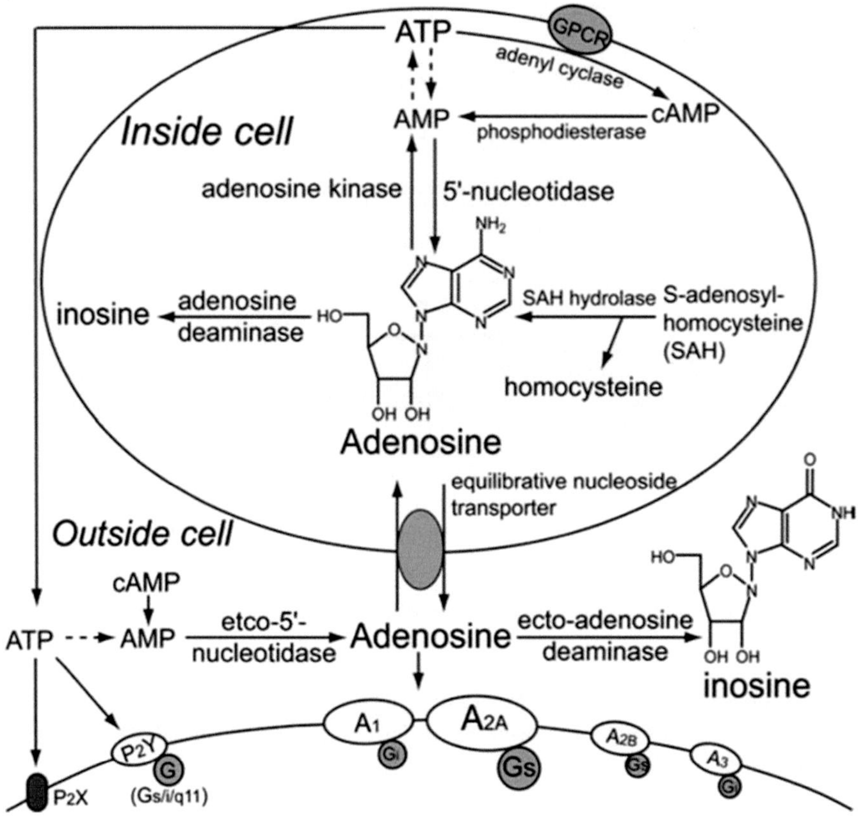

Fig. 3.3 Intracellular and extracellular pathways for the formation and metabolism of adenosine. Inside the cell, adenosine is formed from ATP, cAMP, or SAH, while outside the cell it arises from equilibrating nucleoside transporter-mediated release or metabolism from ATP or cAMP. Adapted from Sawynok and Liu (2003) with modification and permission

cyclic adenosine 3′, 5′-monophosphate (cAMP), either generated inside the cell by a G protein-coupled receptor with subsequent conversion to AMP by phosphodiesterase, or following the efflux of cAMP by a probenecid-sensitive transporter and metabolism by ectoenzyme (Brundege et al. 1997; Rosenberg and Li 1995). However, the conversion of cAMP to AMP by phosphodiesterase is slow, and activation of adenosine receptors following increased availability of cAMP is limited (Dunwiddie and Masino 2001). A further source of adenosine inside the cell is hydrolysis of *S*-adenosyl homocysteine (SAH) (Deussen et al. 1989), but this pathway is not important in the brain (Latini and Pedata 2001).

While in some brain regions, adenosine may act as a neurotransmitter (Burnstock 2007), since it does not accumulate in synaptic vesicles, adenosine is neither stored nor released as a classical neurotransmitter, but is released from the cytoplasm into the extracellular space via a nucleoside transporter. These equilibrating transporters keep the intra- and extracellular adenosine concentrations in equilibrium, which mediate adenosine reuptake, and the concentration gradient on both sides of the membrane determines the direction of the transport (Gu et al. 1995). These equilibrating transporters are abundant in most cells, including astrocytes (Peng et al. 2005).

Extracellular adenosine derives from two major mechanisms: (1) the release of adenosine caused by an increase in the intracellular levels of adenosine through nucleoside transporters (Geiger and Fyda 1991); and (2) the extracellular formation of adenosine through the ectonucleotidase pathway on the release of adenine nucleotides, especially ATP.

Adenosine can be removed by nucleoside transporters and three kinds of enzymes, i.e., adenosine kinase (AK), adenosine deaminase (ADA), and *S*-adenosylhomocysteine hydrolase (SAHH). The clearance of extracellular adenosine mostly occurs through the non-concentrating nucleoside transporters, and ecto-ADA deaminates adenosine to inosine (Fredholm et al. 2005). The major intracellular metabolic pathways of adenosine are the formation of AMP through AK and the irreversible breakdown of inosine via ADA. AK is found enriched in neurons, whereas ADA is more abundant in astrocytes (Fredholm et al. 2005) and histaminergic neurons in the tuberomammillary nuclei (TMN) (Nagy et al. 1984; Oishi et al. 2008). A third enzyme, SAHH, which can convert adenosine to *S*-adenosylhomocysteine in cardiomyocytes, might be of less importance in the CNS (Fredholm et al. 2005).

3.4 Increase in the Extracellular Adenosine Level Promotes Sleep

In 1954, Feldberg and Sherwood (1954) reported that intraventricular injection of micromole quantities of adenosine caused natural sleep for 30 min in cat. Subsequent pharmacological studies by several groups proved that adenosine and its receptor agonists promoted, but antagonists such as caffeine inhibited both NREM and REM sleep for reviews, see Ferre et al. (2007), Basheer et al. (2004), and Monti et al. (2008).

Under physiological conditions, the actions of highly active ADA, adenosine transport or AK are essential, especially when large amounts of adenosine are waiting to be cleared. Thus, inhibition of adenosine metabolism by blocking AK with ABT-702 (Radek et al. 2004) and ADA with (deoxy) coformycin (Oishi et al. 2008; Okada et al. 2003; Radulovacki et al. 1983), or microdialysis perfusion with an adenosine transport inhibitor *S*-(4-nitrobenzyl)-6-thioinosine (NBTI) in the cholinergic basal forebrain (Porkka-Heiskanen et al. 1997), elevates extracellular adenosine levels, increases sleep and induces slow-wave activity (SWA) in the EEG.

These pharmacological data in rats are consistent with genetic findings in mice showing that a genomic region encoding genes that regulate extracellular adenosine levels modify the rate at which the NREM sleep tendency accumulates during prolonged wakefulness (Franken et al. 2001). In humans, a genetic variant of ADA related to the reduced metabolism of adenosine to inosine, is demonstrated to selectively induce deep sleep and SWA during sleep. This finding indicates that the inter-individual variability in brain electrical activity during sleep and wakefulness is associated with the genetic variability in the adenosine system (Retey et al. 2005).

A commonly used method to cause a physiological challenge to promote sleep homeostasis is sleep deprivation. Increased sleep propensity by prolonged wakefulness will be counteracted not only by longer sleep duration, but also by elevated sleep intensity (Borb and Achermann 1999), such as EEG SWA and spindle frequency activity (power within 11–15 Hz). Sleep deprivation can elevate local adenosine levels in the basal forebrain, cortex, and hippocampus in rats and cats during prolonged wakefulness. Enhanced sleep intensity and adenosine levels decline during recovery sleep (Porkka-Heiskanen et al. 1997; Huston et al. 1996; Murillo-Rodriguez et al. 2004). Because the adenosine level changes more significantly in the basal forebrain compared to other cerebral regions (Strecker et al. 2000), the local increase of the extracellular adenosine in the basal forebrain may provide a signal for the homeostatic NREM sleep regulation [see refs. Basheer et al. (2004, 2007) for reviews]. In addition, during sleep deprivation, nitric oxide production in the basal forebrain can increase sleep via adenosine production (Kalinchuk et al. 2010).

The source of extracellular adenosine from neurons and glia cells for sleep regulation in the CNS remains in debate. It has long been thought that homeostatic process regulates sleep through the adenosine originating from neurons (Jones 2009). Astrocytes release ATP and glutamate via many pathways including exocytosis (Zhang et al. 2007; Jourdain et al. 2007) and regulate extracellular adenosine by releasing ATP. Conditional expression of the SNARE domain of the protein synaptobrevin II (dnSNARE) in astrocytes can abolish both tonic and activity-dependent extracellular accumulation of adenosine (Pascual et al. 2005). Halassa et al. (2009) showed that the compensatory response to sleep deprivation disappeared in dnSNARE transgenic mice, such as enhancement of SWA and the rebound in sleep amount that occurs in WT mice, indicating that the glia-dependent accumulation of adenosine is necessary for both sleep drive and homeostasis. However, using a newly developed genetically encoded adenosine sensor, Peng et al. found an activity-dependent rapid increase in the concentration of extracellular adenosine in mouse BF. Although the activity of both BF cholinergic and glutamatergic neurons correlated with changes in the concentration of adenosine, optogenetic activation of these neurons at physiological firing frequencies showed that glutamatergic neurons contributed much more to the adenosine increase. Mice with selective ablation of BF glutamatergic neurons exhibited a reduced adenosine increase and impaired sleep homeostasis regulation (Peng et al. 2020).

3.5 Predominant Roles of $A_{2A}R$ in Sleep Regulation by Adenosine

There are four adenosine receptor subtypes and all of them are G-protein-coupled receptors (GPCR): A_1 and A_3 are primarily coupled to the Gi family of G proteins, whereas A_{2A} and A_{2B} are mostly coupled to Gs, or G_{olf} protein (Peng et al. 2005). Stimulation of A_1Rs inhibits adenylate cyclase through activation of Gi proteins, activates phospholipase C (PLC), opens several types of K^+ channels, and inactivates Q-, P-, and N-type Ca^{2+} channels (Fredholm et al. 2005; Jacobson and Gao 2006). On the other hand, activation of the $A_{2A}R$ subtype increases adenylate cyclase activity through activation of Gs or Golf (in the striatum) proteins, induces the formation of inositol phosphates, and activates protein kinase C (Fredholm et al. 2005; Jacobson and Gao 2006). It has been demonstrated that both A_1 and $A_{2A}R$ participate in sleep induction, whereas $A_{2A}R$ is more important in adenosine-induced sleep. Although $A_{2B}R$ is expressed broadly, it is generally at very low levels; in contrast, the A_3R is expressed at intermediate levels in the hippocampus and cerebellum (Yaar et al. 2005). However, the functional significance of $A_{2B}R$ and A_3R in sleep regulation is still hardly known. The main properties of adenosine receptors are shown in Table 3.1.

Accumulated evidence indicates that the $A_{2A}R$ is critical for the effects of adenosine-induced sleep. The concentrations of A_{2A}Rs are high in the CNS, mainly in the striatum (Yuan et al. 2017), nucleus accumbens (Oishi et al. 2017), and olfactory bulb (Wang et al. 2017; Fredholm et al. 2001). In rats, selective $A_{2A}R$ agonists such as CG-S21680 administered to the subarachnoid space adjacent to the basal forebrain and lateral preoptic area reliably induce NREM sleep, whereas infusion of A_1R agonists produces weak and variable effects (Mohri et al. 2003; Methippara et al. 2005; Satoh et al. 1998; Scammell et al. 2001). When infused into the medial pontine reticular formation in rats, CGS-21680 was tenfold more potent than the A_1R agonist N6-cyclohexyl-adenosine, in inducing REM sleep (Marks et al. 2003). Sleep induced by the $A_{2A}R$ agonist CGS-21680 is followed by a strong rebound of wakefulness after the cessation of CGS-21680 infusion (Gerashchenko et al. 2000). The major region that mediates $A_{2A}R$-induced sleep is thought to be located in or near the rostral basal forebrain, which is proved by the sleep-promoting effect and c-Fos expression after local infusion of CGS-21680 (Satoh et al. 1999). Moreover, CGS-21680-induced sleep is almost completely eliminated in $A_{2A}R$ knockout mice, confirming the specificity of CGS-21680 for A_{2A}Rs (Urade et al. 2003).

A possible neural circuit of $A_{2A}R$-mediated PGD_2-induced sleep was mapped by c-Fos-positive neurons detection (Scammell et al. 2001; Satoh et al. 1999). When PGD_2 or the $A_{2A}R$ agonist CGS-21680 was infused for 2 h into the PGD_2-sensitive zone of the subarachnoid space of the basal forebrain, the number of c-Fos-positive cells was significantly increased in the leptomeningeal membrane as well as in the ventrolateral preoptic (VLPO) area, where increases were concomitant with the induction of NREM sleep (Scammell et al. 2001; Satoh et al. 1999). In contrast,

Table 3.1 Roles of adenosine receptors in sleep–wake regulation

Receptor	A_1R	$A_{2A}R$	$A_{2B}R$	A_3R
Expression High	Cortex, cerebellum, hippocampus	Caudate putamen, nucleus accumbens, tuberculum olfactorium, olfactory bulb		
Intermediate	Other brain regions		Median eminence	Cerebellum, hippocampus
Low		Rest of brain		Most of the brain (rat, mouse)
G protein	Gi, Go	Gs, Golf	Gs, Gq	Gi
Chromosomal location	Chr 1q32.1	Chr 22g11.2	Chr 17p11.2-12	Chr 1p21-13
Selective agonist	CPA, CCPA, CHA	CGS-21680, HE-NECA, CV-1808, CV-1674, ATL146e	None	Cl-IB-MECA
Selective antagonist	DPCPX 8-cyclopentyltheophylline, WRC0571	SCH-58261 moderately: ZM-241385, KF-17387, CSC	MRS1754, enprofylline, 1-butyl-8-[4-(4-benzyl)(piperazino-2-oxyethoxy) phenyl] xanthine	MRS1220, MRE3008-F20, MRS1191; MRS1523
Roles in animal sleep	Activation of A_1R in basal forebrain (Blanco-Centurion et al. 2006), TMN (Oishi et al. 2008), and lateral hypothalamus (Kalinchuk et al. 2010; Thakkar et al. 2002) induces sleep; whereas activation of A_1R in the lateral preoptic area promotes wakefulness (Methippara et al. 2005)	$A_{2A}R$ agonists were administered to the brain induces a dramatic increase in sleep (Satoh et al. 1996, 1998, 1999; Hong et al. 2005); arousal effect of caffeine is seen in A_1R KO, but not in $A_{2A}R$ KO mice (Huang et al. 2005)	None reported	None reported
Roles in human sleep		Variations in $A_{2A}R$ gene	None reported	None reported

(continued)

Table 3.1 (continued)

Receptor	A_1R	$A_{2A}R$	$A_{2B}R$	A_3R
	Prolonged wakefulness induces A_1R up-regulation (Elmenhorst et al. 2007)	contribute to individual sensitivity to caffeine effects on sleep (Retey et al. 2007)		

From Fredholm et al. (2005) and Fredholm (2007) with modification
Abbreviations: *CHA* N6-cyclohexyl adenosine, *CCPA* 2-chloro-N6-cyclopentyladenosine, *CGS21680* 2-*p*-(2-carboxyethyl) phenethylamino-5′-*N*-ethylcarboxamido adenosine hydrochloride, *HE-NECA* 2-hexynyl-5′-(*N*-ethylcarboxamido) adenosine, *CV-1808* 2-phenylaminoadenosine, *CV 1674* 2-(4-methoxyphenyl) adenosine, *ATL-146e* 4-{3-[6-Amino-9-(5-ethylcarbamoyl-3,4-dihydroxy-tetrahydro-furan-2-yl)-9H-purin--2-yl]-prop-2-ynyl}-cyclohexanecarboxylic acid methyl ester, *IB-MECA* 1-deoxy-1-[6-[[(3-iodophenyl)methyl]amino]-9H-purine-9-yl]-*N*-methyl-D-ribofuranuronamide, *DPCPX* 1,3-dipropyl-8-cyclopentylxanthine, *WRC-0571* 8-(*N*-Methylisopropyl)amino-*N*-(5′-endohydroxy endonorbornyl)-9-methyladenine, *SCH-58261* 5-Amino-7-(β-phenylethyl)-2-(8-furyl)pyrazolo(4,3-e)-1,2,4-triazolo(1,5-c)pyrimidine, *ZM241385* 4-(2-[7-Amino-2-(2-furyl)[1,2,4]triazolo[2,3a][1,3,5]t riazin-5-ylamino]ethyl) phenol, *KF 17387* 1,3-dipropyl-8-[3,4-dimethoxystyryl]-7-methylxanthine, *CSC* (8-(3-Chlorostyryl) caffeine, *MRS 1754* *N*-(4-Cyanophenyl)-2-[4-(2,6-dioxo-1,3-dipropyl-2,3,6,7-tetrahydro-1H-purin-8-yl)phenoxy]acetamide, *Enprofylline* 3-npropylxanthine, *MRS-1191* 3-ethyl-5-benzyl-2-methyl-6-phenyl-4-phenylethynyl-1,4-(+)-dihydropridine-3,dicarboxylate, *MRS-1220* 9-chloro-2-(2-furyl)-5-phenylacetylamino[1,2,4]triazolo[1,5c]quinazoline, *MRS 1523* 6-Ethyl-5-(ethylsulfanylcarbonyl)-2-phenyl-4-propylpyridine-3-carboxylic acid propyl ester, *MRE 3008F20* 5N (4 methoxyphenylcarbamoyl) amino-8-propyl-2-(2-furyl) pyrazolo [4,3-e]-1,2,4- triazolo [1,5-c]pyrimidine

the number of c-Fos-positive neurons decreased notably in the TMN of the posterior hypothalamus. The VLPO is known to send specific inhibitory GABAergic and galaninergic projections to the TMN, the neurons of which contain the ascending histaminergic arousal system (Sherin et al. 1998).

Inhibition of the histaminergic system induces sleep. In vivo microdialysis experiments showed that infusion of an adenosine $A_{2A}R$ agonist, CGS-21680, into the subarachnoid space of the basal forebrain inhibited the release of histamine in both the frontal cortex and the medial preoptic area in a dose-dependent manner, and induced the GABA release selectively in the TMN but not in the frontal cortex (Hong et al. 2005). The inhibition of histamine release induced by CGS-21680 can be blocked by perfusion with a $GABA_A$ antagonist, picrotoxin, in the TMN, indicating that the $A_{2A}R$ agonist promotes sleep through inhibiting the histaminergic system by inducing GABA release in the TMN. These results support the original proposal of the flip-flop mechanism, in which sleep is promoted by activating the sleep neurons in the VLPO and meanwhile inhibiting the histaminergic wake neurons in the TMN (Saper et al. 2005).

The local application of CGS-21680 induces c-Fos expression in the VLPO (Satoh et al. 1998), but $A_{2A}R$ seems to be undetectable or very barely expressed in this brain area. Direct activation of sleep-promoting VLPO neurons via postsynaptic stimulation of $A_{2A}R$ was demonstrated in VLPO slices (Gallopin et al. 2005). The intracellular recording of VLPO neurons in rat brain slices uncovered the existence of two different types of VLPO neurons based on their responses to serotonin and adenosine. VLPO neurons were uniformly inhibited by two arousal neurotransmitters, noradrenaline and acetylcholine, and mainly by an adenosine A_1R agonist. Serotonin inhibited the type-1 neurons whereas activated the type-2 neurons.

$A_{2A}R$ agonist excited postsynaptically the type-2, but not the type-1, neurons. These results indicate that the type-2 neurons are involved in the initiation of sleep and that the type-1 neurons contribute to sleep consolidation, since type-1 neurons are activated only when they are released from inhibition by arousal systems (Gallopin et al. 2005). Moreover, the administration of CGS-21680 to the rostral basal forebrain induced substantial c-Fos expression in the shell of the nucleus accumbens and the medial portion of the olfactory tubercle. The microdialysis perfusion of CGS-21680 into the shell of the nucleus accumbens also induced sleep (Satoh et al. 1999). Scammell et al. (2001) reported that activating adenosine $A_{2A}Rs$ in leptomeninges or nucleus accumbens could activate the VLPO. These VLPO neurons may then lead to the inhibition of multiple wake-promoting regions, thereby promoting sleep.

In contrast to adenosine, caffeine promotes wakefulness. Caffeine binds to A_1R and $A_{2A}R$ with similar high affinities and acts as an antagonist for both receptor subtypes (Fredholm et al. 2001). We discovered that caffeine can induce wakefulness in WT and A_1R KO mice but not in $A_{2A}R$ KO mice (Fig. 3.4), suggesting that the wake-promoting effect of caffeine is caused by blocking the $A_{2A}R$, not the A_1R (Huang et al. 2005). Caffeine may also reduce the hypnotic effects of alcohol via $A_{2A}R$ (El Yacoubi et al. 2003). These findings strongly indicate that $A_{2A}R$ plays a critical role in sleep regulation.

$A_{2A}Rs$ are substantially expressed in the caudate–putamen, nucleus accumbens, and the tuberculum olfactorium. Using optogenetic and chemogenetic approaches, we reported that neurons expressing $A_{2A}Rs$ in the caudate–putamen (Yuan et al. 2017), nucleus accumbens (Oishi et al. 2017), and the tuberculum olfactorium (Li et al. 2020) promote sleep in mice, in which dopamine D_2Rs are co-localized (Missale et al. 1998). We found that the D_2R is essential for the maintenance of wakefulness (Qu et al. 2008, 2010; Qiu et al. 2009), whereas activation of $A_{2A}R$ potently induces sleep. Opposing effects of $A_{2A}R$ and D_2R have also been found at neurotransmitter release level, receptor binding, and gene expression (Ferre et al. 2007; Schiffmann et al. 2007), which suggests $A_{2A}R$ and D_2R are involved in sleep–wake regulation in a different and coordinated manner.

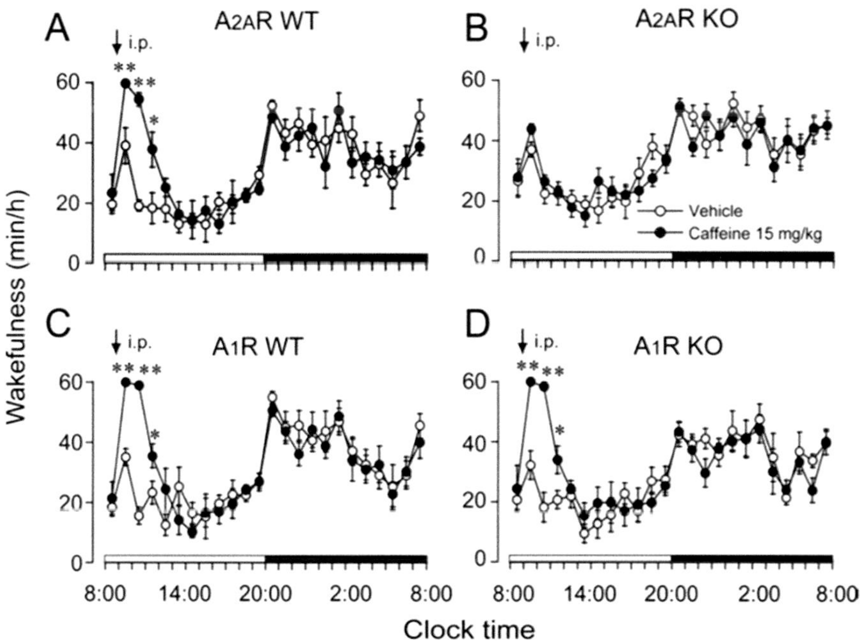

Fig. 3.4 Time course of changes in wakefulness after caffeine 15 mg/kg treatment in WT mice (**a**), $A_{2A}R$ KO (**b**), A_1R WT mice (**c**), and A_1R KO mice (**d**). Each circle represents the hourly mean ± SEM ($n = 5$–7). The arrows indicate the injection time (9 a.m.). $^{*}P < 0.05$; $^{**}P < 0.01$, significantly different from the vehicle, by the paired t-test. Adapted from Huang et al. (2005) with modification and permission

3.6 A_1R-Mediated Effects on Sleep–Wake Cycles Are Brain Region Dependent

The A_1Rs are broadly expressed in the brain cortex, hippocampus, thalamus, lateral hypothalamus, basal ganglia, and TMN (Oishi et al. 2008; Yaar et al. 2005; Thakkar et al. 2002). Because of the extensive distribution of A_1Rs in the cortex and the inhibition of excitatory neurotransmission following presynaptic A_1R activation, it has been generally presumed that adenosine influences sleep mainly by the A_1R. A few findings from pharmacological studies are consistent with this hypothesis. For example, i.p. or i.c.v. administration of the A_1R selective agonist N^6-cyclopentyladenosine (CPA) to rats induces NREM sleep, inhibits REM sleep, and increases changes in the NREM sleep EEG similar to those brought about by prolonged wakefulness (Benington et al. 1995; Schwierin et al. 1996). Furthermore, microdialysis perfusion with A_1R antisense oligonucleotides in the basal forebrain of rats decreases NREM sleep and increases wakefulness (Thakkar et al. 2003). In vitro electrophysiological studies showed that adenosine can postsynaptically inhibit basal forebrain neurons and cholinergic neurons in the laterodorsal tegmental nuclei via A_1R (Arrigoni et al. 2006; Rainnie et al. 1994). Christie et al. reported that sleep loss induces adenosine in the basal forebrain by A_1R, which leads to sleepiness and impaired vigilance (Christie et al. 2008). During the rat Psychomotor Vigilance Task performance, response latencies and performance lapses of rats increased significantly after adenosine was dialyzed in the basal forebrain of rats when compared with baseline (no dialysis) or vehicle dialysis sessions. The codialysis of A_1R antagonist, 8-cyclopentyltheophylline with adenosine completely blocked the effects produced by adenosine alone, resulting in performance equivalent to that of the vehicle sessions. These results suggest that adenosine-induced sleep is mediated via A_1R in the cholinergic neurons in the basal forebrain. In addition, A_1R binding was increased after prolonged wakefulness/sleep deprivation in both humans (Basheer et al. 2007) and rats (Elmenhorst et al. 2009), presumably caused by increases of adenosine, as proved for the basal forebrain (Basheer et al. 2007).

Although local administration of adenosine or A_1R agonist into the basal forebrain induces NREM sleep, infusion of the A_1R agonist CPA into the lateral ventricle does not affect NREM and REM sleep in mice (Urade et al. 2003), indicating that activation of A_1R in other brain areas may promote wakefulness. Methippara et al. (2005) investigated the effects of an adenosine transport inhibitor, NBTI, and A_1R agonists/antagonists on sleep by microdialyzing them into the lateral preoptic area. The results revealed that A_1R activation or inhibition of adenosine transport by NBTI increased wakefulness (Methippara et al. 2005). Moreover, the homeostatic component of sleep–wake regulation is not affected in A_1R knockout animals (Stenberg et al. 2003). These findings indicate that adenosine influences sleep–wake cycles in a site- and receptor-dependent manner and A_1Rs are probably not necessary for sleep homeostasis.

Blanco-Centurion et al. (2006) reported that adenosine levels in the basal forebrain did not increase after 6 h of prolonged wakefulness in rats with 95% cholinergic neurons lesion in the basal forebrain. The lesion rats had an intact sleep drive after 6 and 12 h of prolonged wakefulness. In the absence of cholinergic neurons in the basal forebrain, another selective A_1R agonist, N^6-cyclohexyladenosine, effectively increases sleep after administration to the basal forebrain. Therefore, neither the activity of cholinergic neurons nor the accumulation of adenosine in the basal forebrain during wakefulness is necessary for the sleep drive. However, Kalinchuk et al. (2008) found that lesions of the cholinergic neurons in the basal forebrain eliminated both the increase of adenosine levels and the homeostatic sleep drive. These findings leave open the possibility raised by both studies that A_1R may influence sleep through noncholinergic neurons and that adenosine could affect sleep via the brain regions other than the basal forebrain (Nooralam et al. 2006). To understand the roles of noncholinergic and cholinergic neurons of the basal forebrain in sleep–wake and EEG, as well as in homeostatic sleep regulation, Kaur et al. (2008) ablated noncholinergic neurons in the basal forebrain with ibotenate, and cholinergic neurons with 192-IgG saporin, and found that the noncholinergic neurons in the basal forebrain can activate cortex through inhibiting delta waves, that cholinergic neurons in the basal forebrain are not exclusive in promoting wakefulness, and that both types of neurons in the basal forebrain are critical for the increases in NREM sleep and EEG delta power induced by sleep deprivation.

Inhibition of the adenosine system by A_1R orexin expressing brain areas (Thakkar et al. 2008) and histaminergic TMN (Oishi et al. 2008) are also demonstrated to induce NREM sleep. Thakkar et al. (2002) found that 30% of the orexin-containing neurons were immunoreactive with A_1R antibody. Perfusion with the A_1R agonist CPA significantly inhibited the sleep–wake discharge activity of perifornical-lateral hypothalamic neurons and suppressed wakefulness (Rai et al. 2010). We found that adenosine A_1R is also substantially expressed in the TMN. Bilateral injection of A_1R agonist CPA into the TMN notably promoted NREM sleep in rats. The bilateral injection of adenosine or an inhibitor of ADA, coformycin, into the TMN also increased NREM sleep in rats (Fig. 3.5), which can be completely eliminated by a selective A_1R antagonist, 1, 3-dimethyl-8-cyclopenthylxanthine (Oishi et al. 2008). These findings suggest that endogenous adenosine in the TMN inhibits the histaminergic system by A_1Rs to induce NREM sleep.

3.7 Potential Application of Adenosine Receptor Agonists to Sleep Disorders

Although many hypnotic and antihypnotic drugs are on the market, most of these compounds show various unwanted side effects. The molecular mechanisms underlying sleep–wake regulation by adenosine described in this chapter may provide a valid and practical approach for the development of drugs to mitigate sleep disorders based on the pharmacological use of enzyme inhibitors and receptor-specific therapies. The concept of using adenosine receptor agonists as modulators for sleep disorders is fascinating; however, in practice, this approach could be used in a brain region-dependent manner (Jacobson and Gao 2006). It need to be emphasized that much more work is still necessary to clarify the detailed mechanisms of sleep–wake regulation in terms of these mediators.

3.8 Histaminergic System Is Essential for Wakefulness

The histaminergic neurons are located in the TMN (Lin 2000; Brown et al. 2001) and histamine can induce cortical arousal possibly either through direct cortical projections or by tonic control over the sleep-generating mechanisms in the preoptic anterior hypothalamus (Lin et al. 1990, 1996). It was found that GABA exists in most of the neurons in the TMN. Selective siRNA knockdown of the vesicular GABA transporter (Vgat) in histaminergic neurons induced hyperactive mice that have an extraordinary amount of wakefulness. Ablation of the Vgat gene throughout the TMN sharpened this phenotype even further (Yu et al. 2015). Histamine was found to promote wakefulness by the activation of H1R (Lin et al. 1988, 1990, 1996;

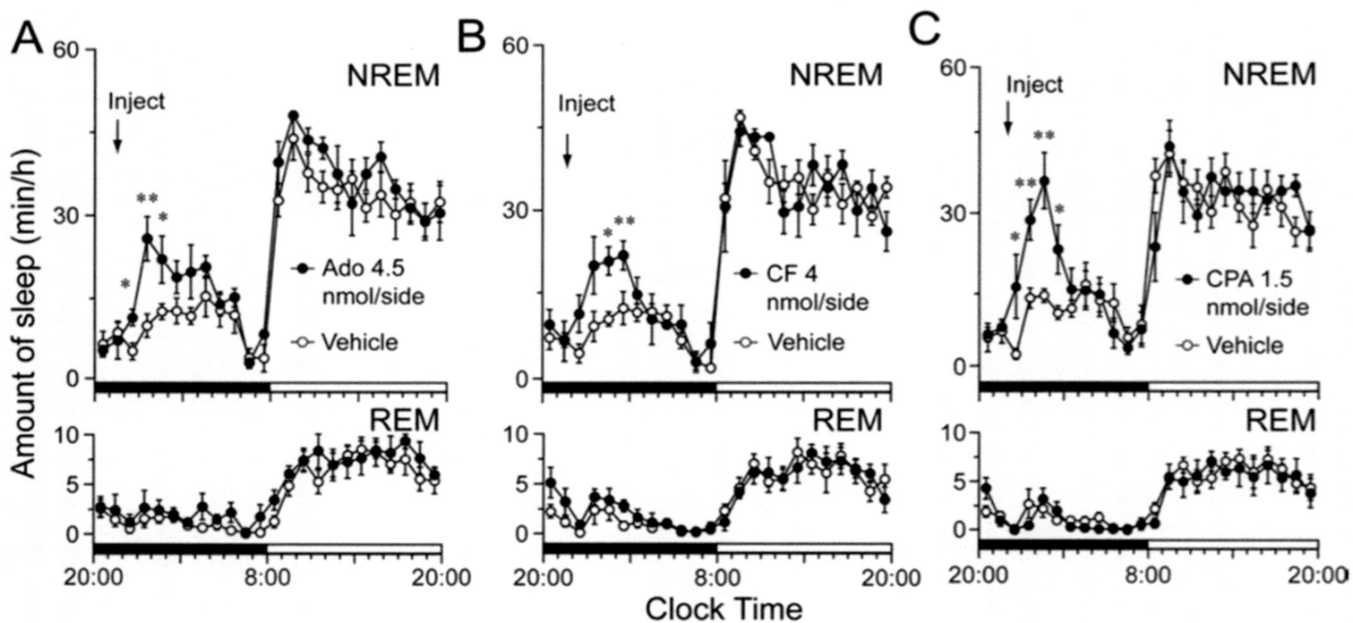

Fig. 3.5 (**a**) Time courses of NREM and REM sleep in rats administered adenosine (Ado) at 4.5 nmol/; (**b**) ADA inhibitor coformycin (CF) at 4 nmol/side; or (**c**) A_1R agonist CPA at 1.5 nmol/side. Values are means ± SEM ($n = 5–8$). $^{*}P < 0.05$; $^{**}P < 0.01$, significantly different from the vehicle injection. Adapted from Oishi et al. (2008) with modification and permission

Monti et al. 1990; Monti 1993). H1R KO mice provide a useful tool to investigate the role of the histaminergic system in the arousal effect induced by orexin A. H1R KO mice were originally generated by Inoue et al. (1996), and their behavior and neuropharmacological characteristics also have been extensively studied (Inoue et al. 1996; Yanai et al. 1998). It is reported that H1R KO mice showed a significant decrease in ambulation in an open field and on an activity wheel, however, no electrophysiological study has been carried out yet. We found that orexin A can significantly promote wakefulness in WT mice but not in H1R KO mice, although both genotypes of mice displayed basically the same amounts of sleep and wakefulness under basal conditions. This suggests that H1R is indispensable for orexin A-induced wakefulness (Huang et al. 2001).

3.9 Conclusions

The roles of adenosine receptors in sleep–wake regulation are summarized in Table 3.1. The strongest endogenous sleep-promoting factor, adenosine, accumulates in the brain during wakefulness and stimulates physiological sleep. Among all the adenosine receptors in sleep–wake regulation, $A_{2A}R$ is predominant in sleep induction because the administration of selective $A_{2A}R$ agonist, CGS-21680, to the subarachnoid space adjacent to the basal forebrain and lateral preoptic area significantly promotes NREM sleep, whereas the infusion of A_1R agonists produces weak and variable effects (Satoh et al. 1996; Methippara et al. 2005; Scammell et al. 2001; Urade et al. 2003; Hong et al. 2005). A_1Rs could induce sleep in a region-dependent manner but may not be necessary for sleep homeostasis. As of now, it is still unclear how and where adenosine derives under physiological conditions or after sleep deprivation. Histaminergic neurons in the TMN, a region within the posterior hypothalamus, contribute to wakefulness maintaining. Wake-active histaminergic neurons generate a paracrine GABAergic signal which may prevent histamine from triggering overactivation.

References

Arrigoni E, Chamberlin N, Saper C, McCarley R. Adenosine inhibits basal forebrain cholinergic and noncholinergic neurons *in vitro*. Neuroscience. 2006;140:403–13.

Basheer R, Strecker RE, Thakkar MM, McCarley RW. Adenosine and sleep–wake regulation. Prog Neurobiol. 2004;73:379–96.

Basheer R, Bauer A, Elmenhorst D, Ramesh V, McCarley RW. Sleep deprivation upregulates A1 adenosine receptors in the rat basal forebrain. Neuroreport. 2007;18:1895–9.

Benington J, Kodali S, Heller H. Stimulation of A1 adenosine receptors mimics the electroencephalographic effects of sleep deprivation. Brain Res. 1995;692:79–85.

Blanco-Centurion C, et al. Adenosine and sleep homeostasis in the basal forebrain. J Neurosci. 2006;26:8092–100.

Borb AA, Achermann P. Sleep homeostasis and models of sleep regulation. J Biol Rhythm. 1999;14:559–70.
Brown RE, Stevens DR, Haas HL. The physiology of brain histamine. Prog Neurobiol. 2001;63: 637–72.
Brundege JM, Diao L, Proctor WR, Dunwiddie TV. The role of cyclic AMP as a precursor of extracellular adenosine in the rat hippocampus. Neuropharmacology. 1997;36:1201–10.
Burnstock G. Physiology and pathophysiology of purinergic neurotransmission. Physiol Rev. 2007;87:659–797.
Christie MA, et al. Microdialysis elevation of adenosine in the basal forebrain produces vigilance impairments in the rat psychomotor vigilance task. Sleep. 2008;31:1393.
Deussen A, Lloyd HG, Schrader J. Contribution of S-adenosylhomocysteine to cardiac adenosine formation. J Mol Cell Cardiol. 1989;21:773–82.
Dunwiddie TV, Masino SA. The role and regulation of adenosine in the central nervous system. Annu Rev Neurosci. 2001;24:31–55.
El Yacoubi M, Ledent C, Parmentier M, Costentin J, Vaugeois J. Caffeine reduces hypnotic effects of alcohol through adenosine A2A receptor blockade. Neuropharmacology. 2003;45:977.
Elmenhorst D, et al. Sleep deprivation increases A1 adenosine receptor binding in the human brain: a positron emission tomography study. J Neurosci. 2007;27:2410–5.
Elmenhorst D, Basheer R, Mccarley RW, Bauer A. Sleep deprivation increases A1 adenosine receptor density in the rat brain. Brain Res. 2009;1258:53–8.
Feldberg W, Sherwood S. Injections of drugs into the lateral ventricle of the cat. J Physiol. 1954;123:148–67.
Ferre S, et al. Adenosine A2A receptors in ventral striatum, hypothalamus and nociceptive circuitry Implications for drug addiction, sleep and pain. Prog Neurobiol. 2007;83:332–47.
Franken P, Chollet D, Tafti M. The homeostatic regulation of sleep need is under genetic control. J Neurosci. 2001;21:2610–21.
Fredholm B. Adenosine, an endogenous distress signal, modulates tissue damage and repair. Cell Death Differ. 2007;14:1315–23.
Fredholm BB, IJzerman AP, Jacobson KA, Klotz K-N, Linden J. International union of pharmacology. XXV Nomenclature and classification of adenosine receptors. Pharmacol Rev. 2001;53: 527–52.
Fredholm BB, Chen J-F, Cunha RA, Svenningsson P, Vaugeois J-M. Adenosine and brain function. Int Rev Neurobiol. 2005;63:191–270.
Gallopin T, et al. The endogenous somnogen adenosine excites a subset of sleep-promoting neurons via A2A receptors in the ventrolateral preoptic nucleus. Neuroscience. 2005;134:1377.
Geiger JD, Fyda DM. Adenosine transport in nervous system tissues. In: Adenosine in the nervous system. New York: Academic Press; 1991. p. 1–23.
Gerashchenko D, Okano Y, Urade Y, Inoué S, Hayaishi O. Strong rebound of wakefulness follows prostaglandin D2-or adenosine A2a receptor agonist-induced sleep. J Sleep Res. 2000;9:81–7.
Gu J, Foga I, Parkinson F, Geiger J. Involvement of Bidirectional Adenosine Transporters in the Release of l-[3H] Adenosine from Rat Brain Synaptosomal Preparations. J Neurochem. 1995;64:2105–10.
Halassa MM, et al. Astrocytic modulation of sleep homeostasis and cognitive consequences of sleep loss. Neuron. 2009;61:213–9.
Hong ZY, et al. An adenosine A2A receptor agonist induces sleep by increasing GABA release in the tuberomammillary nucleus to inhibit histaminergic systems in rats. J Neurochem. 2005;92: 1542–9.
Huang Z-L, et al. Arousal effect of orexin A depends on activation of the histaminergic system. Proc Natl Acad Sci U S A. 2001;98:9965–70. https://doi.org/10.1073/pnas.181330998.
Huang Z-L, et al. Adenosine A2A, but not A1, receptors mediate the arousal effect of caffeine. Nat Neurosci. 2005;8:858–9.
Huang Z-L, Urade Y, Hayaishi O. Prostaglandins and adenosine in the regulation of sleep and wakefulness. Curr Opin Pharmacol. 2007;7:33–8.

Huston J, et al. Extracellular adenosine levels in neostriatum and hippocampus during rest and activity periods of rats. Neuroscience. 1996;73:99–107.

Inoue I, et al. Impaired locomotor activity and exploratory behavior in mice lacking histamine H1 receptors. Proc Natl Acad Sci U S A. 1996;93:13316–20.

Islam F, Watanabe Y, Morii H, Hayaishi O. Inhibition of rat brain prostaglandin D synthase by inorganic selenocompounds. Arch Biochem Biophys. 1991;289:161–6.

Jacobson KA, Gao Z-G. Adenosine receptors as therapeutic targets. Nat Rev Drug Discov. 2006;5: 247–64.

Jones BE. Glia, adenosine, and sleep. Neuron. 2009;61:156–7.

Jordan W, et al. Prostaglandin D synthase (β-trace) in healthy human sleep. Sleep. 2004;27:867–74.

Jourdain P, et al. Glutamate exocytosis from astrocytes controls synaptic strength. Nat Neurosci. 2007;10:331–9.

Kalinchuk AV, McCarley RW, Stenberg D, Porkka-Heiskanen T, Basheer R. The role of cholinergic basal forebrain neurons in adenosine-mediated homeostatic control of sleep: lessons from 192 IgG–saporin lesions. Neuroscience. 2008;157:238–53.

Kalinchuk A, McCarley R, Porkka-Heiskanen T, Basheer R. Sleep deprivation triggers inducible nitric oxide-dependent nitric oxide production in wake-active basal forebrain neurons. J Neurosci. 2010;30:13254.

Kaur S, Junek A, Black MA, Semba K. Effects of ibotenate and 192IgG-saporin lesions of the nucleus basalis magnocellularis/substantia innominata on spontaneous sleep and wake states and on recovery sleep after sleep deprivation in rats. J Neurosci. 2008;28:491–504.

Latini S, Pedata F. Adenosine in the central nervous system: release mechanisms and extracellular concentrations. J Neurochem. 2001;79:463–84.

Li R, et al. Activation of adenosine A2A receptors in the olfactory tubercle promotes sleep in rodents. Neuropharmacology. 2020;168:107923. https://doi.org/10.1016/j.neuropharm.2019.107923.

Lin JS. Brain structures and mechanisms involved in the control of cortical activation and wakefulness, with emphasis on the posterior hypothalamus and histaminergic neurons. Sleep Med Rev. 2000;4:471–503. https://doi.org/10.1053/smrv.2000.0116.

Lin JS, Sakai K, Jouvet M. Evidence for histaminergic arousal mechanisms in the hypothalamus of cat. Neuropharmacology. 1988;27:111–22.

Lin JS, et al. Involvement of histaminergic neurons in arousal mechanisms demonstrated with H3-receptor ligands in the cat. Brain Res. 1990;523:325–30.

Lin JS, Hou Y, Sakai K, Jouvet M. Histaminergic descending inputs to the mesopontine tegmentum and their role in the control of cortical activation and wakefulness in the cat. J Neurosci. 1996;16:1523–37.

Marks G, Shaffery J, Speciale S, Birabil C. Enhancement of rapid eye movement sleep in the rat by actions at A1 and A2a adenosine receptor subtypes with a differential sensitivity to atropine. Neuroscience. 2003;116:913–20.

Matsumura H, Takahata R, Hayaishi O. Inhibition of sleep in rats by inorganic selenium compounds, inhibitors of prostaglandin D synthase. Proc Natl Acad Sci U S A. 1991;88:9046–50.

Methippara MM, Kumar S, Alam MN, Szymusiak R, McGinty D. Effects on sleep of microdialysis of adenosine A1 and A2a receptor analogs into the lateral preoptic area of rats. Am J Phys Regul Integr Comp Phys. 2005;289:R1715–23.

Missale C, Nash SR, Robinson SW, Jaber M, Caron MG. Dopamine receptors: from structure to function. Physiol Rev. 1998;78:189–225.

Mizoguchi A, et al. Dominant localization of prostaglandin D receptors on arachnoid trabecular cells in mouse basal forebrain and their involvement in the regulation of non-rapid eye movement sleep. Proc Natl Acad Sci U S A. 2001;98:11674–9.

Mohri I, Eguchi N, Suzuki K, Urade Y, Taniike M. Hematopoietic prostaglandin D synthase is expressed in microglia in the developing postnatal mouse brain. Glia. 2003;42:263–74.

Monti JM. Involvement of histamine in the control of the waking state. Life Sci. 1993;53:1331–8.

Monti JM, Orellana C, Boussard M, Jantos H, Olivera S. Sleep variables are unaltered by zolantidine in rats: are histamine H2-receptors not involved in sleep regulation? Brain Res Bull. 1990;25:229–31.

Monti J, Pandi-Perumal SR, Sinton CM, Sinton CW. Neurochemistry of sleep and wakefulness. Cambridge: Cambridge University Press; 2008.

Murillo-Rodriguez E, Blanco-Centurion C, Gerashchenko D, Salin-Pascual R, Shiromani P. The diurnal rhythm of adenosine levels in the basal forebrain of young and old rats. Neuroscience. 2004;123:361–70.

Nagy J, LaBella L, Buss M, Daddona P. Immunohistochemistry of adenosine deaminase: implications for adenosine neurotransmission. Science. 1984;224:166–8.

Narumiya S, Ogorochi T, Nakao K, Hayaishi O. Prostaglandin D2 in rat brain, spinal cord and pituitary: basal level and regional distribution. Life Sci. 1982;31:2093.

Nooralam M, Szymusiak R, McGinty D. Adenosinergic regulation of sleep: multiple sites of action in the brain. Sleep. 2006;29:1384–5.

Ogorochi T, et al. Regional distribution of prostaglandins D2, E2, and F2α and related enzymes in postmortem human brain. J Neurochem. 1984;43:71–82.

Oishi Y, Huang Z-L, Fredholm BB, Urade Y, Hayaishi O. Adenosine in the tuberomammillary nucleus inhibits the histaminergic system via A1 receptors and promotes non-rapid eye movement sleep. Proc Natl Acad Sci U S A. 2008;105:19992–7.

Oishi Y, et al. Slow-wave sleep is controlled by a subset of nucleus accumbens core neurons in mice. Nat Commun. 2017;8:734. https://doi.org/10.1038/s41467-017-00781-4.

Okada T, et al. Dominant localization of adenosine deaminase in leptomeninges and involvement of the enzyme in sleep. Biochem Biophys Res Commun. 2003;312:29–34.

Onoe H, et al. Prostaglandin D2, a cerebral sleep-inducing substance in monkeys. Proc Natl Acad Sci U S A. 1988;85:4082–6.

Pandey HP, Ram A, Matsumura H, Hayaishi O. Concentration of prostaglandin D2 in cerebrospinal fluid exhibits a circadian alteration in conscious rats. Biochem Mol Biol Int. 1995;37:431–7.

Pascual O, et al. Astrocytic purinergic signaling coordinates synaptic networks. Science. 2005;310:113–6.

Peng L, et al. Nucleoside transporter expression and function in cultured mouse astrocytes. Glia. 2005;52:25–35.

Peng W, et al. Regulation of sleep homeostasis mediator adenosine by basal forebrain glutamatergic neurons. Science. 2020;369:eabb0556. https://doi.org/10.1126/science.abb0556.

Porkka-Heiskanen T, et al. Adenosine: a mediator of the sleep-inducing effects of prolonged wakefulness. Science. 1997;276:1265–8.

Porkka-Heiskanen T, Strecker R, McCarley R. Brain site-specificity of extracellular adenosine concentration changes during sleep deprivation and spontaneous sleep: an in vivo microdialysis study. Neuroscience. 1999;99:507–17.

Qiu M, et al. D (1)/D (2) receptor-targeting L-stepholidine, an active ingredient of the Chinese herb Stephonia, induces non-rapid eye movement sleep in mice. Pharmacol Biochem Behav. 2009;94:16.

Qu W-M, et al. Lipocalin-type prostaglandin D synthase produces prostaglandin D2 involved in regulation of physiological sleep. Proc Natl Acad Sci U S A. 2006;103:17949–54.

Qu W-M, Huang Z-L, Xu X-H, Matsumoto N, Urade Y. Dopaminergic D1 and D2 receptors are essential for the arousal effect of modafinil. J Neurosci. 2008;28:8462–9.

Qu W-M, et al. Essential role of dopamine D2 receptor in the maintenance of wakefulness, but not in homeostatic regulation of sleep, in mice. J Neurosci. 2010;30:4382–9.

Radek RJ, Decker MW, Jarvis MF. The adenosine kinase inhibitor ABT-702 augments EEG slow waves in rats. Brain Res. 2004;1026:74–83.

Radulovacki M, Virus R, Djuricic-Nedelson M, Green R. Hypnotic effects of deoxycorformycin in rats. Brain Res. 1983;271:392–5.

Rai S, et al. A1 receptor mediated adenosinergic regulation of perifornical-lateral hypothalamic area neurons in freely behaving rats. Neuroscience. 2010;167:40.

Rainnie DG, Grunze HC, McCarley RW, Greene RW. Adenosine inhibition of mesopontine cholinergic neurons: implications for EEG arousal. Science (New York, NY). 1994;263:689.

Ram A, et al. CSF levels of prostaglandins, especially the level of prostaglandin D2, are correlated with increasing propensity towards sleep in rats. Brain Res. 1997;751:81.

Retey J, et al. A functional genetic variation of adenosine deaminase affects the duration and intensity of deep sleep in humans. Proc Natl Acad Sci U S A. 2005;102:15676–81.

Retey J, et al. A genetic variation in the adenosine A2A receptor gene (ADORA2A) contributes to individual sensitivity to caffeine effects on sleep. Clin Pharmacol Ther. 2007;81:692–8.

Rosenberg PA, Li Y. Adenylyl cyclase activation underlies intracellular cyclic AMP accumulation, cyclic AMP transport, and extracellular adenosine accumulation evoked by β-adrenergic receptor stimulation in mixed cultures of neurons and astrocytes derived from rat cerebral cortex. Brain Res. 1995;692:227–32.

Sala-Newby GB, Skladanowski AC, Newby AC. The mechanism of adenosine formation in cells cloning of cytosolic 5′-nucleotidase-I. J Biol Chem. 1999;274:17789–93.

Saper CB, Scammell TE, Lu J. Hypothalamic regulation of sleep and circadian rhythms. Nature. 2005;437:1257–63.

Satoh S, Matsumura H, Suzuki F, Hayaishi O. Promotion of sleep mediated by the A2a-adenosine receptor and possible involvement of this receptor in the sleep induced by prostaglandin D2 in rats. Proc Natl Acad Sci U S A. 1996;93:5980–4.

Satoh S, Matsumura H, Hayaishi O. Involvement of adenosine A2A receptor in sleep promotion. Eur J Pharmacol. 1998;351:155–62.

Satoh S, et al. Region-dependent difference in the sleep-promoting potency of an adenosine A2A receptor agonist. Eur J Neurosci. 1999;11:1587–97.

Sawynok J, Liu XJ. Adenosine in the spinal cord and periphery: release and regulation of pain. Prog Neurobiol. 2003;69:313–40.

Scammell T, et al. An adenosine A2a agonist increases sleep and induces Fos in ventrolateral preoptic neurons. Neuroscience. 2001;107:653–63.

Schiffmann S, Fisone G, Moresco R, Cunha R, Ferre S. Adenosine A2A receptors and basal ganglia physiology. Prog Neurobiol. 2007;83:277–92.

Schwierin B, Borbely A, Tobler I. Effects of N6-cyclopentyladenosine and caffeine on sleep regulation in the rat. Eur J Pharmacol. 1996;300:163–72.

Sherin JE, Elmquist JK, Torrealba F, Saper CB. Innervation of histaminergic tuberomammillary neurons by GABAergic and galaninergic neurons in the ventrolateral preoptic nucleus of the rat. J Neurosci. 1998;18:4705–21.

Stenberg D, et al. Sleep and its homeostatic regulation in mice lacking the adenosine A1 receptor. J Sleep Res. 2003;12:283–90.

Strecker RE, et al. Adenosinergic modulation of basal forebrain and preoptic/anterior hypothalamic neuronal activity in the control of behavioral state. Behav Brain Res. 2000;115:183–204.

Takahata R, et al. Intravenous administration of inorganic selenium compounds, inhibitors of prostaglandin D synthase, inhibits sleep in freely moving rats. Brain Res. 1993;623:65–71.

Thakkar MM, Winston S, McCarley RW. Orexin neurons of the hypothalamus express adenosine A1 receptors. Brain Res. 2002;944:190–4.

Thakkar MM, Winston S, McCarley RW. A1 receptor and adenosinergic homeostatic regulation of sleep-wakefulness: effects of antisense to the A1 receptor in the cholinergic basal forebrain. J Neurosci. 2003;23:4278–87.

Thakkar M, Engemann S, Walsh K, Sahota P. Adenosine and the homeostatic control of sleep: effects of A1 receptor blockade in the perifornical lateral hypothalamus on sleep–wakefulness. Neuroscience. 2008;153:875–80.

Ueno R, Ishikawa Y, Nakayama T, Hayaishi O. Prostaglandin D2 induces sleep when microinjected into the preoptic area of conscious rats. Biochem Biophys Res Commun. 1982;109:576.

Ueno R, Honda K, Inoué S, Hayaishi O. Prostaglandin D2, a cerebral sleep-inducing substance in rats. Proc Natl Acad Sci U S A. 1983;80:1735–7.

Urade Y, Hayaishi O. Crucial role of prostaglandin D2 and adenosine in sleep regulation: experimental evidence from pharmacological approaches to gene-knockout mice. Future Neurol. 2010;5:363–76.

Urade Y, et al. Dominant expression of mRNA for prostaglandin D synthase in leptomeninges, choroid plexus, and oligodendrocytes of the adult rat brain. Proc Natl Acad Sci. 1993;90:9070–4.

Urade Y, et al. Sleep regulation in adenosine A2A receptor-deficient mice. Neurology. 2003;61: S94–6.

Wang YQ, et al. Adenosine A2A receptors in the olfactory bulb suppress rapid eye movement sleep in rodents. Brain Struct Funct. 2017;222:1351–66. https://doi.org/10.1007/s00429-016-1281-2.

Wang P, et al. Lipocalin-type prostaglandin D synthase levels increase in patients with narcolepsy and idiopathic hypersomnia. Sleep. 2021;44:zsaa234. https://doi.org/10.1093/sleep/zsaa234.

Yaar R, Jones M, Chen JF, Ravid K. Animal models for the study of adenosine receptor function. J Cell Physiol. 2005;202:9–20.

Yanai K, et al. Behavioural characterization and amounts of brain monoamines and their metabolites in mice lacking histamine H1 receptors. Neuroscience. 1998;87:479–87.

Yu X, et al. Wakefulness is governed by GABA and histamine cotransmission. Neuron. 2015;87: 164–78. https://doi.org/10.1016/j.neuron.2015.06.003.

Yuan XS, et al. Striatal adenosine A2A receptor neurons control active-period sleep via parvalbumin neurons in external globus pallidus. elife. 2017;6:e29055. https://doi.org/10.7554/eLife.29055.

Zhang Z, et al. Regulated ATP release from astrocytes through lysosome exocytosis. Nat Cell Biol. 2007;9:945–53.

Zimmermann H. Extracellular metabolism of ATP and other nucleotides. Naunyn Schmiedeberg's Arch Pharmacol. 2000;362:299–309.

Zimmermann H, Braun N, Kegel B, Heine P. New insights into molecular structure and function of ecto-nucleotidases in the nervous system. Neurochem Int. 1998;32:421–5.

Chapter 4
Sleep and Neuronal Plasticity

Marcos G. Frank

Abstract Sleep is considered to play an important role in neuronal plasticity yet the underlying mechanisms remain controversial. In the last two decades, scientists have made important advances in understanding these mechanisms in the developing and adult brain. An emergent view is that sleep influences a number of types of plasticity and this is determined by a number of factors, including preceding experience, and ontogenetic status. Several theories of sleep function have also been proposed that integrate older ideas about sleep and more recent discoveries in the field of synaptic plasticity. In this chapter, I discuss these key findings and current theories that posit different roles for sleep in neuronal plasticity.

Keywords Synapse · REM · Rhythm · Scaling · Hebbian · Neurodevelopment · Cortex · Hippocampus · Maturation

4.1 Introduction

Sleep has long been suspected to play an important role in neuronal plasticity. Scientists historically conceptualized and investigated the problem in terms of what was known about classic Hebbian forms of plasticity such as long-term synaptic potentiation (LTP) and depression (LTD) [reviewed in Benington and Frank (2003) and Frank and Benington (2006)]. LTP and LTD refer to use-dependent, persistent alterations in synaptic weights that strengthen (LTP) or weaken (LTD)-specific synapses, respectively (Malenka and Bear 2004). They are considered Hebbian because they are associative, input (synapse) specific and require coordinated pre- and post-synaptic activity (Markram et al. 2011). Today, LTP and LTD are believed to be cellular correlates (if not the substrates) of learning and memory (Malenka and Bear 2004; Bear and Malenka 1994).

M. G. Frank (✉)
Elson S. Floyd College of Medicine, Washington State University Spokane, Spokane, WA, USA
e-mail: marcos.frank@wsu.edu

A. I. Pack, Q. Y. Li (eds.), *Sleep and its Disorders*, Translational Medicine Research,
https://doi.org/10.1007/978-94-024-2168-2_4

More recently sleep has also been proposed to promote non-Hebbian ("homeostatic") forms of plasticity (Tononi and Cirelli 2003, 2006). In contrast to LTP and LTD, these forms of plasticity can adjust all synapses in a neuron or network of neurons upward or downward in response to global changes in activity (Turrigiano 1999, 2008; Pozo and Goda 2010). This type of plasticity is proposed to offset pure Hebbian mechanisms in the brain, that if left unchecked would saturate synaptic strength and prevent further learning. Homeostatic plasticity was originally described in the late 1990s by non-sleep scientists [for review see Nelson and Turrigiano (2008)], and conceptually incorporated into what came to be known as the "synaptic homeostasis hypothesis" (SHY) in 2003 (Tononi and Cirelli 2001, 2003, 2006).

In the following sections, I discuss our current knowledge concerning interactions between sleep and Hebbian and non-Hebbian synaptic plasticity in the developing and adult brain. I also discuss these findings in the context of two theories of sleep function that incorporate Hebbian and non-Hebbian forms of plasticity in different ways.

4.2 Sleep and Developmental Plasticity

In a variety of mammalian species, sleep amounts are highest during developmental periods of rapid brain development and synaptic plasticity than at any other time in life (Roffwarg et al. 1966; Frank and Heller 1997; Jouvet-Mounier et al. 1970). Many of the mechanisms governing developmental plasticity also mediate plasticity in the adult brain. Therefore, studying the role of sleep in developmental plasticity may provide insights more generally into sleep function across the lifespan. Most of what we know about sleep and developmental plasticity comes from studies of the developing visual system, particularly during sensitive or critical periods when visual circuits are highly plastic (Frank 2011). These studies are discussed in the following sections.

4.2.1 Sleep and Ocular Dominance Plasticity

Ocular dominance plasticity (ODP) refers to electrophysiological and anatomical changes in visual cortical circuits in vivo triggered by blocking patterned vision in one [also known as monocular deprivation (MD)]. When performed during a critical period of development (a stage when the brain is most sensitive to experience), MD results in synaptic weakening in circuits serving the deprived eye and synaptic strengthening in circuits serving the open eye (Wiesel and Hubel 1963; Hubel and Wiesel 1970). These mechanisms involve both Hebbian and non-Hebbian forms of plasticity. Although first described in developing animals, ODP shares numerous mechanisms that mediate Hebbian and non-Hebbian plasticity in the adult hippocampus and non-sensory cortex. ODP is considered *physiological* because it occurs in vivo in response to changes in sensory input and the resulting plasticity involves naturally occurring changes in synaptic proteins and molecules. The underlying plasticity is also present without MD as it governs cortical adjustments to visual input that normally occur during the critical period. For these reasons, ODP is recognized as a canonical model of physiological plasticity in vivo [for review see Spolidoro et al. (2009), Tropea et al. (2009), Smith et al. (2009), and Espinosa and Stryker (2012)].

A role for sleep in ODP has been demonstrated in developing cats (Fig. 4.1) and mice. In both species, 6–8 h of sleep significantly enhances the effects of MD on cortical neurons; a process that does not occur when animals are instead sleep deprived (Frank et al. 2001; Dumoulin Bridi et al. 2015; Zhou et al. 2020). The underlying mechanisms appear similar in both species but the type of plasticity that is enhanced is species dependent. In cats, both acute (Aton et al. 2009) and chronic (Aton et al. 2013) recordings of single neurons show that MD in awake animals results in an initial weakening of responses to the deprived eye. After sleep, responses to the non-deprived eye become stronger but there is no further change in the magnitude of depression observed in the deprived eye pathway. Infusing the *N*-methyl-D-aspartate receptor (NMDAR) antagonist APV, the protein kinase A (PKA) inhibitor Rp-8-Cl-cAMPS, the extracellular-regulated kinase (ERK) inhibitor UO126 or the mammalian target of rapamycin (mTOR) inhibitor rapamycin into the visual cortex during post-MD sleep completely abolishes this potentiated response (Aton et al. 2009; Seibt et al. 2012). In addition, post-MD sleep is accompanied by activation of several kinases implicated in LTP and phosphorylation of the α-amino-3-hydroxy-5-methyl-4-isoxazolepropionic acid receptor (AMPAR) that lead to trafficking and insertion of this receptor into the postsynaptic membrane (Aton et al. 2009). Post-MD sleep also promotes the synthesis or phosphorylation of several proteins implicated in LTP (Dumoulin Bridi et al. 2015; Seibt et al. 2012; Renouard et al. 2018).

In mice, however, sleep only enhances the loss of response to the deprived eye (Zhou et al. 2020). As is true in cats, this enhancement of MD is REM sleep and NMDAR dependent (Dumoulin Bridi et al. 2015; Frank 2017). Differences between cats and mice likely reflect differences in the layout of visual pathways in carnivores and rodents. Rodent visual cortex is mostly innervated from the contralateral eye. Therefore, MD of the contralateral eye only results in a weakened response to the deprived eye when measured in the monocular segment of the visual cortex (Frank 2017). Carnivore (and primate) visual cortex instead receive balanced input from both eyes, resulting in a mixture of circuit strengthening and weakening.

Studies in the cat further demonstrate that ODP in wakefulness and sleep may be governed by distinct mechanisms in species with visual cortices more similar to humans. Sleep-dependent ODP is protein synthesis dependent, whereas the initial plasticity triggered during waking MD is not. This was shown by intracortical infusing pharmacological agents that inhibit protein synthesis either during the induction of MD (while animals were awake) or only after they went to sleep. Intracortical blockade of two essential kinases for mRNA translation (mTOR and

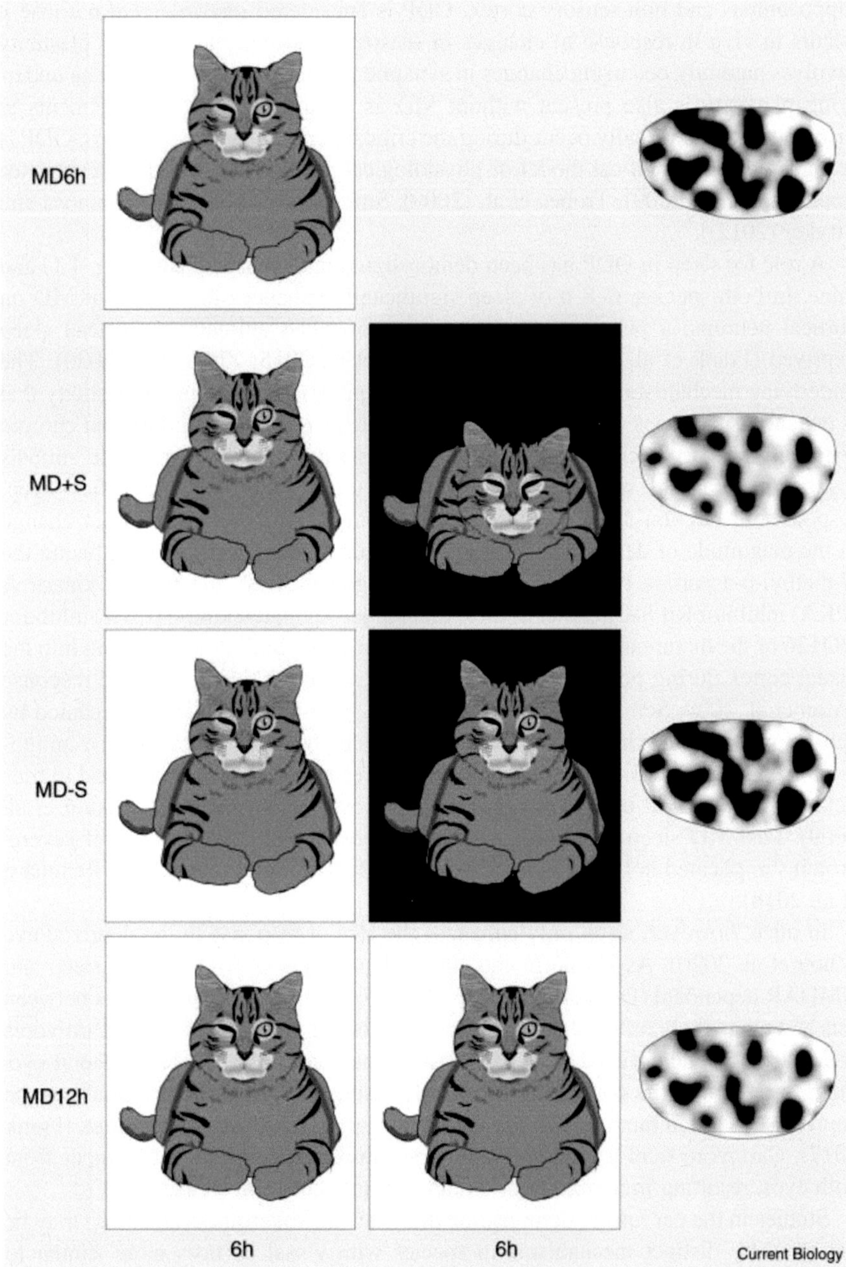

Fig. 4.1 Effect of sleep on the magnitude of the ocular dominance shift induced by monocular deprivation (MD). The first two columns show the experimental conditions of all kittens. The right-most column schematically shows ocular dominance maps obtained from primary visual cortex under various conditions. All kittens were monocularly deprived for 6 h, and one group was tested immediately afterward (MD6h). A second group was allowed to sleep ad-lib during the following 6 h (MD+S), while a third group was kept awake in the dark (MD−S). A fourth group was deprived for 12 h and then tested (MD12h). The ocular dominance maps obtained by intrinsic-signal imaging

ERK) has no effect on circuit weakening in wakefulness, but when conducted during subsequent sleep, this completely blocked sleep-dependent ODP (Seibt et al. 2012; Dumoulin et al. 2015). Additional studies of cortical genes and proteins showed that while plasticity-related mRNAs are upregulated by visual experience, they are not translated into proteins until sleep occurs (Seibt et al. 2012). This suggests that the transcription and translation of plasticity-related mRNAs are divided across sleep and wake.

A two-stage process in ODP is further demonstrated by a study of single-neuron activity in freely behaving cats. Aton et al. (2013) used chronic, stereotrode recording of single visual cortical neurons to track their activity and interactions before, during, and after a period of MD. In contrast to previous studies employing similar longitudinal recording (Mioche and Singer 1989), neuronal activity was also recorded across the sleep–wake cycle. MD in the awake animal caused a large reduction in firing rate in fast-spiking neurons (i.e., putative GABAergic cells) in the visual cortex. This decrease in activity was maintained during the first 6 h of post-MD sleep and accompanied by an increase in firing in regular spiking (i.e., putative excitatory neurons). The decrease in fast-spiking activity was also proportional to plastic changes in regular spiking neurons observed after sleep. This suggests that in addition to changes in the deprived eye pathway, MD alters intracortical inhibition which contributes to sleep-dependent changes in excitatory circuits.

4.2.2 Sleep and Developmental LTP In Vitro

REM sleep has also been shown to influence a form of LTP in vitro that parallels the critical period for ODP in rodents. In this type of LTP, high-frequency white matter stimulation in cortical slices prepared from postnatal (P) day 28–30 rats produces synaptic potentiation in cortical layers II/III. This form of LTP is only observed during these particular ages and not in cortical slices from adult rats (Kirkwood et al. 1995). Shaffery et al. (2002) reported that 1 week of REM sleep deprivation prolonged the critical period for the developmentally regulated form of LTP. Similar manipulations of older animals outside of the critical period did not show the same results. These investigators showed that this plasticity could be partially rescued if REM sleep deprivation was administered near (or overlapping) the end of the critical period (Shaffery et al. 2006; Shaffery and Roffwarg 2003). The effects of REM sleep

Fig. 4.1 (continued) display cortical regions dominated by the deprived eye in black, and those dominated by the non-deprived eye in white. The MD+S group shows a loss of territory dominated by the deprived eye well beyond that observed in the MD6h group, while the sleep-deprived group (MD−S) does not. In fact, the consolidation of the MD shift in the MD+S group amounts to about the same magnitude as is observed after 12 h of monocular deprivation (MD12h). Reproduced with permission from Sengpiel (2001)

deprivation can also be prevented by chronically infusing brain-derived neurotrophic factor (BDNF) into the visual cortex. This indicates that REM sleep may normally promote BDNF synthesis (Shaffery et al. 2012). This idea is supported by work in the developing cat, demonstrating that sleep is accompanied by increased cortical synthesis of BDNF and activity-regulated cytoskeleton-associated protein (Arc) (Seibt et al. 2012).

4.3 Sleep and Plasticity in the Adult Brain

4.3.1 LTP and LTD: In Vitro and In Vivo Studies in Adult Animals

The role of sleep in adult synaptic plasticity has historically been investigated using classic tetany-based forms of Hebbian LTP and LTD [reviewed in Benington and Frank (2003) and Hennevin et al. (2007)] in different brain states, or in slices of brains after periods of sleep or sleep deprivation. Overall, hippocampal LTP can be induced during REM sleep, whereas similar stimulus protocols during NREM sleep have inconsistent effects or produce LTD [reviewed in Benington and Frank (2003) and Hennevin et al. (2007)]. Conversely, sleep deprivation impairs the induction or maintenance of LTP in vivo and in vitro, although this varies depending on the brain area examined. For example, REM sleep deprivation and total sleep deprivation impair the maintenance of LTP in the hippocampus but enhance this process in the medial prefrontal cortex (Romcy-Pereira and Pavlides 2004). The effects of sleep loss on hippocampal LTP in vivo have been replicated in other studies but the timing of this effect varies, with some studies showing delayed impact on LTP (Marks and Wayner 2005; Kim et al. 2005).

A large number of studies also show that in vitro hippocampal LTP (either the induction or the maintenance) is reduced in rodents that undergo varying amounts of REM sleep deprivation, total sleep deprivation, or sleep restriction prior to sacrifice (Kopp et al. 2006; Arrigoni et al. 2009; Campbell et al. 2002; Davis et al. 2003; Ishikawa et al. 2006; McDermott et al. 2003, 2006; Ravassard et al. 2006, 2009; Tartar et al. 2006; Florian et al. 2011; Vecsey et al. 2009; Chen et al. 2006). Interestingly, when REM sleep is restored (after prior deprivation) or increased in rodents, this reverses deficits in hippocampal LTP (Ravassard et al. 2009, 2016).

The underlying mechanisms mediating the effects of sleep loss on LTP are not completely understood. However, they do not appear to be simply due to indirect effects of the sleep deprivation procedures. For example, these deficits can be dissociated from changes in stress hormones (Kopp et al. 2006; Ravassard et al. 2009, 2016). Diminished plasticity may instead be linked to decrements in hippocampal NMDA receptor function (Kopp et al. 2006; McDermott et al. 2006; Chen et al. 2006; Longordo et al. 2009) and ERK/MAPK activation (Ravassard et al. 2009) combined with reductions in plasticity-related mRNAs or proteins (Ravassard et al. 2016; Guzman-Marin et al. 2006; Davis et al. 2006), and elevated concentrations of PDE4 (Vecsey et al. 2009) and extracellular adenosine (Arrigoni et al. 2009; Florian et al. 2011).

4.3.2 *Naturally Occurring Forms of Cortical and Hippocampal Plasticity*

Sleep also promotes naturally occurring forms of synaptic potentiation in the adult visual and motor cortex. Stimulus specific-response plasticity (SRP) is a form of in vivo LTP that manifests as a potentiated response to an experienced (trained) visual stimulus (Cooke and Bear 2010). SRP is only observed after a period of sleep, and suppressed by sleep deprivation (Aton et al. 2014). A follow-up investigation (Durkin and Aton 2016) showed that these changes could not be explained as a form of "relative" synaptic weakening (Cirelli and Tononi 2015).

Interestingly, motor learning in adult mice promotes morphological signs of synaptic potentiation. After the learning experience, sleep promotes the formation of dendritic spines in motor cortex in a dendritic branch-dependent manner (Yang et al. 2014). Similar sleep-dependent changes are reported in the hippocampus. Sleep deprivation reduces structural changes in synapses normally induced by learning. Conversely, during sleep these synaptic structures grow and expand (Havekes et al. 2016). However, these latter effects also appear to be highly dependent on the dendritic branches and hippocampal regions under examination [reviewed in Frank (2021)].

4.4 Models of Sleep-Dependent Plasticity

4.4.1 *Replay-Reactivation of Waking Experience During Sleep*

"Replay-reactivation" refers to the reappearance during sleep of neural activity patterns present in prior wakefulness. Replay was initially suggested by findings from Pavlides and Winson (1989) who showed in rats that hippocampal neurons active during exploration showed increased activity in subsequent sleep. Subsequent studies from the McNaughton laboratory demonstrated that correlational patterns in firing, which matched the order in which cells fired during maze running, also replayed during sleep (Wilson and McNaughton 1994; Skaggs and McNaughton 1996). Collectively these findings led to the theory that replay may be a means of transferring information (or memories) from the hippocampus to the neocortex (Buzsaki 1996; Diekelmann and Born 2010). On a synaptic level, this transfer likely involves LTP as it occurs during rapid bursts of hippocampal activity among specific sets of circuits (ripples and sharp waves) (Buzsaki 1996; Schwindel and McNaughton 2011; Pfeiffer 2020).

The phenomenon appears quite robust, as variants have been found in the rodent hippocampus, ventral striatum, and cortex (Yang et al. 2014; Wilson and McNaughton 1994; Skaggs and McNaughton 1996; Lee and Wilson 2002; Louie and Wilson 2001; Kudrimoti et al. 1999; Pennartz et al. 2004; Ji and Wilson 2007). Forms of replay have been found in an impressive number of animal species, ranging from birds (Dave and Margoliash 2000), cats (Dumoulin Bridi et al. 2015) to primates (Hoffman and McNaughton 2002) and based on brain imaging, humans (Maquet et al. 2000; Peigneux et al. 2004; Deuker et al. 2013). The animal studies are also embedded in well-established paradigms of behavior, cellular physiology, and plasticity [reviewed in Schwindel and McNaughton (2011), Pfeiffer (2020), and Girardeau and Zugaro (2011)]. Although there is some evidence that forms of replay occur during REM sleep (Dumoulin Bridi et al. 2015; Louie and Wilson 2001; Poe et al. 2000), communication between the hippocampus and cortex is generally conjectured to occur during NREM sleep. This is because during this state activity in the hippocampus is consistent with outflow, rather than inflow (Buzsaki 1996; Diekelmann and Born 2010; Graves et al. 2001; Hasselmo 1999). There are indeed interesting correlations between ripples and sharp waves (hippocampal events when a replay is reported) and thalamocortical spindles and cortical slow waves consistent with this hypothesis (Siapas and Wilson 1998; Battaglia et al. 2004; Sirota et al. 2003). In addition, though quite rare, there are instances when hippocampal and cortical replay occurs simultaneously (Ji and Wilson 2007; Qin et al. 1997).

4.4.2 A Closer Look at Replay

Although replay provides a very attractive model for sleep-dependent plasticity, there remain a number of unresolved issues. First, replay is not unique to sleep. Replay can be detected during periods of waking immobility and even during active exploration (Kudrimoti et al. 1999; O'Neill et al. 2006; Foster and Wilson 2006). This in turn suggests that replay may have little to do with central functions of sleep and is instead one of many phenomena that are peripherally modulated by sleep. While it remains possible that replay in sleep is qualitatively different than replay in wake, this has yet to be fully determined (Pfeiffer 2020). Therefore, sleep is sufficient, but not necessary for replay.

Second, replay in sleep is commonly not detected during learning but well after the animal learns the task. Most studies require that animals be pre-trained on a maze for several days to weeks before replay can be detected (Peyrache et al. 2009; Frank 2007). The slow appearance of replay might reflect a gradually developing memory trace that appears after initial learning and contributes to the transfer of memories from short-term stores (hippocampus) to long-term stores (neocortex). However, it could also mean that replay is only a decaying reverberation of a very well-ingrained pattern of neural activity present during wakefulness. This may explain the ephemeral nature of replay. It is typically detectable only within the first 20–30 min of sleep and then fades away. In some measures, it also accounts for only a fraction of total variance in neuronal activity [reviewed in Frank (2007)].

The effects of novel experience on replay are less explored. Some studies show that neuronal activity patterns associated with "novel" experience can appear in sleep, but the novel tasks are often very similar to familiar tasks. For example, in one study there was substantial overlap in cells active in the familiar versus novel maze configurations (between 70 and 77%) (Kudrimoti et al. 1999). This issue seemed to be resolved by studies reporting novelty-induced reactivation of waking activity patterns in the sleeping rat forebrain (Ribeiro et al. 2004; Ribeiro 2007), but these findings have been challenged on technical and methodological grounds (Tatsuno et al. 2006). More recent findings, however, indicate that replay can occur following a novel experience. In one study, rats were exposed to novel learning rules, and medial prefrontal cortex ensemble recordings showed that patterns of activity induced by learning "replayed" in subsequent NREM sleep (Peyrache et al. 2009). Similar results were reported in rats trained on a brain–machine interface. In this study, neuronal ensembles recruited in a learning task showed greater "reactivation" during NREM sleep after only a few learning trials (Gulati et al. 2014).

A final consideration is whether replay in sleep actually has any function. Two independent studies in rodents provide evidence that interrupting the hippocampal bursts that convey replay impairs critically important behavior (learning and memory) (Ego-Stengel and Wilson 2010; Girardeau et al. 2009). These studies must be cautiously interpreted because they involved disruption of the hippocampal ripples and sharp waves, and not replay per se. It is also not clear if similar results would be obtained if disruption were restricted to replay in wakefulness vs. sleep. Hippocampal replay during sleep can also be triggered by presentation of auditory tones present during experience—which suggests that replay represents a memory trace (Bendor and Wilson 2012). The imposition of waking patterns of activity (associated with a conditioned stimulus) in the olfactory bulb during sleep led to better performance in an aversive training task (Barnes and Wilson 2014). Interestingly, similar experiments in humans lead to greater performance on memory tasks (Schonauer et al. 2014), and spontaneous replay can predict future performance (Deuker et al. 2013). These results strongly suggest that replay induces adaptive, functional plastic changes in the brain.

4.4.3 The Synaptic Homeostasis Hypothesis

Sleep has been variously hypothesized to stabilize (Kavanau 1996; Krueger and Obal 1993), strengthen (Datta and Patteron 2003), or remove synapses (Crick and Mitchison 1983; Giuditta et al. 1995). The synaptic Homeostasis Hypothesis (SHY) is the most recent version of the latter idea. SHY proposes that sleep promotes "net" synaptic weakening, which offsets synaptic strengthening during wakefulness (Tononi and Cirelli 2003, 2006, 2014). Theoretically, this preserves the relative strength between synapses, allows for further synaptic changes and prevents maladaptive metabolic costs associated with excessive synaptogenesis or synapse maintenance. Therefore, SHY predicts that, overall, synapses should be weaker, not stronger, after sleep.

As reviewed elsewhere (Tononi and Cirelli 2014), a number of findings are consistent with SHY (but see (Frank 2021; Frank 2012; Frank and Cantera 2014; Timofeev and Chauvette 2017). There are several changes in proteins, synaptic efficacy, and dendrite morphology consistent with predictions of SHY (Vyazovskiy et al. 2008; Maret et al. 2011; Liu et al. 2010). Briefly, markers of synaptic potentiation (e.g., changes in AMPAR subunit number or phosphorylation) are elevated in the brains of adult rats sacrificed at the end of the active phase (or after sleep deprivation), relative to animals sacrificed at the end of the rest phase (Vyazovskiy et al. 2008). Similar results are reported for measures of synaptic efficacy (EPSPs and mini EPSPs), which are also elevated at the end of the active phase (or after sleep deprivation) relative to sleep (Vyazovskiy et al. 2008; Liu et al. 2010). Two imaging studies of cortical dendrite spine morphology showed that the ratio of spines eliminated vs. those formed was greater after a period of sleep than a period of wakefulness (Maret et al. 2011; Yang and Gan 2012). Interestingly, these results were restricted to stages of development when there is an overall pruning of synapses, and were entirely absent in adult mice (Maret et al. 2011). It was then shown using electron microscopy in fixed mouse tissue (layer 2–3 of the cortex) that many synapses shrink in size when examined after a long period of sleep, relative to sleep deprivation or the wake phase (de Vivo et al. 2017). In *Drosophila*, pre- and postsynaptic proteins and proteins involved in neurotransmitter release are elevated in the brain after extended waking periods or sleep deprivation (relative to sleep) (Gilestro et al. 2009). Additional studies showed that presynaptic structures, axonal arbors, and postsynaptic spines in *Drosophila* neurons expanded after extended waking periods (or sleep deprivation); a process also reversed by extended periods of sleep (Bushey et al. 2011). Similar results were observed in a separate study by Donlea et al. (2011).

4.4.4 A Closer Look at SHY

As is true for "replay-reactivation," there are several unresolved aspects concerning SHY, although not in the same areas. Relatively little progress has been made in determining the sleep-dependent mechanisms that purportedly weaken synapses in SHY (Frank 2012, 2013). This stems in part from the shifting definitions of what purportedly occurs during sleep that weakens synapses. For example, this mechanism has been variously called "synaptic downscaling," "synaptic renormalization," and most recently "selective down-selection" (Tononi and Cirelli 2003, 2006, 2012, 2014). Nevertheless, there is little doubt that SHY is influenced by earlier studies of non-Hebbian plasticity that preceded by many years the first scientific presentation of SHY (Tononi and Cirelli 2001; Frank 2012, 2013). For example, the weakening mechanism in SHY has been described *using the same language used by* scientists who discovered synaptic scaling: "SWA, in turn, would promote synaptic down-scaling (Turrigiano 1999)" [pg. 4503 (Cirelli et al. 2005)]. The consequences of unchecked synaptic potentiation in SHY are also similar to the network instability described in synaptic downscaling: "Sleep, and the accompanying downscaling of synapses, would then be needed to interrupt the growth of synaptic strength associated with waking and prevent synaptic overload " [pg. 55 (Tononi and Cirelli 2006)]. The renaming of this process to "synaptic renormalization" (Tononi and Cirelli 2012) did not change its basic similarities to synaptic scaling. Like the original descriptions of synaptic downscaling, synaptic renormalization affects all or most synapses and offsets LTP (or LTP-like plasticity) (Tononi and Cirelli 2003, 2006, 2014). Selective down-selection involves a modest variation in this concept by adding the idea that some synapses are protected against this renormalization process. Therefore, despite the changing names, it is reasonable to ask whether sleep primarily promotes synaptic downscaling or other forms of non-Hebbian synaptic weakening.

As reviewed elsewhere (Frank 2012), many molecular and electrophysiological changes reported across the sleep–wake cycle are inconsistent with a primary synaptic downscaling function for sleep. For example, it has been suggested that global decreases in cortical activity (down-states) that occur during NREM sleep might downscale synapses. However, the basic principle of synaptic scaling is that global decreases in neuronal activity *upscale* synapses, while increases in neuronal activity downscale synapses. Consequently, down-states in NREM sleep should upscale, not downscale, synapses. Similarly, the neural expression of scaling factors (Arc, Homer 1a, and tumor necrosis factor [tnfα]) across the sleep–wake cycle is inconsistent with downscaling during sleep [reviewed in Frank (2012)]. While it has been reported that Homer 1a mediates synaptic downscaling during sleep, this study did not examine sleep per se. It instead measured changes in synapses at two vastly different times of day in a circadian species (mice) in the absence of quantitative measures of sleep or wakefulness or controls for circadian influences (Diering et al. 2017). Therefore, the results may be equally due to sleep or circadian rhythms.

Other mechanisms proposed in SHY to explain state-dependent synaptic strengthening and weakening require greater scrutiny. For example, SHY proposes that the neurotrophin BDNF is a key factor in the synaptic strengthening during wake that increases sleep drive (Cirelli et al. 2005). This idea is supported by several lines of evidence. BDNF promotes LTP (Yoshii and Constantine Paton 2010) which according to SHY increases sleep drive (Tononi and Cirelli 2014). BDNF mRNA and protein levels increase with wakefulness (Huber et al. 2007; Hairston et al. 2004; Taishi et al. 2001), Intraventricular/intracortical administration of exogenous BDNF increases sleep time (Kushikata et al. 1999, 2003), and NREM SWA (Faraguna et al. 2008). The latter effect can be prevented pharmacologically with drugs that inhibit protein kinase activity. However, these studies are principally correlative in nature, involve nonphysiological means of altering NtrkB signaling, or rely on agents that have broad effects on many kinases—not just those activated by BDNF.

More selective experiments, using a chemical-genetic approach to reversibly inhibit BDNF-NtrkB signaling in vivo, found no role for this pathway in sleep drive. In this study, Muheim et al. (2021) used a mutant mouse bearing a point mutation in the endogenous NtrkB gene that creates a high-affinity binding site for a small exogenously delivered molecule. In the absence of this molecule, endogenous BDNF binds normally to NtrkB receptor (which is the primary receptor for mature forms of BDNF). However, in the presence of this molecule (which can be delivered systemically), the downstream kinase activation of the receptor and its signaling cascades are transiently inhibited (Chen et al. 2005). Using this approach, Muheim et al. found that inhibition of the NtrkB receptor had no effect on sleep drive, whether measured by changes in REM or NREM sleep architecture or NREM SWA (Muheim et al. 2021).

In SHY an important role was originally given to NREM SWA, which was proposed to directly downscale synapses (Tononi and Cirelli 2003, 2006). This role has been modified over the years, as SWA is sometimes described instead as an "index" (Tononi 2009) or "sensor" of synaptic potentiation (Tononi and Cirelli 2012). It is not clear when, according to SHY, SWA should be considered a "sensor," "index," or active mechanism for synaptic weakening. There is, also no direct evidence that natural NREM SWA in vivo [as opposed to anesthesia—for discussion see Timofeev and Chauvette (2017) and Timofeev and Chauvette (2018)] weakens synapses (Frank 2012; Steriade and Timofeev 2003; Timofeev and Chauvette 2017). For example, Tsanov and Manahan-Vaughan showed that when measured during the rodent light phase (when rodents sleep), EPSPs do not decline across sleep, and peaks in SWA precede increases in EPSPs; an unlikely situation if NREM SWA principally leads to synaptic weakening (Tsanov and Manahan-Vaughan 2007). Two separate rodent studies used direct estimates of synaptic strength in vivo via optogenetic stimulation of thalamocortical circuits combined with monitoring of cortical EPSPs (Matsumoto et al. 2020; Cary and Turrigiano 2021). Remarkably, both studies failed to show significant decrements in synaptic strength in waking periods preceded by NREM sleep (Matsumoto et al. 2020; Cary and Turrigiano 2021), and no relationship between NREM SWA and synaptic strength (Cary and Turrigiano 2021). In a different study performed on cats (conducted with natural NREM states-not anesthesia), it was found that SWA instead promotes synaptic potentiation (Chauvette et al. 2012). Chauvette et al. (2012) showed that cortical postsynaptic potentials in vivo are potentiated after a period of NREM SWA, but not wakefulness. They also showed that periods of wakefulness did not result in synaptic potentiation. Intriguingly, experiments in vitro that simulated SWA specifically led to synaptic potentiation, while simulations of waking activity did not.

Given the above considerations, it is not clear if the synaptic changes reported after sleep in support of SHY reflect an active sleep-dependent mechanism. They may instead result from other physiological processes that coincide with sleep, but are themselves not sleep-dependent (Frank 2012; Frank and Cantera 2014). These include circadian rhythms in hormone release, brain temperature, and possibly changes mediated by peripheral clocks in neurons and glia [for review, see Frank (2021) and Frank and Cantera (2014)].

There is also no convincing direct evidence that downscaling in sleep actually causes adaptive changes in circuits or behavior (Tononi and Cirelli 2014). The evidence that does exist is based almost entirely on computational models (Hill et al. 2008; Olcese et al. 2010; Nere et al. 2013), not real biological findings. Computational models can inform neurobiology but are not substitutes for direct experimental observations. They depend critically on what variables are included in the model and the assumptions one makes about how actual neurons operate in vivo. Not surprisingly, there are other computational models of memory consolidation which also posit a role for sleep that do not employ "selective down selection" or "renormalization" as described in SHY (O'Donnell and Sejnowski 2014; Blanco et al. 2015). Therefore, *direct* tests of how down-scaled synapses lead to adaptive changes (behaviorally or otherwise) are now needed. One promising approach along these lines is recent work in *Drosophila* (Donlea et al. 2011). It has been shown in fruit flies that certain forms of experience can saturate synapse numbers, which prevent certain forms of learning. Learning can be rescued after a period of sleep, which also reduces synapses. It will therefore be important to determine if these findings generalize to other circuits in *Drosophila*, and to other species.

4.5 Discussion

In the last decade, scientists have made important discoveries about how sleep and sleep loss impact brain plasticity. There also remain several important challenges. One important unanswered question is whether sleep-dependent plasticity in the developing and adult brain is different. It has been suggested, for example, that synaptic downscaling as described in SHY is equally important during early life (Tononi and Cirelli 2012). This seems unlikely because the developmental ages when sleep is maximal coincide with an overall gain of synapses (Frank and Heller 1997; Sur and Leamey 2001; Aghajanian and Bloom 1967; Thurber et al. 2008). There is also no relationship between the developmental decline in NREM SWA and a net pruning of cortical synapses, as measured by synaptic markers and spine morphology in developing mice (de Vivo et al. 2014). Claims that sleep renormalizes (downscales) synapses during these developmental periods (Cirelli and Tononi 2020) have been challenged based on confounds in the experimental design used in these experiments (Frank 2020).

One possibility is that sleep in developing brains promotes synaptic weakening and strengthening at different times, and is partially determined by the kinds of waking experience that precedes sleep (Genzel et al. 2014; Ribeiro 2012). In cats, cortical kinase activation and protein synthesis necessary for LTP only occur in the first 2–3 h of post-MD sleep (Aton et al. 2009; Seibt et al. 2012). After 5–6 h most of these changes return to baseline or even drop below baseline values. This suggests that under these conditions sleep first leads to synaptic potentiation, and then a

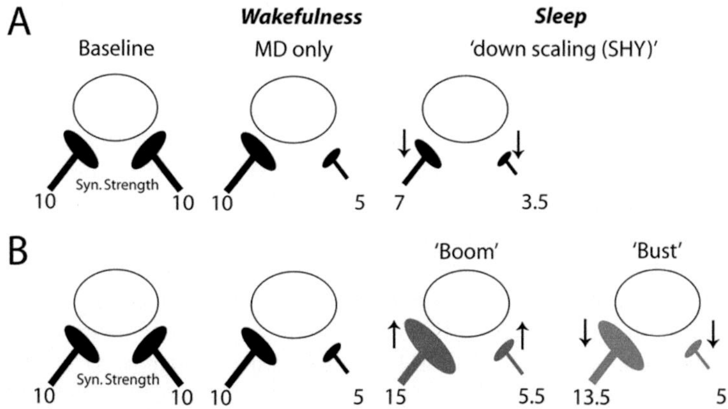

Fig. 4.2 A "*Boom and Bust*" model of sleep-dependent plasticity explains the effects of sleep on ocular dominance plasticity (ODP). The initial effects of monocular deprivation (MD) in the cat are a weakening of responses to the deprived eye during wakefulness. After sleep, there is no further weakening in deprived eye circuits and instead, responses to the non-deprived eye become stronger. (**a**) In the original description of the synaptic homeostasis hypothesis, sleep downscales synaptic strength in a manner proportionate to the strength at each synapse. This produces no net potentiation in the non-deprived circuits and increases depression in the deprived eye pathways. (**b**) According to the Boom and Bust model, sleep immediately after experience leads to synaptic potentiation ("Boom"). This is likely Hebbian, but may involve heterosynaptic changes due to synaptic tagging and capture of plasticity-related proteins in neighboring synapses (Seibt and Frank 2019). As sleep progresses, global downscaling ensues, which reduces synaptic strength proportionately at each synapse ("Bust"). The net result is potentiation in the non-deprived eye pathways, and no further modifications in the deprived eye circuits, which fits empirical data. For illustration purposes, arbitrary units of synaptic strength are shown. Reproduced with permission from Frank (2015)

general synaptic weakening process (Fig. 4.2). This may also explain findings in developing mice, where upscaling and downscaling of synaptic strength are highly dependent on the initial effects of MD (or recovery from MD)—and not necessarily in accordance with predictions of SHY (Cary and Turrigiano 2021; Hengen et al. 2016; Torrado Pacheco et al. 2021).

A second major challenge to the field is reconciling SHY with findings that show that sleep in adult brains also increases synaptic strength or number, without an accompanying "net" downscaling (Frank 2012; Puentes-Mestril and Aton 2017; Havekes and Abel 2017). One possibility is that "replay-reactivation" occurs against a background of global downscaling. For example, sleep during the early part of the rest phase may express high levels of replay (leading to synaptic potentiation) that then declines. Coincident with replay is a slower, non-Hebbian scaling event that progressively asserts greater influence as replay fades. As this downscaling affects all synapses in proportion to their strength, the relative differences in strength are preserved. This is consistent with the time-course of replay during sleep and properties of non-Hebbian synaptic scaling as originally described by Turrigiano (2007). This is also predicted by the "Boom and Bust" model shown in Fig. 4.2 and other theories that posit dual effects of sleep on synaptic strength (Giuditta et al. 1995; Blanco et al. 2015; Genzel et al. 2014; Ribeiro 2012).

A final consideration is that it is critical to conduct direct tests of hypothesized relationships between synaptic plasticity and sleep function. If sleep need arises from synaptic potentiation (or other changes in plasticity), then mutations in fruit flies or mice that reduce synaptic potentiation or plasticity should also reduce sleep need. There are a number of mutant mouse lines with profound reductions in LTP, but these mice have not been examined with respect to sleep (Frank 2012). These mutations can also now be experimentally and reversibly induced, particularly in fruit flies, with increasingly fine temporal and spatial precision. These techniques thus do not suffer from limitations of constitutive mutations (i.e., developmental compensation in embryonic "knock-outs") and can provide potentially powerful and direct tests of current theories.

References

Aghajanian GK, Bloom FE. The formation of synaptic junctions in developing rat brain: a quantitative electron microscopic study. Brain Res. 1967;6(4):716–27.

Arrigoni E, Lu J, Vetrivelan R, Saper CB. Long-term synaptic plasticity is impaired in rats with lesions of the ventrolateral preoptic nucleus. Eur J Neurosci. 2009;30(11):2112–20.

Aton SJ, Seibt J, Dumoulin M, Jha SK, Steinmetz N, Coleman T, et al. Mechanisms of sleep-dependent consolidation of cortical plasticity. Neuron. 2009;61(3):454–66.

Aton SJ, Broussard C, Dumoulin M, Seibt J, Watson A, Coleman T, et al. Visual experience and subsequent sleep induce sequential plastic changes in putative inhibitory and excitatory cortical neurons. Proc Natl Acad Sci U S A. 2013;110(8):3101–6.

Aton SJ, Suresh A, Broussard C, Frank MG. Sleep promotes cortical response potentiation following visual experience. Sleep. 2014;37(7):1163–70.

Barnes DC, Wilson DA. Slow-wave sleep-imposed replay modulates both strength and precision of memory. J Neurosci. 2014;34(15):5134–42.

Battaglia FP, Sutherland GR, McNaughton BL. Hippocampal sharp wave bursts coincide with neocortical "up-state" transitions. Learn Mem. 2004;11(6):697–704.

Bear MF, Malenka RC. Synaptic plasticity: LTP and LTD. Curr Opin Neurobiol. 1994;4(3): 389–99.

Bendor D, Wilson MA. Biasing the content of hippocampal replay during sleep. Nat Neurosci. 2012;15(10):1439–44.

Benington JH, Frank MG. Cellular and molecular connections between sleep and synaptic plasticity. Prog Neurobiol. 2003;69(2):71–101.

Blanco W, Pereira CM, Cota VR, Souza AC, Renno-Costa C, Santos S, et al. Synaptic homeostasis and restructuring across the sleep-wake cycle. PLoS Comput Biol. 2015;11(5):e1004241.

Bushey D, Tononi G, Cirelli C. Sleep and synaptic homeostasis: structural evidence in *Drosophila*. Science. 2011;332(6037):1576–81.

Buzsaki G. The hippocampo-neocortical dialogue. Cereb Cortex. 1996;6(2):81–92.

Campbell IG, Guinan MJ, Horowitz JM. Sleep deprivation impairs long-term potentiation in rat hippocampal slices. J Neurophysiol. 2002;88(2):1073–6.

Cary BA, Turrigiano GG. Stability of neocortical synapses across sleep and wake states during the critical period in rats. elife. 2021;10:e66304.

Chauvette S, Seigneur J, Timofeev I. Sleep oscillations in the thalamocortical system induce long-term neuronal plasticity. Neuron. 2012;75(6):1105–13.

Chen X, Ye H, Kuruvilla R, Ramanan N, Scangos KW, Zhang C, et al. A chemical-genetic approach to studying neurotrophin signaling. Neuron. 2005;46(1):13–21.

Chen C, Hardy M, Zhang J, LaHoste GJ, Bazan NG. Altered NMDA receptor trafficking contributes to sleep deprivation-induced hippocampal synaptic and cognitive impairments. Biochem Biophys Res Commun. 2006;340(2):435–40.

Cirelli C, Tononi G. Sleep and synaptic homeostasis. Sleep. 2015;38(1):161–2.

Cirelli C, Tononi G. Effects of sleep and waking on the synaptic ultrastructure. Philos Trans R Soc Lond Ser B Biol Sci. 2020;375(1799):20190235.

Cirelli C, Huber R, Gopalakrishnan A, Southard TL, Tononi G. Locus ceruleus control of slow-wave homeostasis. J Neurosci. 2005;25(18):4503–11.

Cooke SF, Bear MF. Visual experience induces long-term potentiation in the primary visual cortex. J Neurosci. 2010;30(48):16304–13.

Crick F, Mitchison G. The function of dream sleep. Nature. 1983;304(5922):111–4.

Datta S, Patteron EH. Activation of phasic pontine wave (P-wave): a mechanism of learning and memory processing. In: Maquet P, Smith C, Stickgold R, editors. Sleep and brain plasticity. New York: Oxford University Press; 2003. p. 135–56.

Dave AS, Margoliash D. Song replay during sleep and computational rules for sensorimotor vocal learning. Science. 2000;290(5492):812–6.

Davis CJ, Harding JW, Wright JW. REM sleep deprivation-induced deficits in the latency-to-peak induction and maintenance of long-term potentiation within the CA1 region of the hippocampus. Brain Res. 2003;973(2):293–7.

Davis CJ, Meighan PC, Taishi P, Krueger JM, Harding JW, Wright JW. REM sleep deprivation attenuates actin-binding protein cortactin: a link between sleep and hippocampal plasticity. Neurosci Lett. 2006;400(3):191–6.

de Vivo L, Faraguna U, Nelson AB, Pfister-Genskow M, Klapperich ME, Tononi G, et al. Developmental patterns of sleep slow wave activity and synaptic density in adolescent mice. Sleep. 2014;37(4):689–700. A-B

de Vivo L, Bellesi M, Marshall W, Bushong EA, Ellisman MH, Tononi G, et al. Ultrastructural evidence for synaptic scaling across the wake/sleep cycle. Science. 2017;355(6324):507–10.

Deuker L, Olligs J, Fell J, Kranz TA, Mormann F, Montag C, et al. Memory consolidation by replay of stimulus-specific neural activity. J Neurosci. 2013;33(49):19373–83.

Diekelmann S, Born J. The memory function of sleep. Nat Rev Neurosci. 2010;11(2):114–26.

Diering GH, Nirujogi RS, Roth RH, Worley PF, Pandey A, Huganir RL. Homer1a drives homeostatic scaling-down of excitatory synapses during sleep. Science. 2017;355(6324):511–5.

Donlea JM, Thimgan MS, Suzuki Y, Gottschalk L, Shaw PJ. Inducing sleep by remote control facilitates memory consolidation in *Drosophila*. Science. 2011;332(6037):1571–6.

Dumoulin Bridi MC, Aton SJ, Seibt J, Renouard L, Coleman T, Frank MG. Rapid eye movement sleep promotes cortical plasticity in the developing brain. Sci Adv. 2015;1(6):e1500105.

Dumoulin MC, Aton SJ, Watson AJ, Renouard L, Coleman T, Frank MG. Extracellular signal-regulated kinase (ERK) activity during sleep consolidates cortical plasticity in vivo. Cereb Cortex. 2015;25(2):507–15.

Durkin J, Aton SJ. Sleep-dependent potentiation in the visual system is at odds with the synaptic homeostasis hypothesis. Sleep. 2016;39(1):155–9.

Ego-Stengel V, Wilson MA. Disruption of ripple-associated hippocampal activity during rest impairs spatial learning in the rat. Hippocampus. 2010;20(1):1–10.

Espinosa JS, Stryker MP. Development and plasticity of the primary visual cortex. Neuron. 2012;75 (2):230–49.

Faraguna U, Vyazovskiy VV, Nelson AB, Tononi G, Cirelli C. A causal role for brain-derived neurotrophic factor in the homeostatic regulation of sleep. J Neurosci. 2008;28(15):4088–95.

Florian C, Vecsey CG, Halassa MM, Haydon PG, Abel T. Astrocyte-derived adenosine and A1 receptor activity contribute to sleep loss-induced deficits in hippocampal synaptic plasticity and memory in mice. J Neurosci. 2011;31(19):6956–62.

Foster DJ, Wilson MA. Reverse replay of behavioural sequences in hippocampal place cells during the awake state. Nature. 2006;440(7084):680–3.

Frank MG. Hippocampal dreams, cortical wishes: a closer look at neuronal replay and the hippocampal-neocortical dialogue during sleep. Cell Sci Rev. 2007;3(4):161–71.

Frank MG. Sleep and developmental brain plasticity: not just for kids. Prog Brain Res. 2011;193: 221–32.

Frank MG. Erasing synapses in sleep: is it time to be SHY? Neural Plast. 2012;2012:264378.

Frank MG. Why I'm not SHY: a reply to Tononi and Cirelli. Neural Plast. 2013;2013:394946.

Frank MG. Sleep and synaptic plasticity in the developing and adult brain. Curr Top Behav Neurosci. 2015;25:123–49.

Frank MG. Sleep and plasticity in the visual cortex: more than meets the eye. Curr Opin Neurobiol. 2017;44:8–12.

Frank MG. The ontogenesis of mammalian sleep: form and function. Curr Sleep Med Rep. 2020;6 (4):267–79.

Frank MG. Renormalizing synapses in sleep: the clock is ticking. Biochem Pharmacol. 2021;191: 114533.

Frank MG, Benington JH. The role of sleep in memory consolidation and brain plasticity: dream or reality? Neuroscientist. 2006;12(6):477–88.

Frank MG, Cantera R. Sleep, clocks, and synaptic plasticity. Trends Neurosci. 2014;37(9): 491–501.

Frank MG, Heller HC. Development of REM and slow wave sleep in the rat. Am J Phys. 1997;272 (6 Pt 2):R1792–9.

Frank MG, Issa NP, Stryker MP. Sleep enhances plasticity in the developing visual cortex. Neuron. 2001;30(1):275–87.

Genzel L, Kroes MC, Dresler M, Battaglia FP. Light sleep versus slow wave sleep in memory consolidation: a question of global versus local processes? Trends Neurosci. 2014;37(1):10–9.

Gilestro GF, Tononi G, Cirelli C. Widespread changes in synaptic markers as a function of sleep and wakefulness in *Drosophila*. Science. 2009;324(5923):109–12.

Girardeau G, Zugaro M. Hippocampal ripples and memory consolidation. Curr Opin Neurobiol. 2011;21(3):452–9.

Girardeau G, Benchenane K, Wiener SI, Buzsaki G, Zugaro MB. Selective suppression of hippocampal ripples impairs spatial memory. Nat Neurosci. 2009;12(10):1222–3.

Giuditta A, Ambrosini MV, Montagnese P, Mandile P, Cotugno M, Grassi Zucconi G, et al. The sequential hypothesis of the function of sleep. Behav Brain Res. 1995;69(1–2):157–66.

Graves L, Pack A, Abel T. Sleep and memory: a molecular perspective. Trends Neurosci. 2001;24 (4):237–43.

Gulati T, Ramanathan DS, Wong CC, Ganguly K. Reactivation of emergent task-related ensembles during slow-wave sleep after neuroprosthetic learning. Nat Neurosci. 2014;17(8):1107–13.

Guzman-Marin R, Ying Z, Suntsova N, Methippara M, Bashir T, Szymusiak R, et al. Suppression of hippocampal plasticity-related gene expression by sleep deprivation in rats. J Physiol. 2006;575(Pt 3):807–19.

Hairston IS, Peyron C, Denning DP, Ruby NF, Flores J, Sapolsky RM, et al. Sleep deprivation effects on growth factor expression in neonatal rats: a potential role for BDNF in the mediation of delta power. J Neurophysiol. 2004;91(4):1586–95.

Hasselmo ME. Neuromodulation: acetylcholine and memory consolidation. Trends Cogn Sci. 1999;3(9):351–9.

Havekes R, Abel T. The tired hippocampus: the molecular impact of sleep deprivation on hippocampal function. Curr Opin Neurobiol. 2017;44:13–9.

Havekes R, Park AJ, Tudor JC, Luczak VG, Hansen RT, Ferri SL, et al. Sleep deprivation causes memory deficits by negatively impacting neuronal connectivity in hippocampal area CA1. elife. 2016;5:e13424.

Hengen KB, Torrado Pacheco A, McGregor JN, Van Hooser SD, Turrigiano GG. Neuronal firing rate homeostasis is inhibited by sleep and promoted by wake. Cell. 2016;165(1):180–91.

Hennevin E, Huetz C, Edeline JM. Neural representations during sleep: from sensory processing to memory traces. Neurobiol Learn Mem. 2007;87(3):416–40.
Hill S, Tononi G, Ghilardi MF. Sleep improves the variability of motor performance. Brain Res Bull. 2008;76(6):605–11.
Hoffman KL, McNaughton BL. Coordinated reactivation of distributed memory traces in primate cortex. Science. 2002;297:2070–3.
Hubel DH, Wiesel TN. The period of susceptibility to the physiological effects of unilateral eye closure in kittens. J Physiol. 1970;206(2):419–36.
Huber R, Tononi G, Cirelli C. Exploratory behavior, cortical BDNF expression, and sleep homeostasis. Sleep. 2007;30(2):129–39.
Ishikawa A, Kanayama Y, Matsumura H, Tsuchimochi H, Ishida Y, Nakamura S. Selective rapid eye movement sleep deprivation impairs the maintenance of long-term potentiation in the rat hippocampus. Eur J Neurosci. 2006;24(1):243–8.
Ji D, Wilson MA. Coordinated memory replay in the visual cortex and hippocampus during sleep. Nat Neurosci. 2007;10(1):100–7.
Jouvet-Mounier D, Astic L, Lacote D. Ontogenesis of the states of sleep in rat, cat, and guinea pig during the first postnatal month. Dev Psychobiol. 1970;2(4):216–39.
Kavanau JL. Memory, sleep, and dynamic stabilization of neural circuitry: evolutionary perspectives. Neurosci Biobehav Rev. 1996;20(2):289–311.
Kim EY, Mahmoud GS, Grover LM. REM sleep deprivation inhibits LTP in vivo in area CA1 of rat hippocampus. Neurosci Lett. 2005;388(3):163–7.
Kirkwood A, Lee HK, Bear MF. Co-regulation of long-term potentiation and experience-dependent synaptic plasticity in visual cortex by age and experience. Nature. 1995;375(6529):328–31.
Kopp C, Longordo F, Nicholson JR, Luthi A. Insufficient sleep reversibly alters bidirectional synaptic plasticity and NMDA receptor function. J Neurosci. 2006;26(48):12456–65.
Krueger JM, Obal F. A neuronal group theory of sleep function. J Sleep Res. 1993;2(2):63–9.
Kudrimoti HS, Barnes CA, McNaughton BL. Reactivation of hippocampal cell assemblies: effects of behavioral state, experience, and EEG dynamics. J Neurosci. 1999;19(10):4090–101.
Kushikata T, Fang J, Krueger JM. Brain-derived neurotrophic factor enhances spontaneous sleep in rats and rabbits. AJP. 1999;276(5):R1334–8.
Kushikata T, Kubota T, Fang J, Krueger JM. Neurotrophins 3 and 4 enhance non-rapid eye movement sleep in rabbits. Neurosci Lett. 2003;346(3):161–4.
Lee AK, Wilson MA. Memory of sequential experience in the hippocampus during slow wave sleep. Neuron. 2002;36(6):1183–94.
Liu ZW, Faraguna U, Cirelli C, Tononi G, Gao XB. Direct evidence for wake-related increases and sleep-related decreases in synaptic strength in rodent cortex. J Neurosci. 2010;30(25):8671–5.
Longordo F, Kopp C, Mishina M, Lujan R, Luthi A. NR2A at CA1 synapses is obligatory for the susceptibility of hippocampal plasticity to sleep loss. J Neurosci. 2009;29(28):9026–41.
Louie K, Wilson MA. Temporally structured replay of awake hippocampal ensemble activity during rapid eye movement sleep. Neuron. 2001;29(1):145–56.
Malenka RC, Bear MF. LTP and LTD: an embarrassment of riches. Neuron. 2004;44(1):5–21.
Maquet P, Laureys S, Peigneux P, Fuchs S, Petiau C, Phillips C, et al. Experience-dependent changes in cerebral activation during human REM sleep. Nat Neurosci. 2000;3(8):831–6.
Maret S, Faraguna U, Nelson AB, Cirelli C, Tononi G. Sleep and waking modulate spine turnover in the adolescent mouse cortex. Nat Neurosci. 2011;14(11):1418–20.
Markram H, Gerstner W, Sjostrom PJ. A history of spike-timing-dependent plasticity. Front Synaptic Neurosci. 2011;3:4.
Marks CA, Wayner MJ. Effects of sleep disruption on rat dentate granule cell LTP in vivo. Brain Res Bull. 2005;66(2):114–9.
Matsumoto S, Ohyama K, Diaz J, Yanagisawa M, Greene RW, Vogt KE. Enhanced cortical responsiveness during natural sleep in freely behaving mice. Sci Rep. 2020;10(1):2278.

McDermott CM, LaHoste GJ, Chen C, Musto A, Bazan NG, Magee JC. Sleep deprivation causes behavioral, synaptic, and membrane excitability alterations in hippocampal neurons. J Neurosci. 2003;23(29):9687–95.

McDermott CM, Hardy MN, Bazan NG, Magee JC. Sleep deprivation-induced alterations in excitatory synaptic transmission in the CA1 region of the rat hippocampus. J Physiol. 2006;570(Pt 3):553–65.

Mioche L, Singer W. Chronic recordings from single sites of kitten striate cortex during experience-dependent modifications of receptive-field properties. J Neurophysiol. 1989;62(1):185–97.

Muheim CM, Singletary KG, Frank MG. A chemical-genetic investigation of BDNF-NtrkB signaling in mammalian sleep. Sleep. 2021;45:zsab237.

Nelson SB, Turrigiano GG. Strength through diversity. Neuron. 2008;60(3):477–82.

Nere A, Hashmi A, Cirelli C, Tononi G. Sleep-dependent synaptic down-selection (I): modeling the benefits of sleep on memory consolidation and integration. Front Neurol. 2013;4:143.

O'Donnell C, Sejnowski TJ. Selective memory generalization by spatial patterning of protein synthesis. Neuron. 2014;82(2):398–412.

O'Neill J, Senior T, Csicsvari J. Place-selective firing of CA1 pyramidal cells during sharp wave/ripple network patterns in exploratory behavior. Neuron. 2006;49(1):143–55.

Olcese U, Esser SK, Tononi G. Sleep and synaptic renormalization: a computational study. J Neurophysiol. 2010;104(6):3476–93.

Pavlides C, Winson J. Influences of hippocampal place cell firing in the awake state on the activity of these cells during subsequent sleep. J Neurosci. 1989;9(8):2907–18.

Peigneux P, Laureys S, Fuchs S, Collette F, Perrin F, Reggers J, et al. Are spatial memories strengthened in the human hippocampus during slow wave sleep? Neuron. 2004;44(3):535–45.

Pennartz CM, Lee E, Verheul J, Lipa P, Barnes CA, McNaughton BL. The ventral striatum in off-line processing: ensemble reactivation during sleep and modulation by hippocampal ripples. J Neurosci. 2004;24(29):6446–56.

Peyrache A, Khamassi M, Benchenane K, Wiener SI, Battaglia FP. Replay of rule-learning related neural patterns in the prefrontal cortex during sleep. Nat Neurosci. 2009;12(7):919–26.

Pfeiffer BE. The content of hippocampal "replay". Hippocampus. 2020;30(1):6–18.

Poe GR, Nitz DA, McNaughton BL, Barnes CA. Experience-dependent phase-reversal of hippocampal neuron firing during REM sleep. Brain Res. 2000;855(1):176–80.

Pozo K, Goda Y. Unraveling mechanisms of homeostatic synaptic plasticity. Neuron. 2010;66(3):337–51.

Puentes-Mestril C, Aton SJ. Linking network activity to synaptic plasticity during sleep: hypotheses and recent data. Front Neural Circuits. 2017;11:61.

Qin YL, McNaughton BL, Skaggs WE, Barnes CA. Memory reprocessing in corticocortical and hippocampocortical neuronal ensembles. Philos Trans R Soc Lond Ser B Biol Sci. 1997;352(1360):1525–33.

Ravassard P, Pachoud B, Comte J, Gay N, Touret M, Luppi P, et al. Paradoxical sleep amount modulates neuronal plasticity in adult rat hippocampus. J Sleep Res. 2006;15:191.

Ravassard P, Pachoud B, Comte JC, Mejia-Perez C, Scote-Blachon C, Gay N, et al. Paradoxical (REM) sleep deprivation causes a large and rapidly reversible decrease in long-term potentiation, synaptic transmission, glutamate receptor protein levels, and ERK/MAPK activation in the dorsal hippocampus. Sleep. 2009;32(2):227–40.

Ravassard P, Hamieh AM, Joseph MA, Fraize N, Libourel PA, Lebarillier L, et al. REM sleep-dependent bidirectional regulation of hippocampal-based emotional memory and LTP. Cereb Cortex. 2016;26(4):1488–500.

Renouard L, Bridi MCD, Coleman T, Arckens L, Frank MG. Anatomical correlates of rapid eye movement sleep-dependent plasticity in the developing cortex. Sleep. 2018;41(10):zsy124.

Ribeiro S. Novel experience induces persistent sleep-dependent plasticity in the cortex but not in the hippocampus. Front Neurosci. 2007;1(1):43–55.

Ribeiro S. Sleep and plasticity. Pflugers Arch. 2012;463(1):111–20.

Ribeiro S, Gervasoni D, Soares ES, Zhou Y, Lin SC, Pantoja J, et al. Long-Lasting novelty-induced neuronal reverberation during slow-Wave sleep in multiple forebrain areas. PLoS Biol. 2004;2 (1):E24.

Roffwarg HP, Muzio JN, Dement WC. Ontogenetic development of the human sleep-dream cycle. Science. 1966;152(3722):604–19.

Romcy-Pereira R, Pavlides C. Distinct modulatory effects of sleep on the maintenance of hippocampal and medial prefrontal cortex LTP. Eur J Neurosci. 2004;20(12):3453–62.

Schonauer M, Geisler T, Gais S. Strengthening procedural memories by reactivation in sleep. J Cogn Neurosci. 2014;26(1):143–53.

Schwindel CD, McNaughton BL. Hippocampal-cortical interactions and the dynamics of memory trace reactivation. Prog Brain Res. 2011;193:163–77.

Seibt J, Frank MG. Primed to sleep: the dynamics of synaptic plasticity across brain states. Front Syst Neurosci. 2019;13:2.

Seibt J, Dumoulin MC, Aton SJ, Coleman T, Watson A, Naidoo N, et al. Protein synthesis during sleep consolidates cortical plasticity in vivo. Curr Biol. 2012;22(8):676–82.

Sengpiel F. Cortical plasticity: learning while you sleep? Curr Biol. 2001;11(16):R647–R50.

Shaffery JP, Roffwarg HP. Rapid eye-movement sleep deprivation does not 'rescue' developmentally regulated long-term potentiation in visual cortex of mature rats. Neurosci Lett. 2003;342 (3):196–200.

Shaffery JP, Sinton CM, Bissette G, Roffwarg HP, Marks GA. Rapid eye movement sleep deprivation modifies expression of long-term potentiation in visual cortex of immature rats. Neuroscience. 2002;110(3):431–43.

Shaffery JP, Lopez J, Bissette G, Roffwarg HP. Rapid eye movement sleep deprivation revives a form of developmentally regulated synaptic plasticity in the visual cortex of post-critical period rats. Neurosci Lett. 2006;391(3):96–101.

Shaffery JP, Lopez J, Roffwarg HP. Brain-derived neurotrophic factor (BDNF) reverses the effects of rapid eye movement sleep deprivation (REMSD) on developmentally regulated, long-term potentiation (LTP) in visual cortex slices. Neurosci Lett. 2012;513(1):84–8.

Siapas AG, Wilson MA. Coordinated interactions between hippocampal ripples and cortical spindles during slow-wave sleep. Neuron. 1998;21(5):1123–8.

Sirota A, Csicsvari J, Buhl D, Buzsaki G. Communication between neocortex and hippocampus during sleep in rodents. Proc Natl Acad Sci U S A. 2003;100(4):2065–9.

Skaggs WE, McNaughton BL. Replay of neuronal firing sequences in rat hippocampus during sleep following spatial experience. Science. 1996;271(5257):1870–3.

Smith GB, Heynen AJ, Bear MF. Bidirectional synaptic mechanisms of ocular dominance plasticity in visual cortex. Philos Trans R Soc Lond Ser B Biol Sci. 2009;364(1515):357–67.

Spolidoro M, Sale A, Berardi N, Maffei L. Plasticity in the adult brain: lessons from the visual system. Exp Brain Res. 2009;192(3):335–41.

Steriade M, Timofeev I. Neuronal plasticity in thalamocortical networks during sleep and waking oscillations. Neuron. 2003;37(4):563–76.

Sur M, Leamey CA. Development and plasticity of cortical areas and networks. Nat Rev Neurosci. 2001;2(4):251–62.

Taishi P, Sanchez C, Wang Y, Fang J, Harding JW, Krueger JM. Conditions that affect sleep alter the expression of molecules associated with synaptic plasticity. Am J Phys. 2001;281:R839–R45.

Tartar JL, Ward CP, McKenna JT, Thakkar M, Arrigoni E, McCarley RW, et al. Hippocampal synaptic plasticity and spatial learning are impaired in a rat model of sleep fragmentation. Eur J Neurosci. 2006;23(10):2739–48.

Tatsuno M, Lipa P, McNaughton BL. Methodological considerations on the use of template matching to study long-lasting memory trace replay. J Neurosci. 2006;26(42):10727–42.

Thurber A, Jha SK, Coleman T, Frank MG. A preliminary study of sleep ontogenesis in the ferret (Mustela putorius furo). Behav Brain Res. 2008;189(1):41–51.

Timofeev I, Chauvette S. Sleep slow oscillation and plasticity. Curr Opin Neurobiol. 2017;44:116–26.

Timofeev I, Chauvette S. Sleep, anesthesia, and plasticity. Neuron. 2018;97(6):1200–2.

Tononi G. Slow wave homeostasis and synaptic plasticity. J Clin Sleep Med. 2009;5(2 Suppl): S16–9.

Tononi G, Cirelli C. Some considerations on sleep and neural plasticity. Arch Ital Biol. 2001;139 (3):122–41.

Tononi G, Cirelli C. Sleep and synaptic homeostasis: a hypothesis. Brain Res Bull. 2003;62(2): 143–50.

Tononi G, Cirelli C. Sleep function and synaptic homeostasis. Sleep Med Rev. 2006;10(1):49–62.

Tononi G, Cirelli C. Time to be SHY? Some comments on sleep and synaptic homeostasis. Neural Plast. 2012;2012:415250.

Tononi G, Cirelli C. Sleep and the price of plasticity: from synaptic and cellular homeostasis to memory consolidation and integration. Neuron. 2014;81(1):12–34.

Torrado Pacheco A, Bottorff J, Gao Y, Turrigiano GG. Sleep promotes downward riring rate homeostasis. Neuron. 2021;109(3):530–44.e6.

Tropea D, Van Wart A, Sur M. Molecular mechanisms of experience-dependent plasticity in visual cortex. Philos Trans R Soc Lond Ser B Biol Sci. 2009;364(1515):341–55.

Tsanov M, Manahan-Vaughan D. The adult visual cortex expresses dynamic synaptic plasticity that is driven by the light/dark cycle. J Neurosci. 2007;27(31):8414–21.

Turrigiano GG. Homeostatic plasticity in neuronal networks: the more things change, the more they stay the same. Trends Neurosci. 1999;22(5):221–7.

Turrigiano G. Homeostatic signaling: the positive side of negative feedback. Curr Opin Neurobiol. 2007;17(3):318–24.

Turrigiano GG. The self-tuning neuron: synaptic scaling of excitatory synapses. Cell. 2008;135(3): 422–35.

Vecsey CG, Baillie GS, Jaganath D, Havekes R, Daniels A, Wimmer M, et al. Sleep deprivation impairs cAMP signalling in the hippocampus. Nature. 2009;461(7267):1122–5.

Vyazovskiy VV, Cirelli C, Pfister-Genskow M, Faraguna U, Tononi G. Molecular and electrophysiological evidence for net synaptic potentiation in wake and depression in sleep. Nat Neurosci. 2008;11(2):200–8.

Wiesel TN, Hubel DH. Single cell responses in striate cortex of kittens deprived of vision in one eye. J Neurophysiol. 1963;28:1029–40.

Wilson MA, McNaughton BL. Reactivation of hippocampal ensemble memories during sleep. Science. 1994;265(5172):676–9.

Yang G, Gan WB. Sleep contributes to dendritic spine formation and elimination in the developing mouse somatosensory cortex. Dev Neurobiol. 2012;72(11):1391–8.

Yang G, Lai CS, Cichon J, Ma L, Li W, Gan WB. Sleep promotes branch-specific formation of dendritic spines after learning. Science. 2014;344(6188):1173–8.

Yoshii A, Constantine-Paton M. Postsynaptic BDNF-TrkB signaling in synapse maturation, plasticity, and disease. Dev Neurobiol. 2010;70(5):304–22.

Zhou Y, Lai CSW, Bai Y, Li W, Zhao R, Yang G, et al. REM sleep promotes experience-dependent dendritic spine elimination in the mouse cortex. Nat Commun. 2020;11(1):4819.

Part II
Insufficient Sleep and Its Consequences

Chapter 5
Epidemiology of Insufficient Sleep

Michael A. Grandner

Abstract Insufficient sleep duration has emerged as a key behavioral risk factor for cardiometabolic disease risk, daytime functioning deficits, and other adverse outcomes, including mortality. Epidemiologic estimates of insufficient sleep vary, likely due to variability in how sleep is assessed. Most population-based estimates are based on single item retrospective reports of habitual sleep duration. Based on these reports, approximately 30–35% of the adult population reports 6 h of sleep or less and approximately 8–12% report 9 h or more, with the plurality (approximately 50–60%) reporting the normative 7–8 h. No nationally representative data exist using objective measures, nor do they exist using prospective self-report (diary), nor do they exist using validated questionnaires. These estimates, since they rely on retrospective self-report are likely subject to validity issues, recall biases, and other methodologic problems. They may better reflect time in bed than physiologic sleep. Still, these reports have demonstrated utility. Self-reported habitual sleep duration has been reliably associated in epidemiologic studies with incident mortality, as well as obesity, heart disease, diabetes, and daytime dysfunction across a range of domains. Habitual sleep duration also distinguishes sociodemographic groups, with patterns associated with age (increased sleep duration in younger and older adults), education level (insufficient sleep associated with less education), income (insufficient sleep associated with poverty), and race/ethnicity (insufficient sleep more likely among minority groups).

Keywords Sleep · Insomnia · Insufficient Sleep · Short Sleep · Epidemiology

---

M. A. Grandner (✉)
Sleep and Health Research Program, Department of Psychiatry, University of Arizona College of Medicine, Tucson, AZ, USA
e-mail: grandner@email.arizona.edu

A. I. Pack, Q. Y. Li (eds.), *Sleep and its Disorders*, Translational Medicine Research,
https://doi.org/10.1007/978-94-024-2168-2_5

5.1 Defining Insufficient Sleep

Since as early as 1964 (Hammond 1964), there has been disagreement regarding the definition of "insufficient sleep" as it applies to the general population. Part of the reason for this confusion is due to the various sources of scientific information on "insufficient sleep (Grandner et al. 2010)." In general, two main types of studies have explored this question, including those performed under the controlled conditions of the laboratory (where sleep is systematically manipulated) and those performed in the field, often using survey-based methods.

The laboratory studies that have explored the physiological impacts of alterations in sleep opportunity have explored "total sleep deprivation" (complete loss of sleep for at least 24 h), as well as "partial sleep deprivation" (systematic reduction in sleep opportunity over days or weeks. These studies sometimes characterize this approach as "sleep restriction." Although total sleep deprivation studies are frequently useful for probing sleep loss in extreme scenarios, it is less useful as a model for real-world insufficient sleep. Partial sleep deprivation, or sleep restriction, serves as a better model, because it consists of sleep durations that are frequently seen in real-world settings (e.g., 4–6 h). Although these experimental protocols can be useful approaches to revealing the physiologic effects of acute changes in sleep duration, they often lack external validity. As such, these approaches have improved precision for observing subtle effects but lack generalizability as a consequence (Grandner et al. 2010; Grandner 2016; Consensus Conference Panel et al. 2015a). Therefore, suppositions regarding what is "insufficient" based on laboratory studies may not generalize to real-world settings where issues such as compensation/countermeasures, self-selection, and the presence of confounding variables may cloud predictive accuracy.

In addition to controlled studies in the laboratory, the other primary source of research on sleep duration and its impacts comes from population-based methods. In contrast to the laboratory studies that characterize acute sleep loss relative to a baseline, these studies are better suited for characterizing habitual sleep behaviors in context. Regarding sleep duration, this is often classified as "short sleep duration" or "long sleep duration," as compared to "normal sleep duration." The criteria for classification may vary by the study and population examined. These studies, when longitudinal, can model chronic sleep loss or changes in sleep duration, as well as other aspects of sleep health. These may include sleep quality, sleep continuity, and sleep timing. Sleep duration might be obtained by self-report of a number of hours, or it might be calculated, based on time in bed, subtracting sleep latency and wake time after sleep onset. Although most of these studies are survey-based, these dimensions of sleep may be assessed retrospectively (e.g., through surveys and questionnaires) or prospectively. Prospective assessment strategies can include subjective (e.g., sleep diary) or objective (e.g., wearables) methods. These studies often sacrifice precision for generalizability (Grandner et al. 2010; Grandner 2016; Consensus Conference Panel et al. 2015a), in contrast to the laboratory studies.

Thus, there are many terms that could refer to "insufficient sleep" from laboratory protocols of experimental sleep deprivation to population studies of habitual sleep duration. In addition, research studies variously employ terms interchangeably that nonetheless refer to slightly different measurement strategies and definitions, such as "sleep deprivation," "sleep loss," and "short sleep". In addition, "insufficient sleep" is sometimes used in situations that do not clearly apply to questions about sleep duration, including "sleep deficiency," poor sleep quality," and "insomnia." Even though these concepts do not apply to insufficient sleep (Grandner et al. 2010; Grandner 2016; Consensus Conference Panel et al. 2015a), they are often used in the literature. For these reasons, readers should be aware that these terms are not standardized and specific definitions should be examined prior to any interpretation of results.

Since the label of "insufficient sleep" has been used (and abused) across many or all of these related and unrelated concepts, a consistent definition is lacking in the literature. For the purposes of this chapter, "insufficient sleep" will refer to habitual sleep duration that is likely of duration too brief to meet physiologic needs, as implied by either laboratory or population-level research. Also, it should be noted that the focus of this chapter is on habitual sleep duration in the general population (so terms more commonly used to describe experimental protocols, including "sleep deprivation" are not applied). Still, there is disagreement regarding how much sleep is "insufficient." Various studies use cutoffs of 4, 5, 6, or 7 h as representing insufficient sleep.

In an effort to standardize definitions for insufficient sleep, two parallel, simultaneous efforts were undertaken. Both the National Sleep Foundation and the Healthy Sleep Awareness Project (a collaborative effort between the Sleep Research Society and the American Academy of Sleep Medicine, supported by the Centers for Disease Control and Prevention) engaged in consensus efforts to define healthy (and unhealthy) sleep duration. The results of the effort by the Sleep Research Society and the American Academy of Sleep Medicine indicated a consensus that 7 h of habitual sleep was necessary for optimal health for most adults. No consensus for an upper limit was reached, with the caveat that the recommendation is not that more sleep is necessarily better and that there is likely an upper limit (Watson et al. 2015; Consensus Conference Panel et al. 2015b). A follow-up manuscript points out that 6 h or less was likely insufficient, but it was less clear that sleep durations between 6 and 7 h are associated with suboptimal health (Watson et al. 2015; Consensus Conference Panel et al. 2015b). The effort by the National Sleep Foundation also recommended at least 7 h for adults, but did reach consensus of an upper limit of 9 h (Hirshkowitz et al. 2015a, b). Subsequent documents from the American Thoracic Society (Mukherjee et al. 2015) and the American Heart Association (St-Onge et al. 2016) echoed these consensus guidelines. Therefore, for the purposes of this chapter, "insufficient sleep" will generally refer to a habitual sleep duration of 6 h or fewer.

5.2 Prevalence of Insufficient Sleep[1]

To develop prevalence estimates, sleep duration needs to be sampled in large, representative populations. As there is still limited characterization of sleep in large populations using well-validated measures, it is important to note that most of these prevalence estimates rely on subjective, retrospective self-report, which presents biases in assessing sleep (Kurina et al. 2013; Lauderdale et al. 2008). These estimates may better reflect time in bed than actual physiologic sleep and should be interpreted with this in mind.

5.2.1 Insufficient Sleep in the Population

Perhaps the most current estimates of insufficient sleep come from the Behavioral Risk Factor Surveillance System (BRFSS). The BRFSS is an annual survey conducted by the Centers for Disease Control and Prevention (CDC) (http://www.cdc.gov/brfss). It is state-based, with population-weighted samples representing each strata of age, sex, race/ethnicity, and geographic region. Sleep duration in the BRFSS is assessed with the item, "On average, how many hours of sleep do you get in a 24-hour period?" Responses are coded in whole numbers. Liu and colleagues reported population-weighted prevalence estimates for sleep duration around a cutoff of 7 h (based on the consensus statement (Centers for Disease Control and Prevention 2015) from the 2014 BRFSS ($N = 444{,}306$). Overall, the age-adjusted estimated prevalence of insufficient sleep ($\leq$6 h) was reported to be 35.1% of the US population. Grandner and colleagues (2016a) reported prevalence estimates also using the 2014 BRFSS. Estimated prevalence by hour was calculated, such that the estimated prevalence by hour of sleep duration was 1.12% for $\leq$3 h, 3.19% for 4 h, 7.75% for 5 h, 23.55% for 6 h, 28.72% for 7 h, 27.64% for 8 h, 4.42% for 9 h, 2.35% for 10 h, and 1.27% for $\geq$11 h.

Other prevalence estimates have also been calculated using the National Health and Nutrition Examination Survey (NHANES). The NHANES is a survey that is also conducted by the CDC that includes a nationally representative sample (http://www.cdc.gov/nchs/nhanes). The sample size is much smaller than BRFSS, though the reliability of data may be better since surveys were administered in person rather than over the phone. Similar to the BRFSS, NHANES assesses sleep duration by a whole number (no partial hours). Unlike the BRFSS, though, NHANES assesses sleep duration with the item, "How much sleep do you usually get at night on weekdays or workdays?" Thus, this item may capture modal nighttime sleep, rather than 24-h sleep (which may include naps). Using the 2007–2008 wave of NHANES, Grandner and colleagues calculated prevalence estimates for sleep duration by

[1] This section is adapted from Grandner, M. A. (2019). Epidemiology of insufficient sleep and poor sleep quality. In: M. A. Grandner (Ed.) Sleep and Health. Oxford: Academic Press.

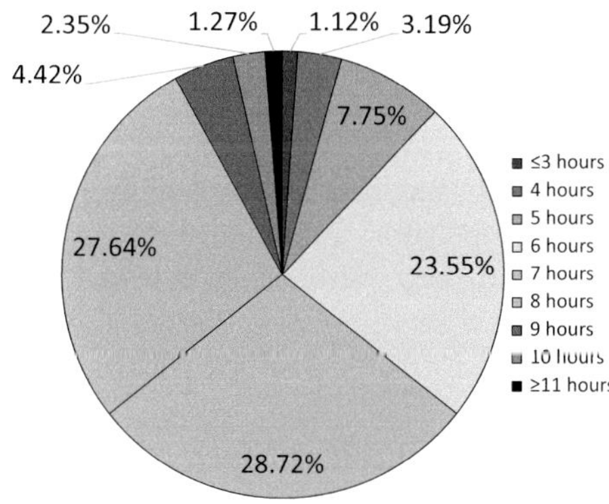

Fig. 5.1 Distribution of sleep duration in the US population using 2014 BRFSS [Data from Grandner et al. (2016a)]

category, with 4.96% reporting ≤4 h, 32.16% reporting 5–6 h, 55.68% reporting 7–8 h, and 7.20% reporting ≥9 h (Grandner et al. 2015a). Thus, insufficient sleep (≤6 h) was reported by 37.12% of the US population. The higher estimate relative to BRFSS may be explained by the wording of the item, which does not include naps or weekends. See Fig. 5.1 for an illustration of these values.

Krueger and Friedman (2009) reported lower estimates of insufficient sleep. This group used data from 2004 to 2007 waves of the National Health Interview Survey (NHIS). The NHIS, like NHANES, is a nationally-representative survey conducted by the CDC that includes in-person interviews (https://www.cdc.gov/nchs/nhis). The sleep duration item included in NHIS is the same as the BRFSS. Based on these NHIS estimates, the prevalence of sleep duration of ≤5 h was 7.8%, and estimates were 20.5% for 6 h, 30.8% for 7 h, 32.5% for 8 h, and 8.5% for ≥9 h (Krueger and Friedman 2009). Thus, based on NHIS data, the population prevalence of insufficient sleep is 28.3%. Even lower estimates of short sleep duration are reported by Basner and colleagues using data from the American Time Use Survey (ATUS) (Basner et al. 2014). The ATUS is a survey conducted annually by the Bureau of Labor Statistics and assigns activity codes to each 15-min increment of the 24-h data in a representative sample of US adults (http://www.bls.gov/tus). Because ATUS does not well distinguish time in bed versus time asleep, values will generally overestimate sleep and understate insufficient sleep (Basner et al. 2014). Using ATUS from 2003 to 2011 ($N = 124{,}517$), the estimated prevalence of insufficient sleep (≤6 h) was 10.6%, compared to 78.4% for 6–11 h and 11.0% for ≥11 h.

Thus, estimates for insufficient sleep (≤6 h) from relatively recent, nationally-representative surveys, are 10.6% from ATUS, 20.5% from NHIS, 35.1% from BRFSS, and 37.12% from NHANES. These may vary as a result of the survey item asked, as well as other factors including the years included and sampling methodologies. Although other studies have examined large samples using more well-validated measures, none of these studies are nationally-representative and thus cannot be used to develop population prevalence estimates.

An alternate way to assess insufficient sleep is, rather than determining insufficiency post hoc, asking individuals how often they experience self-identified insufficient sleep. The 2008 BRFSS asked, "During the past 30 days, for about how many days have you felt that you did not get enough rest or sleep?" Based on this variable, Mcknight-Eily and colleagues (2009) reported prevalence estimates based on responses to this variable. They estimate that 30.7% of the population reports 0/30 days of insufficient sleep, with 1–13 days reported by 41.3% of the population, 14–29 days reported by 16.8% of the population, and 30/30 days reported by 11.1% of the population. Based on these estimates, 27.9% of the US population reports perceived sleep insufficiency at least 2 weeks out of the month.

5.2.2 *Insufficient Sleep by Age*

Table 5.1 reports sleep duration prevalence by age, using population-weighted data from the 2013 BRFSS. Chi-square analysis indicated that sleep duration differed by age group ($p < 0.0001$). Several studies have examined age-related differences. Based on BRFSS data, Liu and colleagues (2016) provided age-based prevalence estimates for insufficient sleep (≤6 h). They reported estimated of 32.2% for those age 18–24, 37.9% for 25–34, 38.3% for 35–44, 37.3% for 45–64, and 26.3% for those 65 years or above. Of note, the lowest rate of insufficient sleep was seen among the oldest adults. This is consistent with other studies that showed that perceived insufficient sleep declines with age (Grandner et al. 2015b), as does self-reported sleep disturbance (Grandner et al. 2012a; Soldatos et al. 2005; Zilli et al. 2009). This is in contrast to more objective sleep disturbances, which are well-characterized to increase in older adults (Ohayon et al. 2004; Lindstrom et al. 2012; Cooke and Ancoli-Israel 2011). There are a number of potential reasons for this, including retirement offering greater sleep opportunities and differing expectations regarding sleep (Grandner et al. 2012b).

Prevalence estimates of sleep duration by age in NHANES were reported by Grandner and colleagues (2015a). Among teenagers aged 16–17 years, prevalence of sleep duration was 0.63% for ≤4 h, 19.38% for 5–6 h, 62.47% for 7–8 h, and 17.52% for ≥9 h. For younger adults aged 18–30 years, prevalence was 4.83% for ≤4 h, 31.02% for 5–6 h, 54.44% for 7–8 h, and 9.81% for ≥9 h. For adults aged 30–50 years, prevalence was 5.86% for ≤4 h, 33.61% for 5–6 h, 55.49% for 7–8 h, and 5.03% for ≥9 h. For adults aged 50–65 years, prevalence was 4.95% for ≤4 h, 35.41% for 5–6 h, 56.04% for 7–8 h, and 3.61% for ≥9 h. For older adults 65 and older, prevalence was 4.17% for ≤4 h, 28.31% for 5–6 h, 55.58% for 7–8 h, and 11.94% for ≥9 h. Thus, prevalence of insufficient sleep (≤6 h) was reported to be 20.01% for those aged 16–17 years, 35.85% for those aged 18–30 years, 39.47% for adults 30–50, 40.36% for adults aged 50–65 years, and 32.48% for older adults over 65 years. Again, the prevalence of insufficient sleep is highest in working age adults.

Using the ATUS data, Basner and colleagues (2014) found that, compared to 15–24 year olds, increased likelihood of insufficient sleep (≤6 h) was seen in those aged 25–34 (OR = 1.38; 95% CI = 1.18;1.61), 35–44 (OR = 1.40; 95% CI = 1.22;1.62), 45–54 (OR = 1.68; 95% CI = 1.44;1.94), and 55–64

Table 5.1 Distribution of sleep duration by age and sex, using the 2013 BRFSS

	Complete Sample	Stratified by age												
		18–24	25–29	30–34	35–39	40–44	45–49	50–54	55–59	60–64	65–69	70–74	75–79	≥80
All														
Very Short (≤4 h) (%)	4.31	3.88	4.73	4.62	4.50	5.04	4.92	5.18	4.93	4.17	3.46	2.76	2.64	2.67
Short (5–6 h) (%)	31.30	29.20	33.76	33.79	34.27	34.35	35.41	34.71	32.72	29.59	26.41	23.65	23.35	22.37
Normal (7–8 h) (%)	56.36	55.42	54.36	54.72	55.28	55.38	54.40	54.31	56.29	58.60	60.33	61.90	61.08	59.10
Long (≥9 h) (%)	8.03	11.49	7.15	6.87	5.96	5.23	5.28	5.80	6.06	7.64	9.79	11.69	12.93	15.85
Men														
Very Short (≤4 h) (%)	4.46	4.60	5.21	4.88	4.77	4.95	4.77	5.22	4.52	4.24	3.56	2.56	2.31	2.48
Short (5–6 h) (%)	31.68	28.86	34.89	34.61	36.57	34.99	37.26	35.04	32.78	29.51	25.54	21.30	21.16	19.87
Normal (7–8 h) (%)	56.34	55.33	53.84	54.76	53.93	55.14	53.48	54.46	57.16	58.82	60.92	64.05	62.41	60.25
Long (≥9 h) (%)	7.52	11.22	6.06	5.76	4.72	4.92	4.50	5.28	5.54	7.43	9.98	12.08	14.12	17.39
Women														
Very Short (≤4 h) (%)	4.17	3.12	4.19	4.37	4.23	5.14	5.06	5.14	5.33	4.10	3.37	2.93	2.87	2.80
Short (5–6 h) (%)	30.93	29.57	32.52	33.01	32.04	33.70	33.57	34.39	32.67	29.67	27.20	25.65	24.86	24.01
Normal (7–8 h) (%)	56.38	55.53	54.94	54.69	56.57	55.63	55.32	54.17	55.45	58.38	59.80	60.07	60.17	58.34
Long (≥9 h) (%)	8.52	11.79	8.35	7.94	7.16	5.53	6.05	6.30	6.55	7.85	9.63	11.36	12.10	14.84

(OR = 1.41; 95% CI = 1.18;1.68), but not those 65 years or older. Similarly, shortest sleep durations were seen in working age adults.

Using self-reported insufficiency from the BRFSS, Mcknight-Eily and colleagues (2009) report that the prevalence of self-reported insufficient sleep at least 14 of the past 30 days was reported by 31.3% of 18–24 year olds. The estimated prevalence was 34.2% for 35–34 year olds, 32.1% for 35–44 year olds, 27.2% for 45–64 year olds, and 15.0% for those 65 years or older.

5.2.3 *Insufficient Sleep by Sex*

Several studies have examined sex relative to insufficient sleep. Liu and colleagues report that based on the 2014 BRFSS data, insufficient sleep ($\leq$6 h) is reported by 35.4% of men and 34.8% of women (Liu et al. 2016). Using data from 2007 to 2008 NHANES, Whinnery and colleagues report no sex differences in the likelihood of insufficient sleep (though they report that women are 35% less likely to report long sleep duration after adjusting for covariates) (Whinnery et al. 2014). Using NHIS data, Kruger and Friedman report that men are 7% less likely to report $\leq$5 vs. 7 h of sleep (Krueger and Friedman 2009). Basner and colleagues report that men are more likely to report insufficient sleep (OR = 1.27; 95% CI = 1.20;1.35) (Basner et al. 2014). McKnight-Eily reports that self-reported insufficient sleep at least 14 out of the past 30 days was reported by 25.5% of men and 30.4% of women (McKnight-Eily et al. 2009). Taken together, sex differences in insufficient sleep are likely small and difficult to observe. This is in contrast to self-reported sleep disturbances, which are much more prevalent in women (Schredl and Reinhard 2011; Subramanian et al. 2011; Zhang and Wing 2006).

See Table 5.1 for population-weighted estimates of habitual sleep duration, broken down by age and sex, derived from the 2013 BRFSS. A chi-square test found that the distribution of sleep duration categories differed between men and women ($p < 0.0001$), with slightly more short sleep in men and slightly more long sleep in women.

5.2.4 *Insufficient Sleep by Race/Ethnicity*

Many studies have documented differences in sleep duration by race/ethnicity. In general, racial/ethnic minorities are more likely to experience insufficient sleep duration. Actigraphic studies have shown that racial/ethnic minorities demonstrate a sleep duration between 40 and 60 min less than non-Hispanic White counterparts (Jean-Louis et al. 2000; Lauderdale et al. 2006; Ertel et al. 2011).

More data are available from survey studies that included larger numbers of people but lack the precision of objective measurements. For example, data from the NHIS has shown that sleep duration of 6 h or less was more prevalent among

Blacks/African-Americans, non-Mexican Hispanics/Latinos, and Asians/Others, compared to non-Hispanic Whites (Hale and Do 2007; Nunes et al. 2008). Longitudinal analysis of NHIS data suggests that Black-White differences in insufficient sleep have persisted, relatively unchanged since 1977 (Jean-Louis et al. 2015a, b).

Other population-level studies have found similar patterns. For example, Stamatakis et al showed in the Alameda County study that African-Americans were about twice as likely to report short sleep duration (Stamatakis et al. 2007). Using NHANES data, Whinnery and colleagues showed that Blacks/African-Americans are about 2.5 times as likely to sleep <5 h and about twice as likely to sleep 5–6 h, compared to non-Hispanic Whites. Non-Mexican Hispanics/Latinos were about 2.7 times as likely to sleep <5 h and Asians/Others were about 4 times as likely to sleep <5 h and about twice as likely to sleep 5–6 h. Mexican-Americans were the only minority group not more likely to report insufficient sleep (Whinnery et al. 2014).

5.2.5 *Insufficient Sleep by Socioeconomic Status*

Perhaps due to environmental stressors, those of lower socioeconomic status are more likely to experience insufficient sleep. Kruger and Friedman used NHIS data to compute mean family income according to sleep duration (Krueger and Friedman 2009). They found that the highest mean income was reported among 7-h sleepers ($48,065), with the lowest income levels in those sleeping 5 h or less ($36,819) or 9 h or more ($34,883). Stamatakis et al. evaluated the likelihood of insufficient sleep relative to income quintiles (Stamatakis et al. 2007). This study reported that compared to the highest income quintile, short sleep duration (6 h or less) was increasingly reported in the 4th (3% more likely), 3rd (11% more likely), 2nd (29% more likely), and 1st quintile (54% more likely). Using BRFSS data, days of perceived insufficient sleep decreased at higher levels of household income (Grandner et al. 2015b).

Using NHANES data, Whinnery and colleagues examined several socioeconomic indices relative to sleep duration (Whinnery et al. 2014). Compared to those with family income over $75,000, increased likelihood of <5 h of sleep ($p < 0.05$) was observed for all categories, including <$20,000 (OR = 5.5), $20,000–25,000 (OR = 2.9), $25,000–35,000 (OR = 4.1), $35,000–45,000 (OR = 2.4), $45,000–55,000 (OR = 2.8), $55,000–65,000 (OR = 2.4), and even $65,000–75,000 (OR = 3.8). Increased likelihood of 5–6 h sleep relative to those earning over $75,000 was only seen in the lowest income group earning <$20,000 (OR = 1.3). Education level was another socioeconomic indicator that was associated with sleep duration in this sample. Those with less than a high school education were approximately 4 times as likely to report <5 h of sleep, compared to college graduates. Similarly, those who completed some high school were more likely than college graduates to report <5 (OR = 5.3) and 5–6 (OR = 1.7) hours of sleep; those who completed high school were more likely than college graduates to report <5

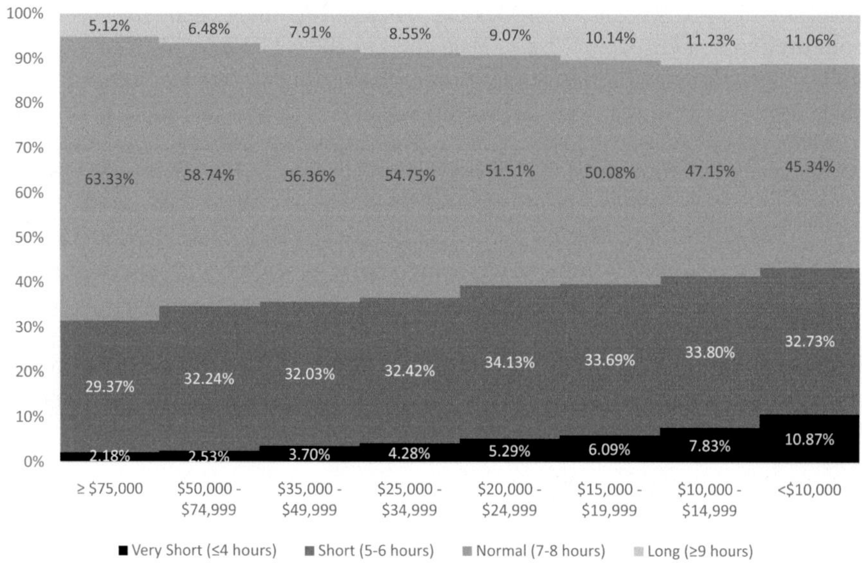

Fig. 5.2 Distribution of sleep duration by income, from BRFSS 2013

(OR = 4.3) or 5–6 (OR = 1.6) hours, and those with some college education were also more likely than college graduates to report <5 (OR = 3.6) or 5–6 (OR = 1.6) hours of sleep (Whinnery et al. 2014). Another socioeconomic indicator evaluated in this study was lack of access to healthcare, which was more common among those reporting <5 h of sleep. Food insecurity—a measure of inability to financially provide healthy access to enough food—was also more common among those reporting <5 and 5–6 h of sleep (Whinnery et al. 2014).

Figure 5.2 depicts the distribution of income categories across sleep duration categories, using BRFSS 2013 data. These values are population weighted. A chi-square test showed that the distribution of sleep duration categories differed across income groups ($p < 0.0001$).

5.2.6 Insufficient Sleep by Geography

Insufficient sleep in the USA is differentially experienced across varying regions of the country. An analysis of self-reported perceived insufficient sleep using BRFSS data was reported (Grandner et al. 2015c). See Fig. 5.3 for a map of the prevalence of insufficient sleep by county, based on the data reported. Using a geospatial hotspot analysis, several key "hotspots" of insufficient sleep were identified in the USA, including parts of the southeast, parts of the Texas/Louisiana border, areas in the Midwest, and the largest hotspot in central Appalachia. "Coldspots" with

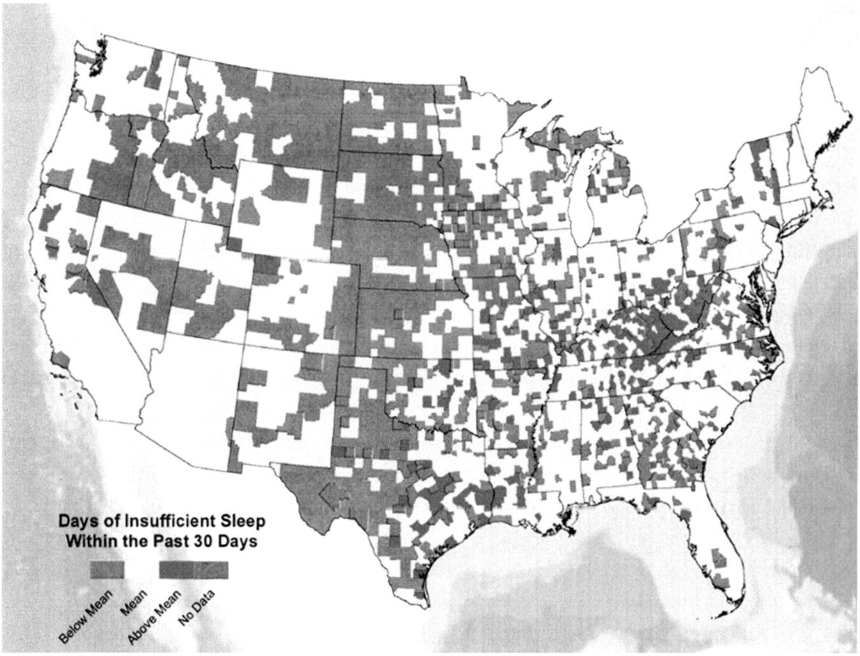

Fig. 5.3 Geographic distribution of insufficient sleep [based on data reported in Grandner et al. (2015c)]

abnormally low levels of insufficient sleep were seen in the northern Midwest (Wisconsin/Minnesota/Iowa), central Texas, central Virginia, and areas along the West Coast.

Rather than examine statistical hotspots of perceived insufficient sleep, researchers at the CDC used BRFSS data to map prevalence of ≤6 h of sleep across the USA (Liu et al. 2016). The US states with the highest prevalence were (in order) Hawaii (43.9%), Kentucky (39.7%), Maryland (38.9%), Alabama (38.8%), Georgia (38.7%), and Michigan (38.7%). The US states with the lowest prevalence were (in order) South Dakota (28.4%), Colorado (28.5%), Minnesota (29.2%), Nebraska (30.4%), and Idaho (30.6%).

5.3 Insufficient Sleep and Epidemiology of Other Domains of Health

Many epidemiologic studies have examined the overlapping incidence and prevalence of insufficient sleep with a number of other health outcomes.

5.3.1 Insufficient Sleep and Mortality

Since 1964 (Hammond 1964), over 50 studies have examined relationships between insufficient sleep and mortality. These have been summarized in narrative reviews (Bixler 2009; Bliwise and Young 2007; Grandner and Patel 2009; Youngstedt and Kripke 2004) and meta-analyses (Gallicchio and Kalesan 2009; Cappuccio et al. 2010). Although the meta-analyses used slightly different methodologies, they generally come to similar conclusions. Gallicchio and Kalesan (2009) found an increased risk for mortality associated with short sleep duration (RR = 1.10; 95% CI [1.06,1.15], $p < 0.05$), as well as longer sleep duration (RR = 1.23; 95%CI [1.17,1.30], $p < 0.05$). Similarly, Cappuccio and colleagues (2010) found significant increased risk associated with both short (RR = 1.12; 95%CI [1.06,1.18]; $p < 0.01$) and long sleep (RR = 1.30; 95%CI [1.22,1.38]; $p < 0.0001$). The analysis by Cappuccio conducted post-tests and found that relationships between mortality and short sleep did not differ by age, sex, socioeconomic status, the definition of sleep duration category, duration of follow-up, or geographic location.

5.3.2 Insufficient Sleep and Epidemiology of Obesity

Many studies have documented associations between insufficient sleep duration and obesity. These have been summarized in both narrative reviews (St-Onge et al. 2016; Grandner et al. 2016a, b; St-Onge 2013; Morselli et al. 2012; Akinnusi et al. 2012; Zimberg et al. 2012; Nielsen et al. 2011; Horne 2011; Chaput 2011; Beccuti and Pannain 2011) and meta-analyses (Cappuccio et al. 2008; Chen et al. 2008). Overall, habitual short sleep duration is associated with obesity prevalence, which persists whether obesity is subjectively or objectively measured. Further, habitual short sleep is associated with increased weight gain and other measures of adiposity over time in epidemiologic studies (Nagai et al. 2013; Watanabe et al. 2010; Chaput et al. 2008; Patel et al. 2006; Ayas et al. 2003). These findings have led to increased epidemiologic study of other cardiometabolic disease outcomes associated with habitual short sleep (see below), as well as laboratory and other studies of mechanisms potentially linking sleep duration and obesity (Grandner et al. 2016a, b; Yi et al. 2013; Bornhorst et al. 2012). Although these are outside the scope of an epidemiology review, this line of research is an example of how research across the translational spectrum can influence work at all other levels. In some cases, more basic science is influencing epidemiologic study and in others, epidemiologic trends are inspiring hypotheses at the basic science level.

5.3.3 Insufficient Sleep and Cardiovascular Epidemiology

Epidemiologic studies of cardiovascular disease have identified insufficient sleep as an important risk factor. Habitual short sleep duration (6 h or less) has been associated cross-sectionally with hypertension (Altman et al. 2012; Buxton and Marcelli 2010; Grandner et al. 2014; Meng et al. 2013), dyslipidemia (Altman et al. 2012; Grandner et al. 2014; Adedayo et al. 2014; Sabanayagam and Shankar 2012), inflammation (Grandner et al. 2013), and history of cardiovascular events (Altman et al. 2012; Grandner et al. 2014; Hoevenaar-Blom et al. 2014). Although fewer studies have examined increased incidence of these conditions, habitual short sleep duration is associated with increased incidence of hypertension (Meng et al. 2013) and cardiovascular events (von Ruesten et al. 2012; Cappuccio et al. 2011; Eguchi et al. 2010). Regarding inflammation, the literature is more inconclusive. A recent review (Grandner et al. 2013) and meta-analysis (Irwin et al. 2016) document that at the population level, detecting an association between habitual sleep duration and inflammation may depend on the sample selected, the marker of inflammation evaluated, and the variability in sleep duration observed. Still, the epidemiologic literature supports experimental studies that suggest that insufficient sleep may result in a pro-inflammatory state.

5.3.4 Insufficient Sleep and Diabetes Epidemiology

Laboratory studies have shown that otherwise healthy adults, when sleep deprived in the laboratory, would demonstrate metabolic dysregulation suggestive of diabetes risk (Van Cauter et al. 2008; Spiegel et al. 2004). Since then, several studies have demonstrated that habitual short sleep duration in the population is associated with diabetes (Grandner et al. 2014, 2016a; Buxton and Marcelli 2010; Perelis et al. 2016). In addition to cross-sectional analyses, meta-analyses suggest that individuals who habitually get 6 h or less of sleep are approximately 30% more likely to develop diabetes over time (Anothaisintawee et al. 2016; Shan et al. 2015). Several reviews have discussed these patterns of findings relative to proposed mechanisms (Grandner et al. 2016a; Perelis et al. 2016; Anothaisintawee et al. 2016; Lee et al. 2017; Rangaraj and Knutson 2016; Upala et al. 2015).

5.3.5 Insufficient Sleep and Epidemiology of Daytime Dysfunction

In addition to cardiometabolic disease risk factors such as obesity, cardiovascular disease, and diabetes, several epidemiologic studies have examined daytime function deficits relative to insufficient sleep. These studies are informed by a large body of laboratory literature that documents with great precision the effects of acute sleep loss on neurocognition. Taken together, sleep deprivation is associated with immediate and cumulative deficits in sustained attention (Banks and Dinges 2007; Dinges 2006; Dinges and Banks 2009; Durmer and Dinges 2005; Lim and Dinges 2008; Rogers et al. 2003; Van Dongen et al. 2005), which can have profound impacts in the domains of vigilance and safety-sensitive activities such as driving. Other studies have shown that acute sleep loss impairs decision-making (Jackson et al. 2013; Killgore et al. 2012; Pace-Schott et al. 2012), planning (Killgore 2010), working memory (Verweij et al. 2014; Drummond et al. 2012; Joo et al. 2012; Lo et al. 2012; Jiang et al. 2011), and other cognitive domains. Although these are difficult to study at a population level, several studies have examined these relationships. For example, Maia and colleagues (2013) found that habitual short sleep duration was associated with drowsy driving, even if those individuals felt fully rested. These findings are supported by work by Abe and colleagues (2012) who found that short sleep duration was associated with increased drowsy driving in a large sample of Japanese adults.

5.4 Methodological Issues for Estimates of Insufficient Sleep in the Population

Several issues continue to limit the robustness and reliability of population estimates of insufficient sleep. First, there are no direct measures of sleep, so all assessment strategies contain some elements of measurement error. Even polysomnography is an indirect measure of sleep, so there is no way to measure sleep duration in a definitive way. For example, sleep diaries are the gold standard for insomnia, which reflects the individual's experience. Yet, it suffers from recall and other biases. Objective methods (e.g., wearables) do not have the same recall biases but may fail to capture important elements of sleep that correlate with outcomes and also have their own inherent limitations. Questionnaires may be easy to administer and efficient for capturing a wide range of outcomes, but their retrospective nature and imprecision limit interpretability. Retrospective assessments of sleep duration may better approximate time in bed than physiologic sleep. There still exists no nationally-representative sample with sampling via prospective, validated measurements. Therefore, all presumptions about population-level estimates should be made with caution.

Second, the definition of insufficient sleep still varies greatly among different studies. Some studies examine sleep by clock hour, but most use categorical groupings. Given the recent consensus statements, some uniformity may be emerging, but all studies should report how cutoffs were determined and interpretations should be cautious when comparing results based on different definitions of insufficient sleep. It is still not clear, for example, whether sleep insufficiency is more reliably determined based on subjective or objective sleep assessment methods.

Third, even if definitions become more standardized, they are still based on population-level recommendations which fail to take into account individual differences in sleep need, sleep ability, and resilience to sleep loss. All of these factors may contribute to individual differences in what is "insufficient." Also, general cutoffs typically fail to resolve insufficiency relative to any specific outcome. For example, the amount of sleep that is sufficient for an individual to experience optimal cardiovascular health may be different than for mental health, cognitive function, immunity, or other outcomes. More information is needed to personalize recommendations of sleep duration, matched with relevant outcomes. It is possible that the amount of sleep needed may differ depending on the outcome assessed.

References

Abe T, Komada Y, Inoue Y. Short sleep duration, snoring and subjective sleep insufficiency are independent factors associated with both falling asleep and feeling sleepiness while driving. Intern Med. 2012;51(23):3253–60.

Adedayo AM, Olafiranye O, Smith D, Hill A, Zizi F, Brown C, et al. Obstructive sleep apnea and dyslipidemia: evidence and underlying mechanism. Sleep Breath = Schlaf Atmung. 2014;18(1): 13–8.

Akinnusi ME, Saliba R, Porhomayon J, El-Solh AA. Sleep disorders in morbid obesity. Eur J Int Med. 2012;23(3):219–26.

Altman NG, Izci-Balserak B, Schopfer E, Jackson N, Rattanaumpawan P, Gehrman PR, et al. Sleep duration versus sleep insufficiency as predictors of cardiometabolic health outcomes. Sleep Med. 2012;13(10):1261–70.

Anothaisintawee T, Reutrakul S, Van Cauter E, Thakkinstian A. Sleep disturbances compared to traditional risk factors for diabetes development: systematic review and meta-analysis. Sleep Med Rev. 2016;30:11–24.

Ayas NT, White DP, Al-Delaimy WK, Manson JE, Stampfer MJ, Speizer FE, et al. A prospective study of self-reported sleep duration and incident diabetes in women. Diabetes Care. 2003;26 (2):380–4.

Banks S, Dinges DF. Behavioral and physiological consequences of sleep restriction. J Clin Sleep Med. 2007;3(5):519–28.

Basner M, Spaeth AM, Dinges DF. Sociodemographic characteristics and waking activities and their role in the timing and duration of sleep. Sleep. 2014;37(12):1889–906.

Beccuti G, Pannain S. Sleep and obesity. Curr Opin Clin Nutr Metab Care. 2011;14(4):402–12.

Bixler E. Sleep and society: an epidemiological perspective. Sleep Med. 2009;10(Suppl 1):S3–6.

Bliwise DL, Young TB. The parable of parabola: what the U-shaped curve can and cannot tell us about sleep. Sleep. 2007;30(12):1614–5.

Bornhorst C, Hense S, Ahrens W, Hebestreit A, Reisch L, Barba G, et al. From sleep duration to childhood obesit—what are the pathways? Eur J Pediatr. 2012;171(7):1029–38.

Buxton OM, Marcelli E. Short and long sleep are positively associated with obesity, diabetes, hypertension, and cardiovascular disease among adults in the United States. Soc Sci Med. 2010;71(5):1027–36.

Cappuccio FP, Taggart FM, Kandala NB, Currie A, Peile E, Stranges S, et al. Meta-analysis of short sleep duration and obesity in children and adults. Sleep. 2008;31(5):619–26.

Cappuccio FP, D'Elia L, Strazzullo P, Miller MA. Sleep duration and all-cause mortality: a systematic review and meta-analysis of prospective studies. Sleep. 2010;33(5):585–92.

Cappuccio FP, Cooper D, D'Elia L, Strazzullo P, Miller MA. Sleep duration predicts cardiovascular outcomes: a systematic review and meta-analysis of prospective studies. Eur Heart J. 2011;32 (12):1484–92.

Centers for Disease Control and Prevention. Behavioral risk factor surveillance system 2014 codebook report. Atlanta, GA: CDC; 2015.

Chaput JP. Short sleep duration as a cause of obesity: myth or reality? Obesity Rev. 2011;12(5): e2–3.

Chaput JP, Despres JP, Bouchard C, Tremblay A. The association between sleep duration and weight gain in adults: a 6-year prospective study from the Quebec Family Study. Sleep. 2008;31 (4):517–23.

Chen X, Beydoun MA, Wang Y. Is sleep duration associated with childhood obesity? A systematic review and meta-analysis. Obesity. 2008;16(2):265–74.

Consensus Conference Panel, Watson NF, Badr MS, Belenky G, Bliwise DL, Buxton OM, et al. Joint consensus statement of the American Academy of Sleep Medicine and Sleep Research Society on the recommended amount of sleep for a healthy adult: methodology and discussion. J Clin Sleep Med. 2015a;11(8):931–52.

Consensus Conference Panel, Watson NF, Badr MS, Belenky G, Bliwise DL, Buxton OM, et al. Recommended amount of sleep for a healthy adult: a joint consensus statement of the American Academy of Sleep Medicine and Sleep Research Society. J Clin Sleep Med. 2015b;11(6):591–2.

Cooke JR, Ancoli-Israel S. Normal and abnormal sleep in the elderly. In: Montagna P, Chokroverty S, editors. Sleep disorders. Handbook of clinical neurology. Edinburgh: Elsevier; 2011. p. 653–65.

Dinges DF. The state of sleep deprivation: From functional biology to functional consequences. Sleep Med Rev. 2006;10(5):303–5.

Dinges DF, Banks S. Sleep deprivation: cognitive performance. In: Amlaner CJ, Fuller PM, editors. Basics of sleep guide. 2nd ed. Westchester, IL: Sleep Research Society; 2009. p. 257–64.

Drummond SP, Anderson DE, Straus LD, Vogel EK, Perez VB. The effects of two types of sleep deprivation on visual working memory capacity and filtering efficiency. PLoS One. 2012;7(4): e35653.

Durmer JS, Dinges DF. Neurocognitive consequences of sleep deprivation. Semin Neurol. 2005;25 (1):117–29.

Eguchi K, Hoshide S, Ishikawa S, Shimada K, Kario K. Short sleep duration is an independent predictor of stroke events in elderly hypertensive patients. J Am Soc Hypertens. 2010;4(5): 255–62.

Ertel KA, Berkman LF, Buxton OM. Socioeconomic status, occupational characteristics, and sleep duration in African/Caribbean immigrants and US White health care workers. Sleep. 2011;34 (4):509–18.

Gallicchio L, Kalesan B. Sleep duration and mortality: a systematic review and meta-analysis. J Sleep Res. 2009;18(2):148–58.

Grandner MA. Sleep deprivation: societal impact and long-term consequences. In: Chokroverty S, Billiard M, editors. Sleep medicine: a comprehensive guide to its development, clinical milestones, and advances in treatment. New York: Springer; 2016. p. 495–509.

Grandner MA, Patel NP. From sleep duration to mortality: implications of meta-analysis and future directions. J Sleep Res. 2009;18(2):145–7.

Grandner MA, Patel NP, Gehrman PR, Perlis ML, Pack AI. Problems associated with short sleep: bridging the gap between laboratory and epidemiological studies. Sleep Med Rev. 2010;14(4): 239–47.

Grandner MA, Martin JL, Patel NP, Jackson NJ, Gehrman PR, Pien G, et al. Age and sleep disturbances among American men and women: data from the U.S. Behavioral Risk Factor Surveillance System. Sleep. 2012a;35(3):395–406.

Grandner MA, Patel NP, Gooneratne NS. Difficulties sleeping: a natural part of growing older? Aging Health. 2012b;8(3):219–21.

Grandner MA, Sands-Lincoln MR, Pak VM, Garland SN. Sleep duration, cardiovascular disease, and proinflammatory biomarkers. Nat Sci sleep. 2013;5:93–107.

Grandner MA, Chakravorty S, Perlis ML, Oliver L, Gurubhagavatula I. Habitual sleep duration associated with self-reported and objectively determined cardiometabolic risk factors. Sleep Med. 2014;15(1):42–50.

Grandner MA, Schopfer EA, Sands-Lincoln M, Jackson N, Malhotra A. Relationship between sleep duration and body mass index depends on age. Obesity. 2015a;23(12):2491–8.

Grandner MA, Jackson NJ, Izci-Balserak B, Gallagher RA, Murray-Bachmann R, Williams NJ, et al. Social and behavioral determinants of perceived insufficient sleep. Front Neurol. 2015b;6: 112.

Grandner MA, Smith TE, Jackson N, Jackson T, Burgard S, Branas C. Geographic distribution of insufficient sleep across the United States: a county-level hotspot analysis. Sleep Health. 2015c;1(3):158–65.

Grandner MA, Seixas A, Shetty S, Shenoy S. Sleep duration and diabetes risk: population trends and potential mechanisms. Curr Diab Rep. 2016a;16(11):106.

Grandner MA, Alfonso-Miller P, Fernandez-Mendoza J, Shetty S, Shenoy S, Combs D. Sleep: important considerations for the prevention of cardiovascular disease. Curr Opin Cardiol. 2016b;31(5):551–65.

Hale L, Do DP. Racial differences in self-reports of sleep duration in a population-based study. Sleep. 2007;30(9):1096–103.

Hammond EC. Some preliminary findings on physical complaints from a prospective study of 1,064,004 men and women. Am J Public Health Nations Health. 1964;54:11–23.

Hirshkowitz M, Whiton K, Albert SM, Alessi C, Bruni O, DonCarlos L, et al. National Sleep Foundation's updated sleep duration recommendations: final report. Sleep Health. 2015a;1(4): 233–43.

Hirshkowitz M, Whiton K, Albert SM, Alessi C, Bruni O, DonCarlos L, et al. National Sleep Foundation's sleep time duration recommendations: methodology and results summary. Sleep Health. 2015b;1(1):40–3.

Hoevenaar-Blom MP, Spijkerman AM, Kromhout D, Verschuren WM. Sufficient sleep duration contributes to lower cardiovascular disease risk in addition to four traditional lifestyle factors: the MORGEN study. Eur J Prev Cardiol. 2014;21(11):1367–75.

Horne J. Obesity and short sleep: unlikely bedfellows? Obes Rev. 2011;12(5):e84–94.

Irwin MR, Olmstead R, Carroll JE. Sleep disturbance, sleep duration, and inflammation: a systematic review and meta-analysis of cohort studies and experimental sleep deprivation. Biol Psychiatry. 2016;80(1):40–52.

Jackson ML, Gunzelmann G, Whitney P, Hinson JM, Belenky G, Rabat A, et al. Deconstructing and reconstructing cognitive performance in sleep deprivation. Sleep Med Rev. 2013;17(3): 215–25.

Jean-Louis G, Kripke DF, Ancoli-Israel S, Klauber MR, Sepulveda RS. Sleep duration, illumination, and activity patterns in a population sample: effects of gender and ethnicity. Biol Psychiatry. 2000;47(10):921–7.

Jean-Louis G, Grandner MA, Youngstedt SD, Williams NJ, Zizi F, Sarpong DF, et al. Differential increase in prevalence estimates of inadequate sleep among black and white Americans. BMC Public Health. 2015a;15:1185.

Jean-Louis G, Youngstedt S, Grandner M, Williams NJ, Sarpong D, Zizi F, et al. Unequal burden of sleep-related obesity among black and white Americans. Sleep Health. 2015b;1(3):169–76.

Jiang F, VanDyke RD, Zhang J, Li F, Gozal D, Shen X. Effect of chronic sleep restriction on sleepiness and working memory in adolescents and young adults. J Clin Exp Neuropsychol. 2011;33(8):892–900.

Joo EY, Yoon CW, Koo DL, Kim D, Hong SB. Adverse effects of 24 hours of sleep deprivation on cognition and stress hormones. J Clin Neurol. 2012;8(2):146–50.

Killgore WDS. Effects of sleep deprivation on cognition. In: Kerkhof GA, Van Dongen HPA, editors. Human sleep and cognition, part I: basic research. Amsterdam: Elsevier; 2010. p. 105–29.

Killgore WD, Grugle NL, Balkin TJ. Gambling when sleep deprived: don't bet on stimulants. Chronobiol Int. 2012;29(1):43–54.

Krueger PM, Friedman EM. Sleep duration in the United States: a cross-sectional population-based study. Am J Epidemiol. 2009;169(9):1052–63.

Kurina LM, McClintock MK, Chen JH, Waite LJ, Thisted RA, Lauderdale DS. Sleep duration and all-cause mortality: a critical review of measurement and associations. Ann Epidemiol. 2013;23 (6):361–70.

Lauderdale DS, Knutson KL, Yan LL, Rathouz PJ, Hulley SB, Sidney S, et al. Objectively measured sleep characteristics among early-middle-aged adults: the CARDIA study. Am J Epidemiol. 2006;164(1):5–16.

Lauderdale DS, Knutson KL, Yan LL, Liu K, Rathouz PJ. Self-reported and measured sleep duration: how similar are they? Epidemiology. 2008;19(6):838–45.

Lee SWH, Ng KY, Chin WK. The impact of sleep amount and sleep quality on glycemic control in type 2 diabetes: a systematic review and meta-analysis. Sleep Med Rev. 2017;31:91–101.

Lim J, Dinges DF. Sleep deprivation and vigilant attention. Ann N Y Acad Sci. 2008;1129:305–22.

Lindstrom V, Andersson K, Lintrup M, Holst G, Berglund J. Prevalence of sleep problems and pain among the elderly in Sweden. J Nutr Health Aging. 2012;16(2):180–3.

Liu Y, Wheaton AG, Chapman DP, Cunningham TJ, Lu H, Croft JB. Prevalence of Healthy Sleep Duration among Adults—United States, 2014. MMWR Morb Mortal Wkly Rep. 2016;65(6): 137–41.

Lo JC, Groeger JA, Santhi N, Arbon EL, Lazar AS, Hasan S, et al. Effects of partial and acute total sleep deprivation on performance across cognitive domains, individuals and circadian phase. PLoS One. 2012;7(9):e45987.

Maia Q, Grandner MA, Findley J, Gurubhagavatula I. Short and long sleep duration and risk of drowsy driving and the role of subjective sleep insufficiency. Accid Anal Prev. 2013;59:618–22.

McKnight-Eily LR, Liu Y, Perry GS, Presley-Cantrell LR, Strine TW, Lu H, et al. Perceived insufficient rest or sleep among adults—United States, 2008. MMWR Morb Mortal Wkly Rep. 2009;58(42):1175–9.

Meng L, Zheng Y, Hui R. The relationship of sleep duration and insomnia to risk of hypertension incidence: a meta-analysis of prospective cohort studies. Hypertens Res. 2013;36(11):985–95.

Morselli LL, Guyon A, Spiegel K. Sleep and metabolic function. Pflugers Arch. 2012;463(1): 139–60.

Mukherjee S, Patel SR, Kales SN, Ayas NT, Strohl KP, Gozal D, et al. An official American Thoracic Society statement: the importance of healthy sleep. Recommendations and future priorities. Am J Respir Crit Care Med. 2015;191(12):1450–8.

Nagai M, Tomata Y, Watanabe T, Kakizaki M, Tsuji I. Association between sleep duration, weight gain, and obesity for long period. Sleep Med. 2013;14(2):206–10.

Nielsen LS, Danielsen KV, Sorensen TI. Short sleep duration as a possible cause of obesity: critical analysis of the epidemiological evidence. Obes Rev. 2011;12(2):78–92.

Nunes J, Jean-Louis G, Zizi F, Casimir GJ, von Gizycki H, Brown CD, et al. Sleep duration among black and white Americans: results of the National Health Interview Survey. J Natl Med Assoc. 2008;100(3):317–22.

Ohayon MM, Carskadon MA, Guilleminault C, Vitiello MV. Meta-analysis of quantitative sleep parameters from childhood to old age in healthy individuals: developing normative sleep values across the human lifespan. Sleep. 2004;27(7):1255–73.

Pace-Schott EF, Nave G, Morgan A, Spencer RM. Sleep-dependent modulation of affectively guided decision-making. J Sleep Res. 2012;21(1):30–9.

Patel SR, Malhotra A, White DP, Gottlieb DJ, Hu FB. Association between reduced sleep and weight gain in women. Am J Epidemiol. 2006;164(10):947–54.

Perelis M, Ramsey KM, Marcheva B, Bass J. Circadian transcription from beta Cell function to diabetes pathophysiology. J Biol Rhythm. 2016;31(4):323–36.

Rangaraj VR, Knutson KL. Association between sleep deficiency and cardiometabolic disease: implications for health disparities. Sleep Med. 2016;18:19–35.

Rogers NL, Dorrian J, Dinges DF. Sleep, waking and neurobehavioural performance. Front Biosci. 2003;8:s1056–67.

Sabanayagam C, Shankar A. Sleep duration and hypercholesterolaemia: results from the National Health Interview Survey 2008. Sleep Med. 2012;13(2):145–50.

Schredl M, Reinhard I. Gender differences in nightmare frequency: a meta-analysis. Sleep Med Rev. 2011;15(2):115–21.

Shan Z, Ma H, Xie M, Yan P, Guo Y, Bao W, et al. Sleep duration and risk of type 2 diabetes: a meta-analysis of prospective studies. Diabetes Care. 2015;38(3):529–37.

Soldatos CR, Allaert FA, Ohta T, Dikeos DG. How do individuals sleep around the world? Results from a single-day survey in ten countries. Sleep Med. 2005;6(1):5–13.

Spiegel K, Tasali E, Penev P, Van Cauter E. Brief communication: sleep curtailment in healthy young men is associated with decreased leptin levels, elevated ghrelin levels, and increased hunger and appetite. Ann Intern Med. 2004;141(11):846–50.

Stamatakis KA, Kaplan GA, Roberts RE. Short sleep duration across income, education, and race/ethnic groups: population prevalence and growing disparities during 34 years of follow-up. Ann Epidemiol. 2007;17(12):948–55.

St-Onge MP. The role of sleep duration in the regulation of energy balance: effects on energy intakes and expenditure. J Clin Sleep Med. 2013;9(1):73–80.

St-Onge MP, Grandner MA, Brown D, Conroy MB, Jean-Louis G, Coons M, et al. Sleep duration and quality: impact on lifestyle behaviors and cardiometabolic health: a scientific statement from the American Heart Association. Circulation. 2016;134(18):e367–e86.

Subramanian S, Guntupalli B, Murugan T, Bopparaju S, Chanamolu S, Casturi L, et al. Gender and ethnic differences in prevalence of self-reported insomnia among patients with obstructive sleep apnea. Sleep Breath = Schlaf Atmung. 2011;15(4):711–5.

Upala S, Sanguankeo A, Congrete S, Romphothong K. Sleep duration and insulin resistance in individuals without diabetes mellitus: a systematic review and meta-analysis. Diabetes Res Clin Pract. 2015;109(3):e11–2.

Van Cauter E, Spiegel K, Tasali E, Leproult R. Metabolic consequences of sleep and sleep loss. Sleep Med. 2008;9(Suppl 1):S23–8.

Van Dongen HP, Vitellaro KM, Dinges DF. Individual differences in adult human sleep and wakefulness: leitmotif for a research agenda. Sleep. 2005;28(4):479–96.

Verweij IM, Romeijn N, Smit DJ, Piantoni G, Van Someren EJ, van der Werf YD. Sleep deprivation leads to a loss of functional connectivity in frontal brain regions. BMC Neurosci. 2014;15:88.

von Ruesten A, Weikert C, Fietze I, Boeing H. Association of sleep duration with chronic diseases in the European Prospective Investigation into Cancer and Nutrition (EPIC)-Potsdam study. PLoS One. 2012;7(1):e30972.

Watanabe M, Kikuchi H, Tanaka K, Takahashi M. Association of short sleep duration with weight gain and obesity at 1-year follow-up: a large-scale prospective study. Sleep. 2010;33(2):161–7.

Watson NF, Badr MS, Belenky G, Bliwise DL, Buxton OM, Buysse D, et al. Recommended amount of sleep for a healthy adult: a joint consensus statement of the American Academy of Sleep Medicine and Sleep Research Society. Sleep. 2015;38(6):843–4.

Whinnery J, Jackson N, Rattanaumpawan P, Grandner MA. Short and long sleep duration associated with race/ethnicity, sociodemographics, and socioeconomic position. Sleep. 2014;37(3):601–11.

Yi S, Nakagawa T, Yamamoto S, Mizoue T, Takahashi Y, Noda M, et al. Short sleep duration in association with CT-scanned abdominal fat areas: the Hitachi Health Study. Int J Obes. 2013;37(1):129–34.

Youngstedt SD, Kripke DF. Long sleep and mortality: rationale for sleep restriction. Sleep Med Rev. 2004;8(3):159–74.

Zhang B, Wing YK. Sex differences in insomnia: a meta-analysis. Sleep. 2006;29(1):85–93.

Zilli I, Ficca G, Salzarulo P. Factors involved in sleep satisfaction in the elderly. Sleep Med. 2009;10(2):233–9.

Zimberg IZ, Damaso A, Del Re M, Carneiro AM, de Sa SH, de Lira FS, et al. Short sleep duration and obesity: mechanisms and future perspectives. Cell Biochem Funct. 2012;30(6):524–9.

Chapter 6
Social Factors in Insufficient Sleep

Mathias Basner

Abstract Insufficient sleep (i.e., not getting adequate amounts of daily sleep relative to individual sleep need on a chronic basis) has not only been linked to neurobehavioral performance decrements and physiological changes considered precursors of disease (e.g., decreased insulin sensitivity), but also to negative health outcomes (e.g., diabetes) and all-cause mortality. Sleep can be regarded as a flexible commodity that can be traded for waking activities considered more important or pressing. The high prevalence of habitual short sleep and its association with morbidity and mortality warrant the identification of social factors and waking activities that predispose to insufficient sleep and that could be targeted in intervention programs. Several demographic (e.g., age, gender, and race) and social (e.g., income, educational attainment, and employment status) factors of insufficient sleep have been identified and are discussed in detail in this chapter. Waking activities predominantly exchanged for less sleep (i.e., working, traveling, socializing and communicating, grooming, and watching TV) are also discussed. The relationships between social factors and insufficient sleep demonstrate complex interactions with psychological, behavioral, health, cultural, and environmental factors. Findings reported in the literature therefore often disagree depending on the study design and the degree of adjustment for the above-mentioned confounders. More research is needed that more comprehensively adjusts for social, behavioral, and economic factors when modeling the relation between sleep and other health or mortality outcomes.

Keywords Sleep · Short sleep · Sleep deprivation · Performance · Demographics · Income · Education · Work

M. Basner (✉)
Unit for Experimental Psychiatry, Division of Sleep and Chronobiology, Department of Psychiatry, Perelman School of Medicine, University of Pennsylvania, Philadelphia, PA, USA
e-mail: basner@pennmedicine.upenn.edu

A. I. Pack, Q. Y. Li (eds.), *Sleep and its Disorders*, Translational Medicine Research,
https://doi.org/10.1007/978-94-024-2168-2_6

6.1 Introduction

Sleep is a biological imperative. Undisturbed sleep of sufficient duration is essential for memory consolidation and for maintaining levels of alertness and cognitive performance required for safe and effective functioning (Banks and Dinges 2007; Diekelmann and Born 2010). Epidemiologic studies consistently find associations between habitual insufficient sleep and physiological changes considered precursors of disease, and with negative health outcomes including obesity (Patel and Hu 2008; Knutson and Cauter 2008), diabetes (Knutson and Cauter 2008; Beihl et al. 2009; Holliday et al. 2013), hypertension (Wang et al. 2012), cardiovascular disease (Shankar et al. 2008), declines in cognitive function (Ferrie et al. 2011), and all-cause mortality (Gallicchio and Kalesan 2009; Cappuccio et al. 2010). Importantly, these studies are increasingly prospective in nature, i.e., they allow inferences about the causal role of insufficient sleep. Experimental studies have demonstrated that acute total and chronic partial sleep restriction produce unfavorable changes in physiologic processes [e.g., decreased insulin sensitivity (Buxton et al. 2010) or changes in appetite-regulating hormones leptin and ghrelin (Taheri et al. 2004)] that strengthen biological plausibility for a causal relationship between chronic insufficient sleep and negative health outcomes as well as all-cause mortality (Colten and Altevogt 2006).

Despite the apparent benefits of sufficient sleep for cognitive performance, safety, and health, current representative surveys indicate that 35–40% of the adult US population report sleeping less than the recommended >7 h (Watson et al. 2015) on weekday nights, and about 15% report sleeping less than 6 h (Centers for Disease Control and Prevention 2011). Several demographic (e.g., age, gender, and race) and social (e.g., income, educational attainment, and employment status) determinants of insufficient sleep have been identified. However, they are often highly correlated, and this confounding and effect modification complicates disentangling the contributions of individual factors. For example, high age is not only associated with biological changes in homeostatic sleep pressure and circadian timing, but also with retirement, income, changes in the social environment, etc. It should be noted that variability in sleep duration can be explained not only by social factors, but also by psychological, behavioral (including health behaviors like exercise and smoking), cultural, and environmental factors and factors related to health conditions that are not the focus of this chapter (Watson et al. 2015). Rarely does a single study account for all the individual factors that can confound or mediate the relationship of other factors with insufficient sleep. Furthermore, sleep can be characterized as a flexible commodity that may be exchanged for waking activities considered more important or pressing (Basner et al. 2007), and both the perceived value of sufficient sleep and the ability to sacrifice other waking activities for more sleep also differ across sociodemographic strata. "As with other luxuries that come at cost of either money or time, sleep may be a resource whose price is beyond the reach of some segments of the population" (Stamatakis et al. 2007). The high prevalence of habitual short sleep and its association with morbidity and mortality warrant the identification of social factors that predispose to insufficient sleep and that could be targeted in intervention programs. Below, several demographic and social factors and their relationship to insufficient sleep will be discussed, as well as the relationship of several waking activities to insufficient sleep. This chapter focuses on sleep duration, but it is acknowledged that sleep quality and the timing and variability of sleep also play important roles in health.

6.2 Age

There are systematic changes in sleep across the lifespan, with a delay in the circadian phase during adolescence and a gradual shift to earlier timing during healthy aging (Skeldon et al. 2016). Homeostatic sleep pressure and slow-wave sleep continuously decline with increasing age. Sleep fragmentation, wake periods, and the amount of superficial sleep stages S1 and S2 increase, while the amount of REM sleep decreases with age (Bonnet and Arand 2007). Data from the American Time Use Survey (ATUS) suggest a U-shaped relationship between age and sleep duration, with long sleep in very young (15–24 years) and older (>64 years) respondents, and the lowest amounts of sleep in the 35–64 year age bracket (Basner et al. 2014). A similar U-shaped relationship was found for long sleep (>9 h relative to 7 h) in the National Health Interview Survey, a nationally representative survey of $N = 110{,}441$ Americans 18 years and older (Krueger and Friedman 2009). The striking difference between weekday and weekend sleep time decreases notably with older age, likely related to retirement (Basner et al. 2007). The finding that weekday sleep time starts to increase again in ≥65-year-old respondents is somewhat at odds with the findings of a meta-analysis of quantitative sleep parameters across the human lifespan, which reported continuously decreasing total sleep time with increasing age (Ohayon et al. 2004). However, this meta-analysis concentrated on polysomnographically measured sleep during the main sleep period, often recorded in laboratory contexts. The ATUS data suggest that once the obligation to arrive at work in the morning is no longer present during retirement, older subjects begin to sleep more, both in the morning and in the afternoon. This strongly supports the concept of social jetlag during the years of employment, and its reversibility during retirement (Wittmann et al. 2006).

6.3 Sex

In an actigraphic study of 669 participants, Lauderdale et al. (2006) found significantly longer sleep duration in females compared to males. This finding is in line with the ATUS study: (Basner et al. 2014) on average and across the whole age range, males slept 9.1 min and 3.0 min less than females on weekdays and weekends/holidays, but they were more likely to be both short sleepers (<6 h) and long sleepers

(>11 h). The latter observation agrees with the National Health Interview Survey, where males had reduced odds of sleeping 5 or fewer hours or 8 or more hours compared to females (Krueger and Friedman 2009). However, sex differences were no longer significant after a more comprehensive adjustment for confounding.

6.4 Race/Ethnicity

In the ATUS survey (Basner et al. 2014), Black, Hispanic, and Asian respondents slept on average significantly longer than white respondents and were also significantly more likely to be long sleepers (defined as ≥11 h per 24 h in this analysis). Only Black respondents were also more likely to be short sleepers (defined as ≤6 h per 24 h in this analysis) than white respondents, while Hispanic and Asian respondents were less likely to be short sleepers, indicating some degree of heterogeneity in Black respondents. Several studies have shown that Black respondents are more likely to report short sleep and sometimes also long sleep compared to White respondents (Stamatakis et al. 2007; Grandner et al. 2014; Maslowsky and Ozer 2014; Jackson et al. 2013; Adenekan et al. 2013; Hale and Do 2007; Knutson et al. 2010). In one prospective study (Stamatakis et al. 2007), the age-adjusted odds ratio for short sleep in Black respondents was reduced by 32% after adjusting for household living conditions, income, and education, and only marginally reduced (12–13%) after adjustment for chronic health conditions, health risk behaviors, and depression. The ATUS data showed that the high odds for a short sleep in Black respondents persisted across nearly all other sociodemographic strata. Future studies are needed to identify in detail what characteristics and behaviors predispose Black respondents to become short or long sleepers, and to what extent these behaviors are driven by sociocultural factors and beliefs about the value of sleep. As Knutson (2013) points out, the broad "racial" or "ethnic" categories typically used in research are likely heterogeneous, and sleep time estimates within racial or ethnic groups accordingly reflect this heterogeneity.

6.5 Education

In ATUS (Basner et al. 2014), sleep duration was negatively correlated with educational attainment, with college graduates or those with a higher degree obtaining on average significantly less sleep than high school graduates. However, higher educational attainment was also associated with lower odds of being a short or long sleeper, suggesting less variability in sleep duration in those with higher education compared to high school graduates. In contrast, respondents with less than a high school degree slept significantly longer than those with a high school degree, and were less likely to be a short sleeper and more likely to be a long sleeper. In the National Health Interview Survey, high levels of education were also associated with lower odds of short or long sleep (Krueger and Friedman 2009). These findings are at odds with the finding of Stamatakis et al. (2007) who found a higher odds of short sleep (<7 h) in those with less than a high school degree. This association was reduced by 31–33% in separate models adjusting for living conditions, health risk behaviors, and depression.

6.6 Family Structure

In ATUS (Basner et al. 2014), divorced/separated, widowed, or never married respondents did not differ significantly from married respondents in terms of average sleep duration. However, widowed subjects were significantly more likely to be short sleepers on weekdays, while those never married were more likely to be long sleepers on both weekdays and weekends/holidays compared to married respondents. Although average sleep time did not differ between interview days whether a spouse or unmarried partner was present or not, respondents without a partner present were more likely to be long sleepers on both weekdays and weekends/holidays.

Respondents with two or more household children obtained less sleep and were significantly less likely to be long sleepers than childless respondents in ATUS. Respondents with three or more children were significantly more likely to be short sleepers on weekdays than those without children. In the National Health Interview Survey, parents with children <2 years of age were more likely to sleep 5 h or less and less likely to sleep 9 h or more compared to parents without children (Krueger and Friedman 2009). Parents with children >2 years were only at lower odds for a long sleep.

6.7 Family Income

Stamatakis et al. (2007) found increased odds for short sleep in the lowest income quintile, but this association was substantially reduced by 69% after adjusting for living conditions, race/ethnicity and education, reduced by 42% after adjustment for depression, and reduced by 31% after adjustment for chronic health conditions. After adjustment for multiple covariates related to health behaviors and health status, a study by Stranges et al. (2008) found a significant association between lower socioeconomic position and short sleep in the UK but not in the USA. In the National Health Interview Survey, high income levels were associated with lower odds of short or long sleep (Krueger and Friedman 2009). In ATUS (Basner et al. 2014), family income and sleep duration were negatively correlated, and the odds of being a short sleeper increased while the odds of being a long sleeper decreased with increasing family income, the former on weekdays only. During weekdays, respondents in the higher income categories were less likely to sleep in the morning between 6 am and 10 am and also in the evening between 9 pm and 11 pm compared to the lower income categories. Those in the lowest income category (<$25,000) were more likely to obtain sleep during the day compared to those making $25,000 or more. These diverse findings suggest a complex nature of the relationship between socioeconomic position and insufficient sleep, which explains the dependence of the direction of the finding on the degree of adjustment for relevant confounders. For example, residents with low income may constitute a diverse population, with some working multiple jobs to make their income, and others working part time or not at all. More detailed studies are needed to disentangle the relationship between socioeconomic position and insufficient sleep.

6.8 Employment

In ATUS (Basner et al. 2014), sleep time and the odds of being a short or long sleeper did not differ between the private-sector and government employees. In contrast, self-employed respondents obtained significantly more sleep, had significantly lower odds of being a short sleeper and also higher odds of being a long sleeper compared to private-sector employees on weekdays. Interestingly, this pattern was reversed on weekends/holidays. Relative to private-sector employees, full-time high school students obtained significantly less sleep (−0.28 h) on weekdays, but obtained significantly more sleep (+0.45 h) on weekends/holidays. Full-time college or university students were more likely to be long sleepers on weekdays, but did otherwise not differ from private-sector employees. Those employed but absent from work obtained almost 1 additional hour of sleep, and were significantly less likely to be short sleepers and more likely to be long sleepers on weekdays. Respondents who were unemployed, retired, or not in the labor force obtained significantly more sleep, were less likely to be short sleepers, and were more likely to be long sleepers. In the National Health Interview Survey, those who worked 41 or more hours were 40% more likely to sleep 5 h or less and 59% less likely to sleep 9 or more hours relative to those working 1–34 h (Krueger and Friedman 2009). Those who were not working had increased odds of both short and long sleep. However, after adjusting for health behaviors and health status, non-working individuals no longer had increased odds of short sleep.

In ATUS (Basner et al. 2014) working multiple jobs was associated with the highest observed odds ratio for being a short sleeper (adjusted OR 1.61 on weekdays and OR 1.72 on weekends/holidays) compared to all other sociodemographic characteristics, and this was true across virtually all sociodemographic strata (approximately 1 out of 10 employed respondents worked more than one job). Sleep restriction and high workload associated with working multiple jobs are known risk factors for increased levels of fatigue that may not only affect job performance but also affect safety both on the job and during the commute. This is extremely troubling in subjects working jobs that immediately affect other people's lives, like medical doctors [so-called moonlighting (McNeeley et al. 2014)] or bus drivers.

Oftentimes, employers do not know about other jobs of their employees, and even if work hour regulations for the primary job are not violated, they would be if the other job was taken into account. ATUS data suggest that reducing the number of those who work multiple jobs could have a profound impact on the amount of sleep obtained.

6.9 Insufficient Sleep in Relation to Waking Activities

The ATUS data (Basner et al. 2014) point to work as the dominant waking activity that is performed instead of sleep in short sleepers (1.55 h more on weekdays and 1.86 h more on weekends/holidays compared to average sleepers), while long sleepers spent much less time working compared to average sleepers (2.66 h on weekdays and 0.90 h on weekends/holidays). Working ranked as the primary waking activity that was performed instead of sleep across all sociodemographic strata, with the exception of respondents retired, unemployed, or otherwise not in the labor force. Furthermore, age 25–64 years, male sex, high income, and employment per se (i.e., sociodemographic characteristics usually associated with paid work) were also consistently associated with short sleep. The timing of work in short sleepers compared to average sleepers suggests that short sleepers stop working later at night and start working earlier in the morning, which directly impacts their ability to obtain sufficient amounts of sleep. Between 2003 and 2011 sleep time and work time were significantly negatively correlated (Basner et al. 2007). The longest sleep times were observed in the economic crisis years 2009, 2010, and 2011, which were characterized by layoffs and a decrease in average work time. Prior research also suggests that respondents working long hours get up earlier in the morning than those not working or working fewer hours, but that these groups do not differ in bedtime (Basner and Dinges 2009). For individuals who need to work long hours, going to bed at an earlier time rather than engaging in other activities (e.g., socializing or watching television) would thus be one way to prolong sleep duration (Basner and Dinges 2009). The association between long work hours and short sleep has been identified in earlier research (Basner et al. 2007; Biddle and Hamermesh 1990). Knutson et al. found a significant increase in the odds of short sleep between 1975 and 2006 for full-time workers only (Knutson et al. 2010).

In terms of intervention strategies, it may be difficult to reduce work time in order to increase sleep time. However, postponing work start time or making it more flexible may help increase sleep time; even if the total time spent working is kept constant. According to ATUS (Basner et al. 2014), with every hour of work or class starting later in the morning, sleep time increased by approximately 20 min (for class after 8 am only). Other studies have shown that later class start times may increase students' sleep time, attention and cognitive performance (Lufi et al. 2011; Boergers et al. 2014), and decrease teen automobile crash rates (Vorona et al. 2011), although one study on college students showed that taking later classes was associated with increased alcohol consumption and lower academic performance (Onyper et al.

2012). More flexible work (and class) start times may be possible without decreasing work time and productivity, and would also accommodate individuals with late circadian preferences who cannot fall asleep early but have to get up before their biological wake time to meet social demands (a condition coined "social jet lag") (Wittmann et al. 2006).

Two other waking activities observed more frequently in short sleepers and less frequently in long sleepers were grooming, socializing, and communicating. These activities are typically performed late at night or early in the morning and thus directly "compete" with sleep for a time. In an analysis that concentrated on 2-h periods pre and post-bed, grooming accounted for 6.5% of the 2 h spent before going to bed in the evening and for 20.2% of the 2 h after getting out of bed in the morning (Basner and Dinges 2009). Although a certain level of body hygiene is important for social and physical well-being, excessive time spent in these activities may reduce sleep time at both ends of the sleep period.

In ATUS (Basner et al. 2014), the role of watching TV during short and long sleep was less straightforward, as both short and long sleepers watched more TV than normal sleepers. However, watching TV in the pre-bed hours was a very prevalent behavior in short, normal, and long sleepers, also in the 2 h pre-bedtime (Basner and Dinges 2009). Although short sleepers only watched an average of 4 min more TV than normal sleepers, they started and stopped watching TV much later at night compared to normal and especially long sleepers. This high prevalence of watching TV late at night in short sleepers suggests that considerable amounts of sleep could be gained by turning the TV off earlier at night. Turning off the TV and other electronic devices may also have the added benefit of reducing exposure to bright light during late evening hours, which has been shown to suppress melatonin excretion and delay melatonin onset, and may even delay circadian phase and thus aggravate social jetlag (Burgess 2013; Gooley et al. 2011). Importantly, the extent to which watching TV was exchanged for less sleep varied greatly depending on sociodemographic characteristics. It was more likely in those ≥45 years, in females, in Black respondents, in those with lower educational attainment, in respondents without a partner, in those with family income <$25,000, and in respondents without work.

6.10 Conclusions

The high prevalence of habitual short sleep and its association with morbidity and mortality warrant the identification of social factors and waking activities that predispose to insufficient sleep and that could be targeted in intervention programs. This chapter illustrates that several demographic and social factors, as well as waking activities, are related to insufficient sleep. However, the relationships often demonstrate complex interactions with psychological, behavioral, health, cultural, and environmental factors. Findings reported in the literature therefore often disagree depending on the study design and the degree of adjustment for the above-mentioned confounders. More research is needed that more comprehensively adjusts for social, behavioral, and economic factors when modeling the relation between sleep and other health or mortality outcomes (Krueger and Friedman 2009).

Acknowledgments Supported by NIH NR004281 and by the National Space Biomedical Research Institute through NASA NCC 9-58. The American Time Use Survey was sponsored by the Bureau of Labor Statistics and conducted by the U.S. Census Bureau.

Disclosure of Financial Support Supported by NIH NR004281 and by the National Space Biomedical Research Institute through NASA NCC 9-58.

References

Adenekan B, Pandey A, McKenzie S, Zizi F, Casimir GJ, Jean-Louis G. Sleep in America: role of racial/ethnic differences. Sleep Med Rev. 2013;17(4):255–62.
Banks S, Dinges DF. Behavioral and physiological consequences of sleep restriction. J Clin Sleep Med. 2007;3(5):519–28.
Basner M, Dinges DF. Dubious bargain: trading sleep for Leno and Letterman. Sleep. 2009;32(6): 747–52.
Basner M, Fomberstein KM, Razavi FM, Banks S, William JH, Rosa RR, et al. American time use survey: sleep time and its relationship to waking activities. Sleep. 2007;30(9):1085–95.
Basner M, Spaeth AM, Dinges DF. Sociodemographic characteristics and waking activities and their role in the timing and duration of sleep. Sleep. 2014;37(12):1889–906.
Beihl DA, Liese AD, Haffner SM. Sleep duration as a risk factor for incident type 2 diabetes in a multiethnic cohort. Ann Epidemiol. 2009;19(5):351–7.
Biddle JE, Hamermesh DS. Sleep and the allocation of time. J Polit Econ. 1990;98(5):922–43.
Boergers J, Gable CJ, Owens JA. Later school start time is associated with improved sleep and daytime functioning in adolescents. J Dev Behav Pediatr. 2014;35(1):11–7.
Bonnet MH, Arand DL. EEG arousal norms by age. J Clin Sleep Med. 2007;3(3):271–4.
Burgess HJ. Evening ambient light exposure can reduce circadian phase advances to morning light independent of sleep deprivation. J Sleep Res. 2013;22(1):83–8.
Buxton OM, Pavlova M, Reid EW, Wang W, Simonson DC, Adler GK. Sleep restriction for 1 week reduces insulin sensitivity in healthy men. Diabetes. 2010;59(9):2126–33.
Cappuccio FP, D'Elia L, Strazzullo P, Miller MA. Sleep duration and all-cause mortality: a systematic review and meta-analysis of prospective studies. Sleep. 2010;33(5):585–92.
Centers for Disease Control and Prevention. Effect of short sleep duration on daily activities—United States, 2005–2008. MMWR Morb Mortal Wkly Rep. 2011;60(8):239–42.
Colten HR, Altevogt BM. In: Colten HR, Altevogt BM, editors. Sleep disorders and sleep deprivation: an unmet public health problem. Washington, DC: National Academic Press; 2006.
Diekelmann S, Born J. The memory function of sleep. Nat Rev Neurosci. 2010;11(2):114–26.
Ferrie JE, Shipley MJ, Akbaraly TN, Marmot MG, Kivimaki M, Singh-Manoux A. Change in sleep duration and cognitive function: findings from the Whitehall II Study. Sleep. 2011;34(5): 565–73.
Gallicchio L, Kalesan B. Sleep duration and mortality: a systematic review and meta-analysis. J Sleep Res. 2009;18(2):148–58.
Gooley JJ, Chamberlain K, Smith KA, Khalsa SB, Rajaratnam SM, Van Reen E, et al. Exposure to room light before bedtime suppresses melatonin onset and shortens melatonin duration in humans. J Clin Endocrinol Metab. 2011;96(3):E463–72.
Grandner MA, Chakravorty S, Perlis ML, Oliver L, Gurubhagavatula I. Habitual sleep duration associated with self-reported and objectively determined cardiometabolic risk factors. Sleep Med. 2014;15(1):42–50.

Hale L, Do DP. Racial differences in self-reports of sleep duration in a population-based study. Sleep. 2007;30(9):1096–103.
Holliday EG, Magee CA, Kritharides L, Banks E, Attia J. Short sleep duration is associated with risk of future diabetes but not cardiovascular disease: a prospective study and meta-analysis. PLoS One. 2013;8(11):e82305.
Jackson CL, Redline S, Kawachi I, Williams MA, Hu FB. Racial disparities in short sleep duration by occupation and industry. Am J Epidemiol. 2013;178(9):1442–51.
Knutson KL. Sociodemographic and cultural determinants of sleep deficiency: implications for cardiometabolic disease risk. Soc Sci Med. 2013;79:7–15.
Knutson KL, Cauter E. Associations between sleep loss and increased risk of obesity and diabetes. Ann N Y Acad Sci. 2008;1129:287–304.
Knutson KL, Van Cauter E, Rathouz PJ, DeLeire T, Lauderdale DS. Trends in the prevalence of short sleepers in the USA: 1975-2006. Sleep. 2010;33(1):37–45.
Krueger PM, Friedman EM. Sleep duration in the United States: a cross-sectional population-based study. Am J Epidemiol. 2009;169(9):1052–63.
Lauderdale DS, Knutson KL, Yan LJL, Rathouz PJ, Hulley SB, Sidney S, et al. Objectively measured sleep characteristics among early-middle-aged adults—the CARDIA study. Am J Epidemiol. 2006;164(1):5–16.
Lufi D, Tzischinsky O, Hadar S. Delaying school starting time by one hour: some effects on attention levels in adolescents. J Clin Sleep Med. 2011;7(2):137–43.
Maslowsky J, Ozer EJ. Developmental trends in sleep duration in adolescence and young adulthood: evidence from a national United States sample. J Adolesc Health. 2014;54(6):691–7.
McNeeley MF, Monroe EJ, Prabhu SJ, Iyer RS. Internal versus external moonlighting by radiology trainees: differences in roles and responsibilities. Acad Radiol. 2014;21(4):546–53.
Ohayon MM, Carskadon MA, Guilleminault C, Vitiello MV. Meta-analysis of quantitative sleep parameters from childhood to old age in healthy individuals: developing normative sleep values across the human lifespan. Sleep. 2004;27(7):1255–73.
Onyper SV, Thacher PV, Gilbert JW, Gradess SG. Class start times, sleep, and academic performance in college: a path analysis. Chronobiol Int. 2012;29(3):318–35.
Patel SR, Hu FB. Short sleep duration and weight gain: a systematic review. Obesity (Silver Spring). 2008;16(3):643–53.
Shankar A, Koh WP, Yuan JM, Lee HP, Yu MC. Sleep duration and coronary heart disease mortality among Chinese adults in Singapore: a population-based cohort study. Am J Epidemiol. 2008;168(12):1367–73.
Skeldon AC, Derks G, Dijk DJ. Modelling changes in sleep timing and duration across the lifespan: changes in circadian rhythmicity or sleep homeostasis? Sleep Med Rev. 2016;28:96–107.
Stamatakis KA, Kaplan GA, Roberts RE. Short sleep duration across income, education, and race/ethnic groups: population prevalence and growing disparities during 34 years of follow-up. Ann Epidemiol. 2007;17(12):948–55.
Stranges S, Dorn JM, Shipley MJ, Kandala NB, Trevisan M, Miller MA, et al. Correlates of short and long sleep duration: a cross-cultural comparison between the United Kingdom and the United States the Whitehall II Study and the Western New York Health Study. Am J Epidemiol. 2008;168(12):1353–64.
Taheri S, Lin L, Austin D, Young T, Mignot E. Short sleep duration is associated with reduced leptin, elevated ghrelin, and increased body mass index. PLoS Med. 2004;1(3):e62.

Vorona RD, Szklo-Coxe M, Wu A, Dubik M, Zhao Y, Ware JC. Dissimilar teen crash rates in two neighboring southeastern Virginia cities with different high school start times. J Clin Sleep Med. 2011;7(2):145–51.

Wang Q, Xi B, Liu M, Zhang Y, Fu M. Short sleep duration is associated with hypertension risk among adults: a systematic review and meta-analysis. Hypertens Res. 2012;35(10):1012–8.

Watson NF, Badr MS, Belenky G, Bliwise DL, Buxton OM, Buysse D, et al. Joint consensus statement of the American Academy of Sleep Medicine and Sleep Research Society on the recommended amount of sleep for a healthy adult: methodology and discussion. Sleep. 2015;38 (8):1161–83.

Wittmann M, Dinich J, Merrow M, Roenneberg T. Social jetlag: misalignment of biological and social time. Chronobiol Int. 2006;23(1–2):497–509.

Chapter 7
Sleep Loss and the Unfolded Protein Response

Nirinjini Naidoo

Abstract Sleep loss leads to activation of the unfolded protein response (UPR) not only in the brain but also in peripheral organs (heart, lung, and pancreas). This has been shown in multiple species including mice, rats, *Drosophila*, and migratory birds. The unfolded protein response to sleep loss changes with age. In older mice, there is activation of the maladaptive response to sleep loss with increased expression of genes in the pro-apoptotic pathway. UPR is not simply a consequence of sleep loss but also affects sleep behavior. Alteration of the molecular machinery of the UPR alters baseline sleep as well as the degree of sleep recovery following sleep deprivation. Moreover, administration of drugs that alter the UPR can reduce the sleep fragmentation that occurs with age. UPR response to sleep loss has implications for neurodegenerative disorders and other medical conditions.

Keywords Unfolded protein response · Protein homeostasis/proteostasis · Chaperone · BiP (Immunoglobulin Binding Protein) · Neurodegeneration · Metabolism · Apoptosis · Inflammation

7.1 Introduction

Sleep loss is common in the American population. Sleep deprivation can result from a period of acute sleep loss or from insufficient sleep day after day. Some professional groups, such as health care workers (physicians and nurses) and investment banking analysts/interns (http://news.efinancialcareers.com/us-en/196881/10-worst-banks-working-hours/), (ABC News http://abcnews.go.com/Business/bank-america-investment-banking-analysts-jumping-joy-firms/story; http://www.businessinsider.com/investment-banking-internship-nightmare-2013-8) are particularly at risk for sleep loss because of their work schedules. Insufficient sleep has been the focus of two IOM reports; Sleep Disorders and Sleep Deprivation: An Unmet

N. Naidoo (✉)
Division of Sleep Medicine, Department of Medicine, Perelman School of Medicine, University of Pennsylvania, Philadelphia, PA, USA
e-mail: naidoo@pennmedicine.upenn.edu

A. I. Pack, Q. Y. Li (eds.), *Sleep and its Disorders*, Translational Medicine Research,
https://doi.org/10.1007/978-94-024-2168-2_7

Public Health Problem and Optimizing Graduate Medical Trainee (Resident) Hours and Work Schedule to Improve Patient Safety (Ulmer et al. 2009; Colten et al. 2006). Sleep loss has a number of consequences. It leads to what has been termed wake-state instability (Chee et al. 2006), in which individuals are unable to maintain stable wakefulness and instead drift in and out of sleep. This results in lapses in cognitive performance and compromises aspects of cognitive function such as executive attention and working memory (Dinges 1992; Goel et al. 2009). It is estimated that almost 20% of motor vehicle crashes are attributed to driver sleepiness independent of alcohol effects (Connor et al. 2002). In addition to behavioral consequences, sleep loss/deprivation also has important metabolic and cardiovascular repercussions. Epidemiological studies indicate an association between sleep loss and increased rates of obesity, type 2 diabetes, and an increased risk of cardiovascular disease (Grandner et al. 2014; Knutson et al. 2010; Knutson 2012; Grandner 2014). People reporting short sleep duration (typically less than 6 h/night) display an increased prevalence of type 2 diabetes, hypertension, obesity, cardiovascular disease, and stroke (Qureshi et al. 1997; Elliott et al. 2014; Ayas et al. 2003; Spiegel et al. 2005; Chen et al. 2008). Several microarrays and transcriptomic—and to a lesser extent proteomic studies—over the past few years have begun to elucidate some of the molecular correlates of sleep loss. For example, downregulation of macromolecular synthetic processes with acute sleep loss has been described (Mackiewicz et al. 2007). Concomitantly, the upregulation of immediate early genes and molecules involved in energy regulation and metabolism and an adaptive cellular stress response to acute sleep loss is consistently observed among all studies (for details and references see Table 7.1). Specifically, the molecular chaperone BiP (Immunoglobulin Binding Protein) is upregulated in all studied species in response to sleep loss (Naidoo 2009). BiP is a sentinel marker of the unfolded protein response (UPR), which is a cytoprotective cellular stress response. Upregulation of other components of the UPR signaling pathways (described below) during sleep loss have also been described by several groups (see Table 7.1). This chapter will provide an overview of the UPR from its initial cytoprotective response to the later pro-apoptotic signaling pathway. The chapter will also summarize data from sleep deprivation and intermittent hypoxia studies that demonstrate a role of the UPR in sleep. Understanding the pathways activated by sleep loss and the mechanisms by which they occur will aid in the development of therapies to protect the brain during sleep loss and to treat sleep disorders, including those associated with aging.

7.2 Unfolded Protein Response

The unfolded protein response (UPR) is a coordinated set of signaling pathways that are triggered when endoplasmic reticulum (ER) homeostasis is perturbed. The ER is an organelle within which all secretory and integral membrane proteins are folded and post-translationally modified in ATP-dependent chaperone-mediated processes (Walter and Ron 2011). The ER is also the site of steroid, cholesterol, and lipid

Table 7.1 UPR associated genes that change with sleep loss and sleep fragmentation

Gene name	Function	References
BiP/HSPA5/ GRP78	ER chaperone, folding, ERAD, ATPase activity, anti-apoptotic	Mackiewicz et al. (2007), Naidoo et al. (2005, 2008), Maret et al. (2007), Terao et al. (2006), Jones et al. (2008), Cirelli et al. (2006), and Shaw et al. (2000b)
GRP94	Heat shock 90 family, ER chaperone, folding	Maret et al. (2007), Cirelli and Tononi (2000), and Terao et al. (2003)
CHOP/ GADD153	Apoptotic signaling	Cirelli and Tononi (2000)
ERP72	ER chaperone, folding	Terao et al. (2006) and Cirelli and Tononi (2000)
PERK	Kinase, protein translation inhibition, antioxidant response	Cirelli et al. (2004)
Calcineurin	Calcium activated phosphatase	Cirelli et al. (2004)
FK506 binding protein12	Peptidyl propyl cis/trans isomerases, conformational change, translational control	Cirelli et al. (2004)
IP3 receptor	Calcium receptor signaling	Cirelli et al. (2004)
XBP-1	Transcription factor, ER chaperone induction	Mackiewicz et al. (2007) and Maret et al. (2007)
Calreticulin	Calcium binding, ER chaperone of glycoproteins	Mackiewicz et al. (2007) Maret et al. (2007), and Cirelli et al. (2006)
eIF4B	Translation initiation factor	Mackiewicz et al. (2007)
Ribosomal S6 kinase	Protein translation	Mackiewicz et al. (2007)
Dnajc1	DnaJ (Hsp40) homolog, ER chaperone)—Protein synthesis and folding—ERAD, translocation, HSP70 assistance, ATPase activity	Mackiewicz et al. (2007)
Dnajb5	HSP40; binds unfolded ER proteins	Mackiewicz et al. (2007)
Dnajc3	HSP40 family	Mackiewicz et al. (2007)
Dnajb11	HSP40 family	Mackiewicz et al. (2007)
Gadd45a	(Demethylation—DNA repair)	Mackiewicz et al. (2007)
Gadd45b		Mackiewicz et al. (2007)
Calpain 5	ER protease, caspase cleavage	Mackiewicz et al. (2007)
Mannosidase 2, alpha B1	ER degradation enhancing—EDEM/ ERAD	Mackiewicz et al. (2007)
Hsp90ab1	Signal transduction, protein folding and degradation, and morphological evolution	Maret et al. (2007)
Hsp60	Heat shock protein family	Cirelli and Tononi (2000) and Cirelli (2002)
Hsp70	Heat shock protein family	Cirelli and Tononi (2000) and Cirelli (2002)
Hspb1	Stress resistance and actin organization	Maret et al. (2007) and Cirelli et al. (2006), and Conti et al. (2007)

(continued)

Table 7.1 (continued)

Gene name	Function	References
Hsp105	Member of the Hsp70 superfamily of molecular chaperones, serves as a nucleotide exchange factor for Hsc70/BiP	Mackiewicz et al. (2007)
Hspa1a	Stabilizes existing proteins against aggregation and mediates the folding of newly translated proteins in the cytosol and in organelles	Mackiewicz et al. (2007) and Cirelli et al. (2006)
Hspa1b	Stabilizes existing proteins against aggregation and mediates the folding of newly translated proteins in the cytosol and in organelles	Mackiewicz et al. (2007)
Hspa9	Cell proliferation, stress response and maintenance of the mitochondria	Cirelli and Tononi (2000) and Terao et al. (2003)
Ppp3	Similar to calcineurin	Cirelli et al. (2004)
Mrp14	Calcium-binding myeloid-associated protein 14	Cirelli et al. (2006)
Taf9b	TATA-binding protein	Cirelli et al. (2006)
Cort	Somatostatin homolog: Depression of neuronal activity, induction of slow-wave sleep, reduction of locomotor activity, and activation of cation selective currents	Cirelli et al. (2006)
Cryab	Chaperone protein	Cirelli et al. (2006)
Mgst1	Catalyzes the conjugation of glutathione to electrophiles and the reduction of lipid hydroperoxides	Cirelli et al. (2006)
Gpx3	Detoxification of hydrogen peroxide	Cirelli et al. (2006)
CYP4F4	Encodes a member of the cytochrome P450 superfamily of enzymes	Cirelli et al. (2006)
HSC70	A heat shock cognate 70 and chaperone, member of HSP70 family	Williams et al. (2007)
ERO1L	Member of ER oxidoreductin family—localized to the ER and promotes the formation of disulfide bonds	Williams et al. (2007)

biosynthesis and is the major signal-transducing organelle in the cell that continuously responds to environmental cues to release calcium (Kaufman 2002). Since the endoplasmic reticulum is a complex membranous network that extends throughout the cytoplasm and is contiguous with the nuclear envelope, it can sense and transmit signals that originate in any cellular sub-compartment. Thus, perturbing ER homeostasis disrupts protein folding and leads to the accumulation of unfolded proteins and protein aggregates, which are detrimental to cell survival. The UPR conveys signals from the ER to the nucleus and cytosol through the activation of three signal transducers; PERK (PKR like ER kinase), ATF6 (Activating Transcription Factor 6), and IRE1 (Inositol Requiring Element 1) (see Fig. 7.1). These three molecules are

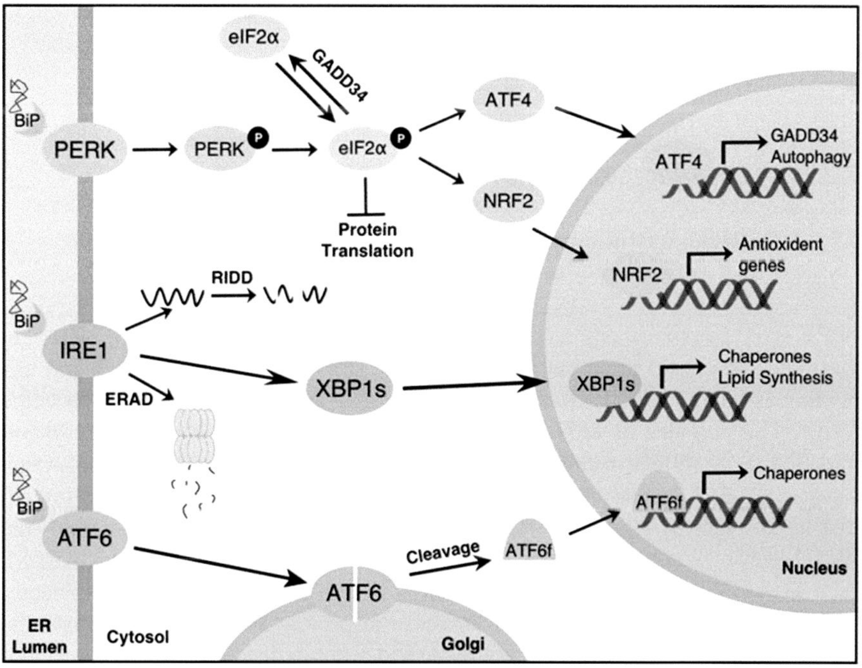

Fig. 7.1 Schematic showing the three major pathways of the unfolded protein response. Misfolded or unfolded proteins titrate BiP away from the three transducers of ER stress: PERK, IRE1, and ATF6. Activated PERK phosphorylates eIF2α to attenuate protein translation and phosphorylates Nrf-2 to upregulate the antioxidant response. Cleaved activated ATF6 leads to induction of molecular chaperones like BiP and GRP94. IRE1 activation leads to XBP-1 splicing, transcriptional activation of chaperones, and stimulation of protein and transcript degradation through ERAD and RIDD, respectively. The various ER chaperones, such as BiP and GRP94 are protective and control protein folding and components of the UPR, while ATF4 induction leads to GADD34 production as well as autophagy

held in an inactive state by binding to a molecular chaperone, BiP on the luminal side of the ER. BiP, also known as GRP78 and Hspa5, is an ATPase and member of the heat shock 70 family of proteins that binds preferentially to nascent and misfolded proteins. Perturbation of ER homeostasis caused by events such as reduced energy, changes in calcium flux, redox changes, ischemia, hyperhomocysteinemia, viral infections, and mutations (Kaufman 2002; Ron 2002) leads to protein misfolding. When this occurs BiP dissociates from PERK, IRE1 and ATF6 bind to the misfolded proteins and assist in their refolding or to escort these proteins out of the ER for degradation. The dissociation of BiP from these three molecules (PERK, IRE1, and ATF6) leads to the activation of their three respective signaling cascades that transduce the ER stress signal to the cytosol and nucleus. The duration and response of each signaling cascade are dependent on the duration of the ER stress signal. The response is initially adaptive, however, sustained ER stress eventually leads to a maladaptive response with inflammatory signaling that if not resolved leads to apoptosis.

7.2.1 The Adaptive Unfolded Protein Response

7.2.1.1 PERK Activation Leads to an Inhibition of Protein Translation and Activation of an Antioxidant Response

PERK is a type I transmembrane serine-threonine kinase that appears to be present in most cells. It is held in an inactive monomeric state by binding to BiP. When this binding is disrupted, PERK homodimerizes and autophosphorylates to become active. This initiates its eIF2α kinase activity. Phosphorylation of the translation initiation factor, eIF2α, results in the formation of a stalled 43S ternary complex that causes a general decrease in translation of most proteins. The attenuation in protein translation serves to reduce the client protein load and stress within the ER. However, some selected proteins with internal ribosomal entry sites (IRES), such as ATF4 and the chaperones BiP and GRP94 are translated more efficiently (Harding et al. 2000) leading to an *increase* in protein levels. ATF4 controls the levels of pro-survival genes that are related to redox balance, amino acid metabolism, protein folding, and autophagy (Ameri and Harris 2008) (Fig. 7.1). This branch of the UPR also regulates the expression of several microRNAs, which may contribute to the attenuation of protein translation or protein synthesis (Behrman et al. 2011).

Inducing ER stress also causes PERK to phosphorylate Nuclear Factor-E2 related factor 2 (Nrf2), a molecule that plays a significant role in the adaptive stress response to oxidative stress (He et al. 2001; Itoh et al. 1999; Venugopal and Jaiswal 1996) and xenobiotic detoxification (Motohashi and Yamamoto 2004). Nrf2 regulates the inducible expression of ARE-containing target genes, such as enzymes involved in glutathione biosynthesis and chemical detoxification (Chan et al. 2001; Ishii et al. 2000) which are induced during the UPR. Nrf2 belongs to the cap "n" collar (CNC) subfamily of basic leucine zipper transcription factors, and is one of the multiple substrates for PERK kinase activity. It is distributed ubiquitously throughout the cytoplasm through its association with Keap-1 (Kelch-like ECH-associated protein 1), its specific repressor (Itoh et al. 1999). Phosphorylation of Nrf2 leads to disassociation from Keap-1, leading to the nuclear recruitment of Nrf2 (Itoh et al. 1999; Motohashi and Yamamoto 2004). PERK/Nrf2 translocation into the nucleus leads to the upregulation of genes involved in redox maintenance (Cullinan et al. 2003). Nrf2 is activated by PERK independent of translational inhibition through eIF2α (Cullinan et al. 2003).

7.2.1.2 IRE1 Activation Leads to Upregulation of Chaperones, ER Expansion and Degradation of Transcripts, and Misfolded Proteins

Once activated, the cytoplasmic domain of IRE1α containing endoribonuclease activity excises an intron from the mRNA encoding an UPR-specific transcription factor, X-box binding protein (XBP) 1, generating the spliced variant xbp1s. Spliced xbp1 encodes XBP1, a potent transcriptional transactivator of genes involved in ER expansion, protein maturation, folding, and export from the ER, as well as export and degradation of misfolded proteins (Yoshida et al. 2001, 2003; Calfon et al. 2002; Lee et al. 2002, 2003). ER-bound mRNAs are also degraded in an IRE1-dependent manner via a process called RIDD ("regulated IRE1-dependent decay") and may serve to limit protein influx and unfolded protein load into the ER lumen after prolonged UPR induction (Walter and Ron 2011; Hollien and Weissman 2006; Pirot et al. 2007). Specifically, mRNAs for secretory proteins that are predicted to be difficult to fold are degraded first (Hollien and Weissman 2006; Maurel et al. 2014). RIDD is conserved in mammals, yeast, and plants and is cell-type specific (Dufey et al. 2014). Ire1 is also implicated in the degradation of microRNAs involved in apoptosis, energy metabolism, and inflammation (Maurel et al. 2014; Upton et al. 2012).

7.2.1.3 Activated ATF6 Upregulates Chaperone Production

ATF6 represents a group of ER stress transducers that encode basic leucine zipper (bZIP) transcription factors, including ATF6α, ATF6β, LUMAN (also known as CREB3), old astrocyte specifically induced substance (OASIS; also known as CREB3L1), BBF2 human homologue on chromosome 7 (BBF2H7; also known as CREB3L2), cyclic AMP-responsive element-binding protein hepatocyte (CREBH; also known as CREB3L3) and CREB4 (also known as CREB3L4) (Asada et al. 2011). Under ER stress conditions ATF6 dissociates from BiP and is exported to the Golgi where it is cleaved by site-1 protease (S1P) and S2P releasing its cytosolic domain which is a potent transcription factor. The 50-kDa cleaved ATF6α then translocates to the cell nucleus, where it binds to the ER stress response element CCAAT(N)9CCACG (Yoshida et al. 1998) in genes encoding ER chaperone proteins such as BiP and GRP94. GRP94 is a member of the heat shock90 family of chaperones. This binding results in increased transcription of these proteins and hence increased protein folding activity in the ER (Yoshida et al. 1998; Okada et al. 2002). Other important targets regulated by ATF6 include XBP-1, CHOP, HERP (hyperhomocysteinemia-induced ER stress-responsive protein), and PDI (Protein disulfide isomerase).

7.2.2 *Prolonged ER Stress Leads to an Inflammatory Response and Apoptotic Signaling*

UPR signaling merges with several components of other well-known stress responses through a series of bidirectional crosstalk points (Dufey et al. 2014) (Fig. 7.2). Activation of IRE1α engages "alarm" genes by recruiting the adaptor protein TRAF2 (TNF receptor-associated factor 2), which results in the activation of the apoptosis signal-regulating kinase 1 (ASK1; also known as MAP3K5) pathway and its downstream target JUN N-terminal kinase (JNK) (Urano et al. 2000; Hu et al. 2006; Hetz et al. 2011). NF-kappa B (NF-κB), which is also known to play a role in sleep (Kuo et al. 2010; Kuo and Williams 2014), is increased in two ways during ER stress. First, I kappa K (IKK), which has a shorter half-life, is reduced when protein translation is attenuated. This changes the stoichiometric ratio of NF-κB: IKK and frees NF-κ B to translocate to the nucleus (Zhang and Kaufman 2008). Secondly, the

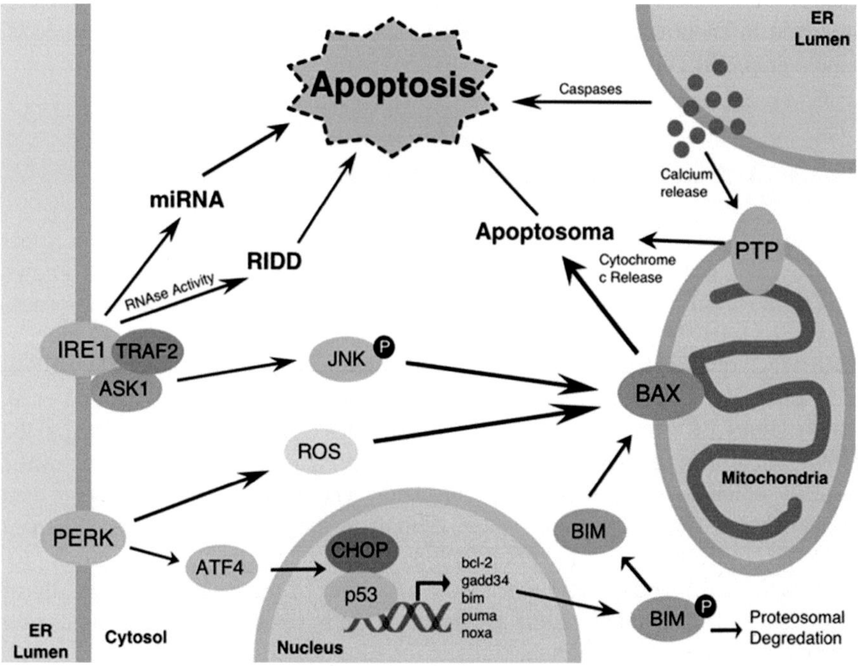

Fig. 7.2 Sustained ER stress leads to pro-apoptotic signaling. Prolonged UPR activation leads to ER calcium release and cell death signaling. Activated IRE-1 complexes with TRAF2 and ASK1 to activate JNK and caspases. ATF4-dependent transcription leads to increases in CHOP. CHOP is a pro-apoptotic transcription factor. CHOP inhibits BCl-2 leading to calcium release; higher calcium levels sensitize mitochondria to other insults inducing cell death. BCl-2 exerts an anti-apoptotic function in the ER.CHOP and JNK also promote the translocation of Bax to the mitochondria where it facilitates the release of cytochrome c required for caspase activation and apoptosis

IRE1-TRAF2 complex recruits I kappa B (IKB) kinase that phosphorylates IKB leading to its degradation (Hu et al. 2006).

JNK activation is an important pro-apoptotic signal in response to IRE1α activation, although its mechanism of action during instances of ER stress is not well understood. IRE1α–JNK signaling can also trigger macroautophagy that is induced by ER stress and nutrient starvation by activating beclin 1 (Urano et al. 2000; Hu et al. 2006; Hetz et al. 2011), an essential autophagy regulator11. IRE1α also engages pathways involving p38, extracellular signal-regulated kinase (ERK), and nuclear factor-κB (NF-κB) through the binding of distinct adaptor proteins (Hu et al. 2006; Nguyen et al. 2004).

Apoptosis in response to ER stress is mediated largely by C/EBP homologous protein (CHOP) also known as growth arrest and DNA damage 153 (GADD 153). CHOP which is downstream of the PERK and ATF6 pathways induces the expression of a number of pro-apoptotic factors including Tribbles 3, and GADD34. CHOP mediates apoptosis through various mechanisms including (1) inhibition of protective anti-apoptotic factors like Bcl-2 and perturbation of cellular redox state by depletion of the antioxidant glutathione (McCullough et al. 2001), (2) promotion of apoptotic caspase activity (McCullough et al. 2001), and (3) the translocation of Bax from the cytosol to the mitochondria (Gotoh and Mori 2004). Insertion of Bax into the mitochondrial membrane is essential for cytochrome c release and mitochondrial-mediated apoptosis (Nechushtan et al. 1999).

7.3 UPR Pathways and Factors Induced by Sleep Loss in the Brain

The induction of the molecular chaperone BiP by sleep loss is conserved across species. Several studies have shown that acute sleep deprivation increases BiP/GRP78 expression in the brains of mice (Mackiewicz et al. 2007; Naidoo et al. 2005; Maret et al. 2007), rats (Cirelli et al. 2004; Terao et al. 2006), birds (Jones et al. 2008), and fruitflies (Shaw et al. 2000a; Naidoo et al. 2007; Williams et al. 2007). Sleep loss activates the PERK pathway in the *Drosophila* brain (Brown et al. 2014) and also in the cerebral cortex of mice (Naidoo et al. 2005, 2008). PERK cerebellar transcript levels were also found to be higher in wakefulness than in sleep (Cirelli et al. 2004). Activation of IRE1 activity through xbp1 mRNA splicing has been observed in sleep-deprived fly brains (Brown et al. 2014); Naidoo et al. unpublished observations). Xbp 1 transcript levels have also been reported to increase in mouse brain (Mackiewicz et al. 2007). Transcripts of several molecular chaperones besides BiP are also increased in brain following sleep loss. ERP72, GRP94, HSP27, HSP70-1, and HSP84 mRNA levels are all increased in cortex, basal forebrain, hypothalamus cerebellum, and medulla during sleep deprivation, whereas increased mRNA levels during recovery sleep were limited to the cortex and medulla (Terao et al. 2006). These chaperones are downstream targets of UPR transcription factors XBP1 and ATF6. Other UPR-specific transcripts that change with sleep deprivation include DNA-J which is a co-chaperone of BiP, calreticulin, caspase-9, ATF4, ATF6 (Mackiewicz et al. 2007), and ERo1L (Williams et al. 2007). Several UPR-activated pro-inflammatory molecules are also induced by sleep deprivation. These include NfkB and JNK (Williams et al. 2007). For a complete list of UPR factors upregulated by sleep loss, see Table 7.1.

7.3.1 Changes in ER Stress Response with Age

Aged animals exhibit more fragmented sleep (Naidoo et al. 2008; Welsh et al. 1986; Shiromani et al. 2000) and display basal levels of ER stress in tissues examined (Brown et al. 2014; Naidoo et al. 2011). The adaptive ER stress response to sleep deprivation is impaired in aged mice cerebral cortices (Naidoo et al. 2008) as well as in aged *Drosophila* brains (Brown et al. 2014). There is a decrease in the adaptive UPR and an increase in inflammatory/pro-apoptotic signaling (Brown et al. 2014). Wake-active neurons in aged mice exhibit considerable ER stress and PERK pathway activation when compared with similar regions in young mice (Naidoo et al. 2011). In a study comparing wake in young and old mice, we found wake instability and impaired wake responses to novelty in older mice that were accompanied by ER stress in orexinergic and noradrenergic wake neurons (Naidoo et al. 2011). The ER stress response in orexin and noradrenergic neurons was evidenced by the presence of activated phosphorylated PERK, nuclear translocation of CHOP, and increased GADD34 expression. The specific wake impairments identified in aged mice were consistent with orexinergic and noradrenergic neuronal injury. Surprisingly, recovery sleep following sleep deprivation is less in older animals than in young. This has been shown in humans (Bonnet 1985; Carskadon and Dement 1987) and in rats (Shiromani et al. 2000; Mendelson and Bergmann 2000). It is not known whether the UPR plays a role in the mammalian recovery sleep response to sleep deprivation and is currently an area of investigation.

7.3.2 Chronic Sleep Loss

While acute sleep deprivation leads to induction of the adaptive UPR, it appears that chronic sleep loss or long-term sleep deprivation as assessed by an increase in BiP transcript levels does not. A study by Cirelli et al. (2006) showed that rat cerebral cortex BiP mRNA levels do not increase after long-term (7 days) sleep deprivation as much as after short-term (8 h) sleep deprivation. It is possible that 7 days of sleep deprivation results in sustained ER stress much like that experienced by aged animals, which results in a shutdown of the adaptive ER stress response. Thus, it is likely to be more injurious. Further studies are needed to address this. A more recent study indicates that long-term REM sleep loss (6–10 days) does lead to increased apoptosis in several regions of the rat brain (Biswas et al. 2006). Using amino cupric staining as a marker of neuronal degeneration, TUNEL (TdT-mediated dUPT nick end labeling) assays, and the ratio of Bcl-2 to Bax as indices of apoptosis this study demonstrates that neurons in locus coeruleus (LC), laterodorsal tegmentum (LDT), and medial preoptic area (MPO) but not in the lateral septum undergo degeneration with REM sleep loss (Biswas et al. 2006). The increase in Bax positive neurons over BCl-2 positive neurons observed in this study suggests that the apoptotic phase of the UPR is activated in the REM sleep-deprived animals. The absence of any apoptotic factors in the lateral septum following REM sleep loss illustrates that there is differential vulnerability between neuronal groups to stress.

7.4 UPR Induction in Peripheral Tissues with Sleep Loss

Most studies have focused on UPR induction in the brain as a result of sleep loss. There are a few studies that indicate that sleep loss does activate the UPR in peripheral tissues. BiP is upregulated in several peripheral tissues with acute sleep deprivation; these include liver (Maret et al. 2007), skeletal muscle (Cirelli et al. 2006), heart (Anafi et al. 2013), lung (Anafi et al. 2013), and pancreas (Naidoo et al. 2014). A transcriptomics study on heart and lung examined the temporal profile of gene expression during 3, 6, 9, and 12 h of sleep deprivation (Anafi et al. 2013). They found several ER stress and UPR transcripts that were repressed during sleep and enhanced during sleep loss. Notably, protein folding and the UPR was the major pathway identified in this study. In addition to BiP, other transcripts identified included XBP1, ATF4, GADD34, GRP94, DNAjb, ER Mannosidase I, Calreticulin, HSP40, IRE1, ATF6, and UGGT (Anafi et al. 2013) (Table 7.1). A later study in the pancreas demonstrated that BiP protein expression was significantly increased with acute sleep deprivation (Naidoo et al. 2014). Induction of the UPR was confirmed using additional markers, including cleavage of ATF6 and phosphorylation of eIF2a, both of which were significantly increased following sleep loss. Expression of CHOP also trended higher with sleep loss, though CHOP expression exhibited a high degree of variation between animals. This study also demonstrated that there is a loss of the adaptive UPR with age and that this affects insulin sensitivity in aged animals providing a link between age-related sleep disturbances and metabolic dysfunction (Naidoo et al. 2014).

7.5 Other Sleep Disturbances and the UPR

Sleep fragmentation that occurs with aging, disease, and sleep apnea also induces the UPR. Exposure to intermittent cyclical hypoxia/reoxygenation similar to that which occurs in obstructive sleep apnea results in ER stress in select brainstem motor neurons (Zhu et al. 2008). Motor neurons process large amounts of secretory and membrane proteins that must be properly folded within the ER (Shaw et al. 2000b), and as such are prone to ongoing ER stress and UPR activation. Both short-term (3 days) and longer-term intermittent hypoxia over 8 weeks selectively activates the PERK pathway of the UPR in the hypoglossal and facial motor nuclei (Zhu et al. 2008). Additionally, pro-apoptotic proteins, CHOP, GADD34, cleaved caspase-7, and caspase-3, are all increased with longer-term intermittent hypoxia in these motor neurons. As a result, these motor neurons undergo ER stress even at baseline which is then exacerbated by long-term intermittent hypoxia. The presence of CHOP and subsequently GADD34 leads to dephosphorylation of p-eIF2α, increased protein synthesis, and greater ER stress in these neurons. The inability of these neurons to relieve the ER stress leads to a neural injury that can be observed at the ultrastructural level; the ER is swollen and distorted and there is disaggregation of ribosomes and degranulation of rough ER (Zhu et al. 2008).

A recent study from the Gozal group showed that chronic sleep fragmentation also induced temporal changes in ER stress in the hypothalamus, across the three major UPR pathways (Hakim et al. 2015). There is an increase in cleaved ATF6 expression, splicing of XBP1 mRNA (indicative of IRE1 activation), and induction of the PERK pathway evidenced by increased p-eIF2α expression. The UPR chaperones BiP, HSP70, and HSP90 also exhibit increased expression levels in hypothalamic extracts after sleep fragmentation compared with sleep control conditions. This study also found that chronic sleep fragmentation leads to sustained ER stress and induction of leptin resistance (Hakim et al. 2015) identifying a possible mechanism by which sleep fragmentation impacts metabolism.

Whether or not the effect of sleep loss on UPR induction in the periphery is a direct effect or occurs via the brain is not known and remains to be determined.

7.6 UPR Role in Sleep Regulation

Not only is ER stress and the UPR activated with sleep loss, but this pathway also appears to be involved in the sleep homeostatic response. In *Drosophila*, there is an increase in BiP with sleep loss and a diminution of expression with recovery sleep (Naidoo et al. 2007). BiP protein levels return to baseline levels over 24 h with recovery sleep following an almost threefold increase with 6 h of sleep deprivation. Overexpression of BiP through genetic means leads to an increase in the amount of sleep recovered after sleep loss (Naidoo et al. 2007). Whether the altered amounts of recovery sleep when BiP levels are manipulated due to BiP itself or more indirectly through other effects on the UPR remains to be determined. Recent data indicates that reducing ER stress in aged animals improves sleep quality. While inducing ER stress fragments sleep (Brown et al. 2014), treatment with 4-phenyl butyrate (PBA)—a chemical chaperone with properties similar to BiP—consolidates sleep in aging *Drosophila* (Brown et al. 2014). Aged flies, like aged mice, display reduced expression of BiP. Thus, supplementing chaperone levels ameliorates fragmented sleep that is typically observed during aging. PBA treatment also improves the recovery of sleep response to sleep deprivation in aged flies recapitulating the effect of BiP overexpression in young flies (Brown et al. 2014). The effect of the chemical chaperone on sleep is not limited to its effect in aged flies. PBA improves sleep quality in the short sleeping mutant, *sleepless*. Sleep in this extreme short sleeping mutant is also very fragmented (Koh et al. 2006); treatment with PBA both consolidated and increased sleep in the *sleepless* mutant (Brown et al. 2014). In all of the studies described, the chemical chaperone acted analogously to BiP to reduce activation of the PERK and IRE1 pathways. Recent data indicates that the PERK pathway itself has a role in sleep regulation. Pharmacological knockdown of PERK has been shown to reduce sleep in zebrafish and *Drosophila* indicating an evolutionarily conserved mechanism (Ly et al. 2020). This effect on sleep is recapitulated by genetic pan-neuronal knockdown of PERK and more specifically in wake-promoting PDF (pigment dispersing factor) neurons. PERK overexpression within the same PDF circuit increases sleep during the night (Ly et al. 2020). Further, genetic manipulation of PERK within the PDF neurons alters PDF expression suggesting that PERK signaling directly impacts wake-promoting neuropeptide expression, revealing a mechanism through which proteostasis pathways can affect sleep and wake behavior. The impact of the direct manipulation of the IRE1 pathway upon sleep is currently being investigated.

7.7 Concluding Remarks: Implications for Human Diseases

The UPR is an integral part of the cell's protein homeostatic machinery and is critical for cellular integrity. Protein folding, processing, and secretion are central to cell function. The ER is exquisitely sensitive to changes in the cell's milieu. The upregulation of the UPR by sleep disturbances indicates that losing sleep causes a perturbation in the cellular environment of the various tissues of affected organisms and that sleep loss is a cellular stressor. The duration of cellular stress/sleep loss also determines the type of response. Prolonged or chronic sleep loss and fragmentation lead to inflammatory and pro-apoptotic signaling which are detrimental to cell survival.

Sleep loss induces the unfolded protein response in the brain as well as peripheral organs and the implications of UPR induction by sleep loss are multifold. First, ER stress and the UPR are known to be the mechanism underlying B-cell death in diabetes (Hotamisligil 2005). ER stress and the UPR could be the link between metabolic dysfunction and sleep deprivation (see model in Fig. 7.3). Many epidemiological studies have indicated that sleep deprivation leads to insulin resistance. Our study in aged mice indicates that chronic sleep loss reduces insulin sensitivity (Naidoo et al. 2014). ER stress and induction of the UPR have also been implicated in abnormal protein processing and neuronal death in age-associated diseases, as well as neurodegenerative diseases [see reviews Forman et al. (2003), Johnson et al. (2008), Rumpf and Pazos (2013), Hetz and Mollereau (2014), and Scheper and Hoozemans (2015)]. Accumulation of misfolded proteins that lead to alterations in

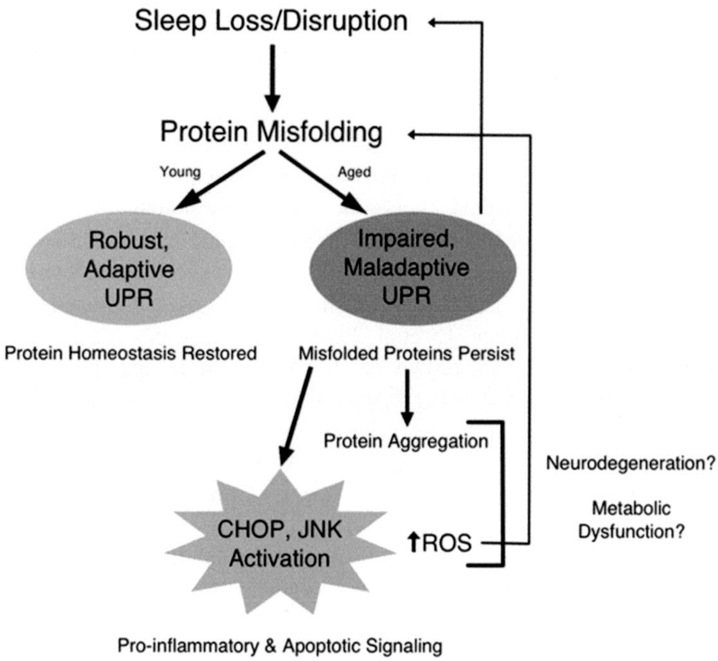

Fig. 7.3 Model of interaction between sleep loss and protein misfolding. Sleep loss/disruption leads to an adaptive robust UPR response in young animals while in aged animals the UPR is impaired. This leads to protein misfolding persisting, activation of pro-inflammatory and pro-apoptotic signaling, and increased oxidative stress that promotes more ER stress and protein misfolding creating a vicious cycle

organelle structure—including the ER—has been described in transgenic models of amyotrophic lateral sclerosis (ALS), Alzheimer's and Huntington's diseases (Rao et al. 2002; Reddy et al. 1999). In addition, markers of ER stress-induced UPR activation have been found in postmortem samples from affected patients as well as in animal models of Alzheimer's, Parkinson's, amyotrophic lateral sclerosis, Huntington's disease, and transmissible spongiform encephalopathies [for reviews, see Rumpf and Pazos (2013) and Hetz and Mollereau (2014)]. Like many other signaling pathways, the UPR suffers from age-related impairments and becomes less effective over the course of the lifespan (Naidoo et al. 2008).

Data from several studies indicate that ER stress and the UPR can mediate the pathogenesis of atherosclerosis and vascular inflammation (Zhang and Kaufman 2008; Santos et al. 2009). Further, UPR activation in hyperhomocysteinemia (HHcy), a common, independent risk factor for cardiovascular disease, has been previously described (Huang et al. 2001; Outinen et al. 1999; Zhang et al. 2001). HHcy activates cleavage of the sterol regulatory element-binding protein (SREBP), which leads to intracellular accumulation of cholesterol (Ron 2001). Overexpression of BiP, which attenuates ER stress, suppresses this activation, implicating the UPR in the process (Kammoun et al. 2009; Basseri and Austin 2012). The role of ER stress in atherosclerosis and other forms of cardiovascular disease likely involves an integrated network of multiple signaling pathways, including, but not limited to inflammation and lipid metabolism.

There is a large body of literature on ER stress and the UPR in cancer (Vandewynckel et al. 2013; Wang and Kaufman 2014; Lee and Hendershot 2006). The adaptive arm of the UPR provides pro-survival mechanisms that have been shown to be conducive to the growth of tumors while suppressing the apoptotic arm of the UPR would contribute to cell death and normal growth. Cancer cells evade the apoptotic pathways by differentially activating the UPR branches (Hersey and Zhang 2008; Pyrko et al. 2007). BiP has been shown to be upregulated in several different types of cancers (Zhang and Zhang 2010) and is implicated in playing a critical cytoprotective role in oncogenesis (Healy et al. 2009; Li and Lee 2006). BiP expression levels have been positively correlated with cerebral tumor malignancy; i.e., the higher the BiP levels, the more malignant the tumor (Zhang and Zhang 2010). BiP has been shown to afford protection against a variety of chemotherapeutic drugs that included: adriamycin, etoposide, 5-FU, and temozolomide (Pyrko et al. 2007; Fu et al. 2007; Lee 2007; Reddy et al. 2003). The role of sleep loss-induced UPR in cancer is not known.

Besides the well-known diseases and disorders discussed above ER stress and the UPR have been implicated in several chronic diseases involving inflammation [for detailed commentary/review see Hotamisligil (2010)]. These include neuromuscular inflammatory diseases, arthritis, and spondyloarthropathies, multiple forms of respiratory inflammation and inflammatory bowel diseases (Mhaille et al. 2008; Hybiske et al. 2007; Colbert et al. 2010; McGuckin et al. 2010). Increasing evidence links ER stress to inflammatory bowel disease; secretory epithelial cells that produce antimicrobial molecules and the mucus barrier, which separate the epithelium from the luminal microbes, are very vulnerable to ER stress (Hasnain et al. 2012). These cells produce high molecular weight cysteine-rich mucins that are prone to misfolding. Genetic studies in rodent models indicate that deficiencies in the UPR pathway lead to spontaneous intestinal inflammation (Heazlewood et al. 2008).

The unfolded protein response comprises a complex set of signaling pathways that serve to maintain ER and protein homeostasis in response to genetic, host (hypoxia, ATP, calcium alterations), microbial and inflammatory stressors. As described above, unresolved ER stress leads to inflammatory signaling that is implicated in a host of human disorders and diseases. Sleep represses activation of ER stress and the UPR and thus serves as a modifiable risk factor for many of the diseases/pathologies downstream of the UPR.

Acknowledgments Thanks to Sarah Ly for helpful comments and edits during the writing of the manuscript and Michael Paolini for assistance with figures. This study was supported by NIH/AG17628.

References

Ameri K, Harris AL. Activating transcription factor 4. Int J Biochem Cell Biol. 2008;40(1):14–21.

Anafi RC, Pellegrino R, Shockley KR, Romer M, Tufik S, Pack AI. Sleep is not just for the brain: transcriptional responses to sleep in peripheral tissues. BMC Genomics. 2013;14:362.

Asada R, Kanemoto S, Kondo S, Saito A, Imaizumi K. J Biochem. 2011;149(5):507–518. https://doi.org/10.1093/jb/mvr041

Ayas NT, White DP, Manson JE, Stampfer MJ, Speizer FE, Malhotra A, et al. A prospective study of sleep duration and coronary heart disease in women. Arch Intern Med. 2003;163(2):205–9.

Basseri S, Austin RC. Endoplasmic reticulum stress and lipid metabolism: mechanisms and therapeutic potential. Biochem Res Int. 2012;2012:841362.

Behrman S, Acosta-Alvear D, Walter P. A CHOP-regulated microRNA controls rhodopsin expression. J Cell Biol. 2011;192(6):919–27.

Biswas S, Mishra P, Mallick BN. Increased apoptosis in rat brain after rapid eye movement sleep loss. Neuroscience. 2006;142(2):315–31.

Bonnet MH. Effect of sleep disruption on sleep, performance, and mood. Sleep. 1985;8(1):11–9.

Brown M, Chan M, Zimmerman J, Pack A, Jackson N, Naidoo N. ER stress alters sleep and sleep homeostasis during aging. Neurobiol Aging. 2014;35(6):1431–41.

Calfon M, Zeng H, Urano F, Till JH, Hubbard SR, Harding HP, et al. IRE1 couples endoplasmic reticulum load to secretory capacity by processing the XBP-1 mRNA. [erratum appears in Nature 2002 Nov 14;420(6912):202]. Nature. 2002;415(6867):92–6.

Carskadon MA, Dement WC. Daytime sleepiness: quantification of a behavioral state. Neurosci Biobehav Rev. 1987;11(3):307–17.

Chan K, Han XD, Kan YW. An important function of Nrf2 in combating oxidative stress: detoxification of acetaminophen. Proc Natl Acad Sci U S A. 2001;98(8):4611–6.

Chee MW, Chuah LY, Venkatraman V, Chan WY, Philip P, Dinges DF. Functional imaging of working memory following normal sleep and after 24 and 35 h of sleep deprivation: correlations of fronto-parietal activation with performance. NeuroImage. 2006;31(1):419–28.

Chen JC, Brunner RL, Ren H, Wassertheil-Smoller S, Larson JC, Levine DW, et al. Sleep duration and risk of ischemic stroke in postmenopausal women. Stroke. 2008;39(12):3185–92.

Cirelli C. How sleep deprivation affects gene expression in the brain: a review of recent findings. J Appl Physiol (1985). 2002;92(1):394–400.

Cirelli C, Tononi G. Gene expression in the brain across the sleep-waking cycle. Brain Res. 2000;885(2):303–21.

Cirelli C, Gutierrez CM, Tononi G. Extensive and divergent effects of sleep and wakefulness on brain gene expression. Neuron. 2004;41(1):35–43.

Cirelli C, Faraguna U, Tononi G. Changes in brain gene expression after long-term sleep deprivation. J Neurochem. 2006;98(5):1632–45.

Colbert RA, DeLay ML, Klenk EI, Layh-Schmitt G. From HLA-B27 to spondyloarthritis: a journey through the ER. Immunol Rev. 2010;233(1):181–202.

Colten HR, Altevogt BM, Institute of Medicine Committee on Sleep Medicine and Research. Sleep disorders and sleep deprivation: an unmet public health problem. Washington, DC: Institute of Medicine, National Academies Press; 2006.

Connor J, Norton R, Ameratunga S, Robinson E, Civil I, Dunn R, et al. Driver sleepiness and risk of serious injury to car occupants: population based case control study. BMJ. 2002;324(7346): 1125.

Conti B, Maier R, Barr AM, Morale MC, Lu X, Sanna PP, et al. Region-specific transcriptional changes following the three antidepressant treatments electro convulsive therapy, sleep deprivation and fluoxetine. Mol Psychiatry. 2007;12(2):167–89.

Cullinan SB, Zhang D, Hannink M, Arvisais E, Kaufman RJ, Diehl JA. Nrf2 is a direct PERK substrate and effector of PERK-dependent cell survival. Mol Cell Biol. 2003;23(20):7198–209.

Dinges D. Probing the limits of functional capability: the effects of sleep loss on short-duration tasks. In: Broughton RJ, Ogilvie RD, editors. Sleep, arousal, and performance. Boston, MA: Birkhäuser; 1992. p. 177–88.

Dufey E, Sepulveda D, Rojas-Rivera D, Hetz C. Cellular mechanisms of endoplasmic reticulum stress signaling in health and disease. 1. An overview. Am J Physiol Cell Physiol. 2014;307(7): C582–94.

Elliott AS, Huber JD, O'Callaghan JP, Rosen CL, Miller DB. A review of sleep deprivation studies evaluating the brain transcriptome. Springerplus. 2014;3:728.

Forman MS, Lee VMY, Trojanowski JQ. 'Unfolding' pathways in neurodegenerative disease. Trends Neurosci. 2003;26(8):407–10.

Fu Y, Li J, Lee AS. GRP78/BiP inhibits endoplasmic reticulum BIK and protects human breast cancer cells against estrogen starvation-induced apoptosis. Cancer Res. 2007;67(8):3734–40.

Goel N, Rao H, Durmer JS, Dinges DF. Neurocognitive consequences of sleep deprivation. Semin Neurol. 2009;29(4):320–39.

Gotoh T, Mori M. Regulation of apoptosis by molecular chaperones. Tanpakushitsu Kakusan Koso. 2004;49(7 Suppl):1010–3.

Grandner MA. Addressing sleep disturbances: an opportunity to prevent cardiometabolic disease? Int Rev Psychiatry. 2014;26(2):155–76.

Grandner MA, Chakravorty S, Perlis ML, Oliver L, Gurubhagavatula I. Habitual sleep duration associated with self-reported and objectively determined cardiometabolic risk factors. Sleep Med. 2014;15(1):42–50.

Hakim F, Wang Y, Carreras A, Hirotsu C, Zhang J, Peris E, et al. Chronic sleep fragmentation during the sleep period induces hypothalamic endoplasmic reticulum stress and PTP1b-mediated leptin resistance in male mice. Sleep. 2015;38(1):31–40.

Harding HP, Zhang YH, Bertolotti A, Zeng HQ, Ron D. Perk is essential for translational regulation and cell survival during the unfolded protein response. Mol Cell. 2000;5(5):897–904.

Hasnain SZ, Lourie R, Das I, Chen AC, McGuckin MA. The interplay between endoplasmic reticulum stress and inflammation. Immunol Cell Biol. 2012;90(3):260–70.

He CH, Gong P, Hu B, Stewart D, Choi ME, Choi AM, et al. Identification of activating transcription factor 4 (ATF4) as an Nrf2-interacting protein. Implication for heme oxygenase-1 gene regulation. J Biol Chem. 2001;276(24):20858–65.

Healy SJ, Gorman AM, Mousavi-Shafaei P, Gupta S, Samali A. Targeting the endoplasmic reticulum-stress response as an anticancer strategy. Eur J Pharmacol. 2009;625(1–3):234–46.

Heazlewood CK, Cook MC, Eri R, Price GR, Tauro SB, Taupin D, et al. Aberrant mucin assembly in mice causes endoplasmic reticulum stress and spontaneous inflammation resembling ulcerative colitis. PLoS Med. 2008;5(3):e54.

Hersey P, Zhang XD. Adaptation to ER stress as a driver of malignancy and resistance to therapy in human melanoma. Pigment Cell Melanoma Res. 2008;21(3):358–67.

Hetz C, Mollereau B. Disturbance of endoplasmic reticulum proteostasis in neurodegenerative diseases. Nat Rev Neurosci. 2014;15(4):233–49.

Hetz C, Martinon F, Rodriguez D, Glimcher LH. The unfolded protein response: integrating stress signals through the stress sensor IRE1alpha. Physiol Rev. 2011;91(4):1219–43.

Hollien J, Weissman JS. Decay of endoplasmic reticulum-localized mRNAs during the unfolded protein response. Science. 2006;313(5783):104–7.

Hotamisligil GS. Role of endoplasmic reticulum stress and c-Jun NH2-terminal kinase pathways in inflammation and origin of obesity and diabetes. Diabetes. 2005;54(Suppl 2):S73–8.

Hotamisligil GS. Endoplasmic reticulum stress and the inflammatory basis of metabolic disease. Cell. 2010;140(6):900–17.

Hu P, Han Z, Couvillon AD, Kaufman RJ, Exton JH. Autocrine tumor necrosis factor alpha links endoplasmic reticulum stress to the membrane death receptor pathway through IRE1alpha-mediated NF-kappaB activation and down-regulation of TRAF2 expression. Mol Cell Biol. 2006;26(8):3071–84.

Huang RF, Huang SM, Lin BS, Wei JS, Liu TZ. Homocysteine thiolactone induces apoptotic DNA damage mediated by increased intracellular hydrogen peroxide and caspase 3 activation in HL-60 cells. Life Sci. 2001;68(25):2799–811.

Hybiske K, Fu Z, Schwarzer C, Tseng J, Do J, Huang N, et al. Effects of cystic fibrosis transmembrane conductance regulator and DeltaF508CFTR on inflammatory response, ER stress, and Ca2+ of airway epithelia. Am J Physiol Lung Cell Mol Physiol. 2007;293(5): L1250–60.

Ishii T, Itoh K, Takahashi S, Sato H, Yanagawa T, Katoh Y, et al. Transcription factor Nrf2 coordinately regulates a group of oxidative stress-inducible genes in macrophages. J Biol Chem. 2000;275(21):16023–9.

Itoh K, Wakabayashi N, Katoh Y, Ishii T, Igarashi K, Engel JD, et al. Keap1 represses nuclear activation of antioxidant responsive elements by Nrf2 through binding to the amino-terminal Neh2 domain. Genes Dev. 1999;13(1):76–86.

Johnson JA, Johnson DA, Kraft AD, Calkins MJ, Jakel RJ, Vargas MR, et al. The Nrf2-ARE pathway: an indicator and modulator of oxidative stress in neurodegeneration. Ann N Y Acad Sci. 2008;1147:61–9.

Jones S, Pfister-Genskow M, Benca RM, Cirelli C. Molecular correlates of sleep and wakefulness in the brain of the white-crowned sparrow. J Neurochem. 2008;105(1):46–62.

Kammoun HL, Chabanon H, Hainault I, Luquet S, Magnan C, Koike T, et al. GRP78 expression inhibits insulin and ER stress-induced SREBP-1c activation and reduces hepatic steatosis in mice. J Clin Invest. 2009;119(5):1201–15.

Kaufman RJ. Orchestrating the unfolded protein response in health and disease. J Clin Invest. 2002;110(10):1389–98.

Knutson KL. Does inadequate sleep play a role in vulnerability to obesity? Am J Hum Biol. 2012;24(3):361–71.

Knutson KL, Van Cauter E, Rathouz PJ, DeLeire T, Lauderdale DS. Trends in the prevalence of short sleepers in the USA: 1975-2006. Sleep. 2010;33(1):37–45.

Koh K, Evans JM, Hendricks JC, Sehgal A. A *Drosophila* model for age-associated changes in sleep: wake cycles. Proc Natl Acad Sci U S A. 2006;103(37):13843–7.

Kuo TH, Williams JA. Acute sleep deprivation enhances post-infection sleep and promotes survival during bacterial infection in *Drosophila*. Sleep. 2014;37(5):859–69.

Kuo TH, Pike DH, Beizaeipour Z, Williams JA. Sleep triggered by an immune response in *Drosophila* is regulated by the circadian clock and requires the NFkappaB Relish. BMC Neurosci. 2010;11:17.

Lee AS. GRP78 induction in cancer: therapeutic and prognostic implications. Cancer Res. 2007;67 (8):3496–9.

Lee AS, Hendershot LM. ER stress and cancer. Cancer Biol Ther. 2006;5(7):721–2.

Lee K, Tirasophon W, Shen X, Michalak M, Prywes R, Okada T, et al. IRE1-mediated unconventional mRNA splicing and S2P-mediated ATF6 cleavage merge to regulate XBP1 in signaling the unfolded protein response. Genes Dev. 2002;16(4):452–66.

Lee K, Neigeborn L, Kaufman RJ. The unfolded protein response is required for haploid tolerance in yeast. J Biol Chem. 2003;278(14):11818–27.

Li J, Lee AS. Stress induction of GRP78/BiP and its role in cancer. Curr Mol Med. 2006;6(1): 45–54.

Ly S, Lee DA, Strus E, Prober DA, Naidoo N. Evolutionarily conserved regulation of sleep by the protein translational regulator PERK. Curr Biol. 2020;30(9):1639–48 e3.

Mackiewicz M, Shockley KR, Romer MA, Galante RJ, Zimmerman JE, Naidoo N, et al. Macromolecule biosynthesis: a key function of sleep. Physiol Genomics. 2007;31(3):441–57.

Maret S, Dorsaz S, Gurcel L, Pradervand S, Petit B, Pfister C, et al. Homer1a is a core brain molecular correlate of sleep loss. Proc Natl Acad Sci U S A. 2007;104(50):20090–5.

Maurel M, Chevet E, Tavernier J, Gerlo S. Getting RIDD of RNA: IRE1 in cell fate regulation. Trends Biochem Sci. 2014;39(5):245–54.

McCullough KD, Martindale JL, Klotz LO, Aw TY, Holbrook NJ. Gadd153 sensitizes cells to endoplasmic reticulum stress by down-regulating Bcl2 and perturbing the cellular redox state. Mol Cell Biol. 2001;21(4):1249–59.

McGuckin MA, Eri RD, Das I, Lourie R, Florin TH. ER stress and the unfolded protein response in intestinal inflammation. Am J Physiol Gastrointest Liver Physiol. 2010;298(6):G820–32.

Mendelson WB, Bergmann BM. Age-dependent changes in recovery sleep after 48 hours of sleep deprivation in rats. Neurobiol Aging. 2000;21(5):689–93.

Mhaille AN, McQuaid S, Windebank A, Cunnea P, McMahon J, Samali A, et al. Increased expression of endoplasmic reticulum stress-related signaling pathway molecules in multiple sclerosis lesions. J Neuropathol Exp Neurol. 2008;67(3):200–11.

Motohashi H, Yamamoto M. Nrf2-Keap1 defines a physiologically important stress response mechanism. Trends Mol Med. 2004;10(11):549–57.

Naidoo N. Cellular stress/the unfolded protein response: relevance to sleep and sleep disorders. Sleep Med Rev. 2009;13(3):195–204.

Naidoo N, Giang W, Galante RJ, Pack AI. Sleep deprivation induces the unfolded protein response in mouse cerebral cortex. J Neurochem. 2005;92(5):1150–7.

Naidoo N, Casiano V, Cater J, Zimmerman J, Pack AI. A role for the molecular chaperone protein BiP/GRP78 in *Drosophila* sleep homeostasis. Sleep. 2007;30(5):557–65.

Naidoo N, Ferber M, Master M, Zhu Y, Pack AI. Aging impairs the unfolded protein response to sleep deprivation and leads to proapoptotic signaling. J Neurosci. 2008;28(26):6539–48.

Naidoo N, Zhu J, Zhu Y, Fenik P, Lian J, Galante R, et al. Endoplasmic reticulum stress in wake-active neurons progresses with aging. Aging Cell. 2011;10(4):640–9.

Naidoo N, Davis JG, Zhu J, Yabumoto M, Singletary K, Brown M, et al. Aging and sleep deprivation induce the unfolded protein response in the pancreas: implications for metabolism. Aging Cell. 2014;13(1):131–41.

Nechushtan A, Smith CL, Hsu YT, Youle RJ. Conformation of the Bax C-terminus regulates subcellular location and cell death. EMBO J. 1999;18(9):2330–41.

Nguyen DT, Kebache S, Fazel A, Wong HN, Jenna S, Emadali A, et al. Nck-dependent activation of extracellular signal-regulated kinase-1 and regulation of cell survival during endoplasmic reticulum stress. Mol Biol Cell. 2004;15(9):4248–60.

Okada T, Yoshida H, Akazawa R, Negishi M, Mori K. Distinct roles of activating transcription factor 6 (ATF6) and double-stranded RNA-activated protein kinase-like endoplasmic reticulum kinase (PERK) in transcription during the mammalian unfolded protein response. Biochem J. 2002;366(Pt 2):585–94.

Outinen PA, Sood SK, Pfeifer SI, Pamidi S, Podor TJ, Li J, et al. Homocysteine-induced endoplasmic reticulum stress and growth arrest leads to specific changes in gene expression in human vascular endothelial cells. Blood. 1999;94(3):959–67.

Pirot P, Naamane N, Libert F, Magnusson NE, Orntoft TF, Cardozo AK, et al. Global profiling of genes modified by endoplasmic reticulum stress in pancreatic beta cells reveals the early degradation of insulin mRNAs. Diabetologia. 2007;50(5):1006–14.

Pyrko P, Schonthal AH, Hofman FM, Chen TC, Lee AS. The unfolded protein response regulator GRP78/BiP as a novel target for increasing chemosensitivity in malignant gliomas. Cancer Res. 2007;67(20):9809–16.

Qureshi AI, Giles WH, Croft JB, Bliwise DL. Habitual sleep patterns and risk for stroke and coronary heart disease: a 10-year follow-up from NHANES I. Neurology. 1997;48(4):904–11.

Rao RV, Peel A, Logvinova A, del Rio G, Hermel E, Yokota T, et al. Coupling endoplasmic reticulum stress to the cell death program: role of the ER chaperone GRP78. FEBS Lett. 2002;514(2–3):122–8.

Reddy PH, Williams M, Tagle DA. Recent advances in understanding the pathogenesis of Huntington's disease. Trends Neurosci. 1999;22(6):248–55.

Reddy RK, Mao C, Baumeister P, Austin RC, Kaufman RJ, Lee AS. Endoplasmic reticulum chaperone protein GRP78 protects cells from apoptosis induced by topoisomerase inhibitors:

role of ATP binding site in suppression of caspase-7 activation. J Biol Chem. 2003;278(23): 20915–24.
Ron D. Hyperhomocysteinemia and function of the endoplasmic reticulum. J Clin Invest. 2001;107 (10):1221–2.
Ron D. Translational control in the endoplasmic reticulum stress response. J Clin Invest. 2002;110 (10):1383–8.
Rumpf RC, Pazos JJ. Optimization of planar self-collimating photonic crystals. J Opt Soc Am A Opt Image Sci Vis. 2013;30(7):1297–304.
Santos CX, Tanaka LY, Wosniak J, Laurindo FR. Mechanisms and implications of reactive oxygen species generation during the unfolded protein response: roles of endoplasmic reticulum oxidoreductases, mitochondrial electron transport, and NADPH oxidase. Antioxid Redox Signal. 2009;11(10):2409–27.
Scheper W, Hoozemans JJ. The unfolded protein response in neurodegenerative diseases: a neuropathological perspective. Acta Neuropathol. 2015;130(3):315–31.
Shaw PJ, Cirelli C, Greenspan RJ, Tononi G. Correlates of sleep and waking in *Drosophila* melanogaster. Science. 2000a;287(5459):1834–7.
Shaw MK, He CY, Roos DS, Tilney LG. Proteasome inhibitors block intracellular growth and replication of *Toxoplasma gondii*. Parasitology. 2000b;121(Pt 1):35–47.
Shiromani PJ, Lu J, Wagner D, Thakkar J, Greco MA, Basheer R, et al. Compensatory sleep response to 12 h wakefulness in young and old rats. Am J Physiol Regul Integr Comp Physiol. 2000;278(1):R125–33.
Spiegel K, Knutson K, Leproult R, Tasali E, Van Cauter E. Sleep loss: a novel risk factor for insulin resistance and Type 2 diabetes. J Appl Physiol (1985). 2005;99(5):2008–19.
Terao A, Steininger TL, Hyder K, Apte-Deshpande A, Ding J, Rishipathak D, et al. Differential increase in the expression of heat shock protein family members during sleep deprivation and during sleep. Neuroscience. 2003;116(1):187–200.
Terao A, Wisor JP, Peyron C, Apte-Deshpande A, Wurts SW, Edgar DM, et al. Gene expression in the rat brain during sleep deprivation and recovery sleep: an Affymetrix GeneChip study. Neuroscience. 2006;137(2):593–605.
Ulmer CS, Calhoun PS, Edinger JD, Wagner HR, Beckham JC. Sleep disturbance and baroreceptor sensitivity in women with posttraumatic stress disorder. J Trauma Stress. 2009;22(6):643–7.
Upton JP, Wang L, Han D, Wang ES, Huskey NE, Lim L, et al. IRE1alpha cleaves select microRNAs during ER stress to derepress translation of proapoptotic Caspase-2. Science. 2012;338(6108):818–22.
Urano F, Bertolotti A, Ron D. IRE1 and efferent signaling from the endoplasmic reticulum. J Cell Sci. 2000;113(Pt 21):3697–702.
Vandewynckel YP, Laukens D, Geerts A, Bogaerts E, Paridaens A, Verhelst X, et al. The paradox of the unfolded protein response in cancer. Anticancer Res. 2013;33(11):4683–94.
Venugopal R, Jaiswal AK. Nrf1 and Nrf2 positively and c-Fos and Fra1 negatively regulate the human antioxidant response element-mediated expression of NAD(P)H: quinone oxidoreductase1 gene. Proc Natl Acad Sci U S A. 1996;93(25):14960–5.
Walter P, Ron D. The unfolded protein response: from stress pathway to homeostatic regulation. Science. 2011;334(6059):1081–6.
Wang M, Kaufman RJ. The impact of the endoplasmic reticulum protein-folding environment on cancer development. Nat Rev Cancer. 2014;14(9):581–97.
Welsh DK, Richardson GS, Dement WC. Effect of age on the circadian pattern of sleep and wakefulness in the mouse. J Gerontol. 1986;41(5):579–86.
Williams JA, Sathyanarayanan S, Hendricks JC, Sehgal A. Interaction between sleep and the immune response in *Drosophila*: a role for the NFkappaB relish. Sleep. 2007;30(4):389–400.
Yoshida H, Haze K, Yanagi H, Yura T, Mori K. Identification of the cis-acting endoplasmic reticulum stress response element responsible for transcriptional induction of mammalian glucose-regulated proteins. Involvement of basic leucine zipper transcription factors. [erratum appears in J Biol Chem 1999 Jan 22;274(4):2592]. J Biol Chem. 1998;273(50):33741–9.

Yoshida H, Matsui T, Yamamoto A, Okada T, Mori K. XBP1 mRNA is induced by ATF6 and spliced by IRE1 in response to ER stress to produce a highly active transcription factor. Cell. 2001;107(7):881–91.

Yoshida H, Matsui T, Hosokawa N, Kaufman RJ, Nagata K, Mori K. A time-dependent phase shift in the mammalian unfolded protein response. Dev Cell. 2003;4(2):265–71.

Zhang K, Kaufman RJ. From endoplasmic-reticulum stress to the inflammatory response. Nature. 2008;454(7203):455–62.

Zhang LH, Zhang X. Roles of GRP78 in physiology and cancer. J Cell Biochem. 2010;110(6):1299–305.

Zhang C, Cai Y, Adachi MT, Oshiro S, Aso T, Kaufman RJ, et al. Homocysteine induces programmed cell death in human vascular endothelial cells through activation of the unfolded protein response. J Biol Chem. 2001;276(38):35867–74.

Zhu Y, Fenik P, Zhan G, Sanfillipo-Cohn B, Naidoo N, Veasey SC. Eif-2a protects brainstem motoneurons in a murine model of sleep apnea. J Neurosci. 2008;28(9):2168–78.

Part III
Sleep Apnea

Chapter 8
Biological and Genetic Mechanisms of Sleepiness in Obstructive Sleep Apnea and Cardiovascular Disease

Victoria M. Pak

Abstract This chapter discusses biological and genetic mechanisms of sleepiness within the oxidative stress and inflammatory pathways focusing on the link to cardiovascular disease risk and future directions in translational medicine. Specifically, the focus is on the underlying hypothesis that mechanisms of sleepiness and cardiovascular disease share common molecular pathways; thus, biological and genetic risk factors for sleepiness may also predict cardiovascular disease risk. Based on the biological evidence, emphasis will be on oxidative stress and the resulting downstream inflammation. Genetic variation may also be involved in the etiology of inflammation and oxidative stress which may impact sleepiness symptoms and cardiovascular disease risk. As the mechanisms of excessive daytime sleepiness associated with obstructive sleep apnea and how this plays a role in cardiovascular disease risk is unknown, exploring the potential mechanisms will be an important avenue to guide treatment options based on data from the molecular level.

Keywords Obstructive sleep apnea · Sleepiness · Biomarkers · Genetics · Cardiovascular disease

8.1 Introduction

OSA is characterized by repeated prolonged pauses in breathing during sleep and is defined by the number of episodes of obstructive apnea (cessation of breathing) and hypopnea (transient reduction in airflow) per hour of sleep, known as the Apnea-Hypopnea Index, which provides a measure of the degree of departure from normal sleep physiology (Young et al. 2002). In patients with OSA, approximately 23% of

V. M. Pak (✉)
Nell Hodgson Woodruff School of Nursing, Emory University, Atlanta, GA, USA

Department of Epidemiology, Rollins School of Public Health, Emory University, Atlanta, GA, USA
e-mail: Victoria.m.pak@emory.edu

A. I. Pack, Q. Y. Li (eds.), *Sleep and its Disorders*, Translational Medicine Research,
https://doi.org/10.1007/978-94-024-2168-2_8

women and 16% of men experience excessive daytime sleepiness (EDS) (Young et al. 1993). EDS can lead to substantial impairment in quality of life and cognitive function (Findley et al. 1986). However, not all OSA patients develop EDS at any level of disease severity (Engleman et al. 1997), which suggests biological and genetic factors may be involved.

EDS is defined in the International Classification of Sleep Disorders (ICSD), based on behavior of falling asleep, or difficulty maintaining alertness or wakefulness and unintentionally falling asleep. EDS is the most common daytime symptom of OSA (Pagel 2009). Daytime sleepiness associated with OSA has been found to be the only sleep disturbance symptom associated with total and cardiovascular mortality in adults, although the mechanism is unidentified (Newman et al. 2000). The mechanism for the development of EDS in OSA and how this may play a role in cardiovascular risk is unknown. Understanding mechanisms of EDS associated with OSA have great significance for public health in order to improve treatment options, symptom management, and reduce cardiovascular risk.

8.2 Genetic and Biological Markers of Oxidative Stress and Inflammation in OSA

I review selected genetic and biological markers of oxidative stress and inflammation that show promise in translational medicine. Exploration of these select pathways will identify future molecular targets in order to improve treatment options and reduce cardiovascular disease risk. There is a need for further studies to examine the utility of the most promising biomarkers to predict sleepiness phenotype and response to treatment.

8.2.1 Oxidative Stress in OSA

Oxidative stress is characterized by an imbalance between oxidant and antioxidant mechanisms. An increased generation of ROS in vivo can lead to the depletion of antioxidants, which can then be measured as an index of oxidative stress (Bast et al. 1991). Sleep disorders, such as OSA, have been shown to cause low-grade inflammation and oxidative stress (Tsaluchidu et al. 2008; Patel et al. 2009). Intermittent hypoxia (repeated episodes of hypoxia followed by reoxygenation) occurs in the context of OSA and is proposed to result in oxidative stress (Lavie et al. 2004; Kim et al. 2000). It will be important for future studies to explore biomarkers of oxidative stress, for instance measuring urinary F2-isoprostane, which is a specific end product of arachidonic acid peroxidation catalyzed by free radicals, and considered a reliable marker of oxidative stress (Morrow and Roberts 2002; Halliwell and Whiteman 2004). An efficient antioxidant defense system is also important in the control of oxidative stress caused by free radicals continuously generated in the body. It is uncertain whether increased antioxidant nutrient intake impacts oxidative stress in OSA patients, as studies in this area are scarce. The effects of oral administration of antioxidants on polysomnographic parameters and plasma lipid peroxidation (a marker of oxidative stress) have been explored in OSA patients, demonstrating reduced oxidation and decreased subjective sleepiness as measured by Epworth Sleepiness Scale (Singh et al. 2009). In addition, some studies have demonstrated that increased antioxidant levels limit the clinical expression of coronary artery disease, but this has not been explored in OSA patients (Solfrizzi et al. 2003; Gray et al. 2003). It is unknown whether an increase in antioxidant activity will protect against the cardiovascular consequences of OSA. No prospective studies have explored antioxidant intake and the impact on adhesion molecules and cardiovascular outcomes in patients with OSA. However, if the endothelial dysfunction characteristic of OSA is a result of oxidative stress, it can potentially be reversed by administration of antioxidants (Pak et al. 2014), which is an area that warrants further studies.

8.2.2 Select Candidate Gene Studies on Oxidative Stress and Sleepiness

Several candidate genes may be involved in oxidative stress pathway and sleepiness symptoms.

NOX-2 (CYBB Gene) Measurable amounts of reactive oxygen species (ROS) in the serum can be largely attributed to NOX-2 (Violi et al. 2006). The observed variability in ROS might be partly due to genetic variability of the NOX-2 enzymatic complex (Bedard et al. 2009). Increased levels of ROS in rodent models are associated with the presence of intermittent hypoxia-induced dysfunction of the central nervous system (Wang et al. 2010). Association studies exploring genetic variability in this gene and the link to sleep symptoms and cardiovascular risk will be important.

NOX p22phox Gene Overproduction of ROS is associated with neurodegenerative disorders and cardiovascular impairments (Tabner et al. 2005). The major sources of ROS in the vasculature are the NOX oxidases whose sole function is to generate ROS (Selemidis et al. 2008). Several SNPs related to NOX expression or activity have been identified (Gozal et al. 2012; Pierola et al. 2011). SNPs in the NOX p22phox gene may account for differences among OSA children with and without cognitive deficits (Gozal et al. 2012). A previous study has shown that the SNP rs4673 was associated with reduced levels of NOX activity and 8-OH-dG urinary concentrations, and accounted for part of the discrepant phenotypic expression in cognitive functioning in the context of pediatric OSA (Gozal et al. 2012). Thus, the differential cognitive symptoms in the context of OSA could partly be explained by the presence of significantly higher levels of oxidative stress among children with cognitive deficits. Future studies should consider the potential link between oxidative stress and sleepiness symptoms and explore SNPs in the NOX p22phox gene.

8.2.3 Inflammation in OSA

Inflammation is known to be upregulated by oxidative stress (Pak et al. 2014). Specifically, oxidative stress causes upregulation of inflammatory markers adhesion molecules such as Intercellular Adhesion Molecule-1 (ICAM-1) and cytokines (e.g., TNF-α) (Kim et al. 2000; Pak et al. 2014; Xu et al. 2004; Yamauchi and Kimura 2008; Sawa et al. 2007; Arnaud et al. 2011). Inflammation is recognized as playing a role in all stages of the atherosclerotic disease process. Thus, the evaluation of circulating biomarkers of inflammation (ICAM-1, TNF-α) will be important to aid in identifying patients at high risk for future cardiovascular events (Blankenberg et al. 2003). The few studies conducted have demonstrated higher levels of ICAM-1 in OSA patients compared to controls (Pak et al. 2014; Ursavas et al. 2007; Ohga et al. 1999; El-Solh et al. 2002; Carpagnano et al. 2010). Higher levels of ICAM-1 are a consistent predictor of cardiovascular risk within initially healthy populations (Blankenberg et al. 2001, 2003). Thus, future studies exploring sleep apneic patients and sleepiness should also consider incorporating markers of inflammation such as ICAM-1 and TNF-α.

8.2.4 Relevant Candidate Gene Studies on Inflammation and Sleepiness

Tumor Necrosis Factor (TNF)-α Gene TNF-α is a pro-inflammatory cytokine that plays a role in initiating sleep and regulating time spent in restorative sleep (Krueger 2008). Increased production of TNF-α in vitro and in vivo in response to specific challenges has been associated with a functional variant in the TNF-α gene at position −308 in the promoter region. Gozal et al. (2010) discovered that TNF-α levels are increased in OSA children harboring this TNF-α variant (Gozal et al. 2010). Further, those with this SNP have been shown to demonstrate significant increases in excessive daytime sleepiness symptoms compared to individuals with OSA who do not have this variant (Khalyfa et al. 2011). TNF-α also enhances the production of reactive oxygen species, as well as inducible nitric oxide, and decreases myocardial contractility (Das 2001). It is plausible that genetic variation in the TNF-α gene increases inflammation and also oxidative stress, thus increasing sleepiness symptoms.

PDE4D Gene A prior genome-wide association (GWAS) study exploring sleep and circadian phenotypes in 749 Framingham Heart Study participants, found SNP (rs12522161) with genome-wide significance on the intron of PDE4D associated with sleepiness (Gottlieb et al. 2007). A candidate gene analysis in 918 adults from the general population of the São Paulo Epidemiologic Sleep Study (EPISONO) in São Paulo, Brazil, found a novel association between the C allele of the rs12522161 SNP on PDE4D and a decreased likelihood of sleepiness (Pak et al. 2018a). PDE4D is located on chromosome 5 and encodes a cAMP-specific phosphodiesterase (found in inflammatory and immune cells) and is a potential target for treating inflammatory diseases. Phosphodiesterase 4 (PDE4) is also a family of enzymes highly distributed in the hippocampus, frontal cortex, olfactory bulb, and cerebellum (Xu et al. 2011). As such, it plays a significant role in cellular communication and has been identified as a prominent regulator of mood, cognition, and inflammatory pathways (Zhang et al. 2000, 2002; Sekut et al. 1995).

8.2.5 Cardiovascular Sequelae of OSA and Sleepiness

Although the mechanism for the initiation of cardiovascular disease in OSA has not been fully established, the generally accepted theory is the intermittent hypoxia (IH) produced by frequent respiratory events (Pak et al. 2014). Pre-atherosclerotic remodeling of large arteries with enlarged intima media thickness under intermittent hypoxic conditions were found to be inflammatory in nature with biochemical evidence (greater nuclear factor [NF]-kB expression) (Arnaud et al. 2011). The link of OSA to cardiovascular sequelae is demonstrated in rodent models, where intermittent hypoxia produces a moderate BP elevation starting from 5 to 8 days after onset (Dematteis et al. 2009). Although daytime sleepiness associated with OSA is the only sleep disturbance symptom associated with total and cardiovascular mortality in adults, the factors involved in this link remain unidentified (Newman et al. 2000). In an exploratory case control study of 36 subjects exploring associations between subjective sleepiness and metabolite concentrations within the oxidative and inflammatory pathways, choline was found to be significantly lower in sleepy subjects (ESS $\geq$ 10) compared with non-sleepy subjects. Other markers with suggestive differences ($P < 0.1$) included isovalerylcarnitine, alpha-amino adipic acid, sphingosine 1 phosphate, aspartic acid, propionylcarnitine, and ceramides (fatty acids; C14–C16 and C–18) (Pak et al. 2018b). One prior study has specifically measured sleepiness and objective cardiovascular risk in OSA (Choi et al. 2006; Empana et al. 2009). Choi et al. found sleepiness independently associated with decreased cardiac function as assessed by impedance cardiography in 86 patients with suspected OSA who then underwent confirmatory diagnostic polysomnography (Choi et al. 2006). However, this study was limited by a small sample size, self-report of sleepiness, and not controlling for obesity or hypertension. Furthermore, impedance cardiography is not easily reproducible as the results are highly dependent on the skill of the operator. In another study by Empana et al., investigators found that elderly people with excessive daytime sleepiness had a 49% increase in relative risk of cardiovascular death and a 33% increase in relative risk of overall

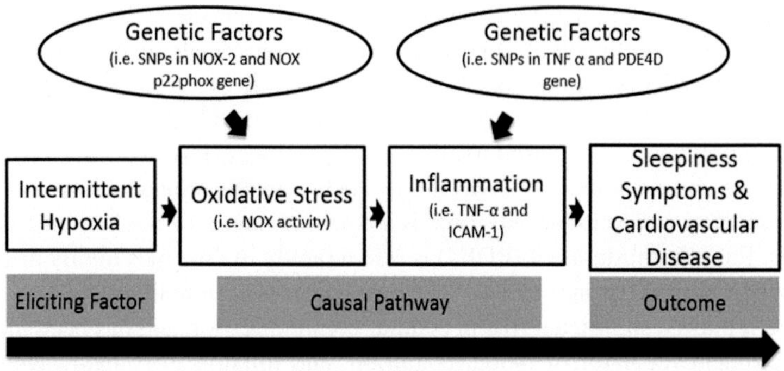

Fig. 8.1 Schematic illustration of the proposed role of oxidative stress and inflammation in OSA, potential molecular targets, and genetic factors in the pathophysiology of sleepiness and cardiovascular disease

death (Empana et al. 2009). This study is limited by self-reported patient responses and the use of ultrasonography of the carotid arteries, which are highly operator dependent. In addition, this study did not specifically examine OSA. Thus, there may be a confounding effect of underlying sleep apnea syndrome.

Future studies are needed to extend these study findings using more robust measures of both sleepiness and cardiovascular risk. The Psychomotor Vigilance Test (PVT) is a gold standard for the assessment of neurobehavioral impairment associated with sleep loss (Dinges et al. 1994). This is a simple test (10-min test) used to classify subjects as sleepy (PVT $\geq$ 2 lapses on systematic 3 trials) vs. non-sleepy (PVT $<$ 2 on systematic 3 trials) by objective criteria. PVT is a simple, portable reaction time test designed to evaluate the ability to sustain attention and measures reaction time to signals presented at random intervals over a brief period of testing (Dinges and Powell 1985). Ambulatory Blood Pressure Monitoring is increasingly recognized as a valuable tool to refine prediction of cardiovascular risk related to blood pressure (Verdecchia et al. 2007). The measurement of Pulse Wave Velocity is accepted as a simple and reproducible method that is a "gold standard" index to measure arterial stiffness along with 24-h ambulatory blood pressure (Kohler et al. 2011). The use of robust measures of sleepiness and cardiovascular disease risk will be important in clarifying the cardiovascular sequelae associated with sleepiness symptoms. See Fig. 8.1 for schematic and biological pathways.

8.3 Potential Therapies for Sleepiness in Sleep Apnea

In understanding how sleepiness associated with sleep apnea is related to cardiovascular disease, the utility of markers of inflammation should be considered. In the development of atherosclerosis and cardiovascular disease, Leukocyte adhesion to

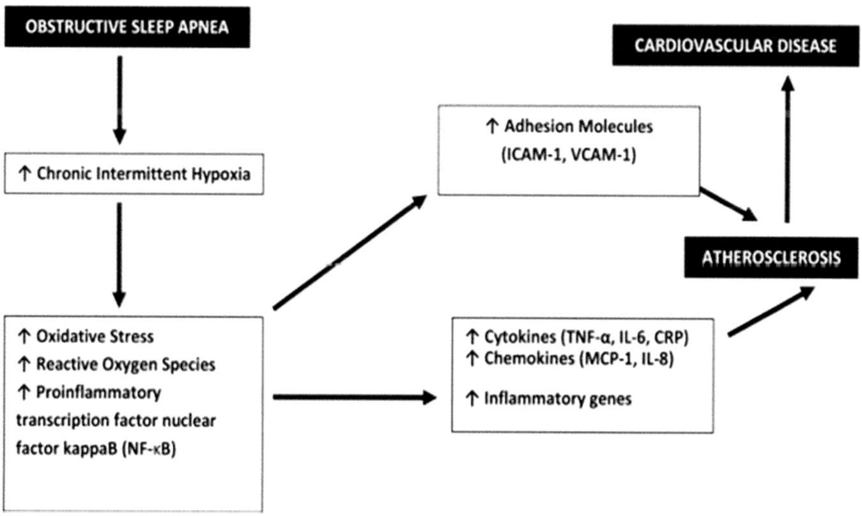

Fig. 8.2 Schematic illustration of obstructive sleep apnea and the link to atherosclerosis and cardiovascular disease, including the role of adhesion molecules. *CRP* C-reactive protein, *ICAM-1* intercellular adhesion molecule 1, *IL-6* interleukin-6, *IL-8* interleukin-8, *MCP-1* monocyte chemoattractant protein-1, *NF-κ B* nuclear factor-kappa B, *TNF-α* tumor necrosis factor α, *VCAM-1* vascular cell adhesion molecule-1. Reproduced from Pak et al. (2014)

vascular endothelial cells and migration into the vessel wall is critical in the development of atherosclerosis (Pak et al. 2014). The repeated episodes of hypoxia followed by reoxygenation that is characteristic of OSA is proposed to result in oxidative stress and increased production of reactive oxygen species (Lavie et al. 2004), see Fig. 8.2.

Continuous positive airway pressure treatment has been shown to have a beneficial impact on blood pressure only in patients with OSA who were sleepy and not in non-sleepy patients (Robinson et al. 2004). These results suggest that daytime sleepiness may be a significant factor in the pathogenesis of cardiovascular disease. This finding also reinforces the theory that elevated inflammation and oxidative stress in sleep apnea patients lead to sleepiness, thus increasing cardiovascular disease risk.

The logical focus of potential therapies would be to target oxidative stress and inflammation which causes the increase in cardiovascular disease risk. For instance, potential therapies for reducing circulating adhesion molecules to diminish cardiovascular disease in OSA include CPAP and antioxidant supplementation (Pak et al. 2014). Specific molecular targets include intercellular adhesion molecule-1 (ICAM-1) and vascular cell adhesion molecule-1 (VCAM-1), which are expressed on cell surfaces and found in their soluble forms in the plasma (Ballantyne and Entman 2002). Leukocyte adhesion to vascular endothelial cells and migration into the vessel wall is critical in the development of atherosclerosis, and elevated levels of adhesion molecules have been demonstrated in subjects with OSA (Ursavas et al. 2007; Ohga

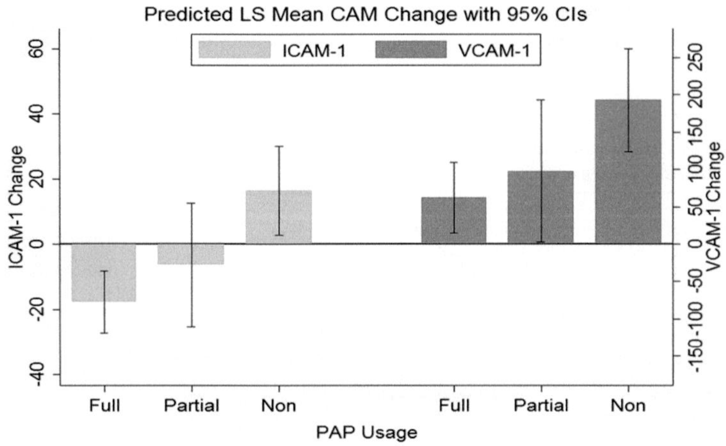

Fig. 8.3 Predicted least squares mean change from baseline in entire population. The predicted least squares mean change in ICAM-1 and VCAM-1 levels for each PAP usage group are presented in the overall population, along with the associated 95% confidence intervals. Results are adjusted for baseline ICAM-1 or VCAM-1 levels, BMI, change in BMI, hypertension at baseline and follow-up and statin use at baseline and follow-up (for VCAM-1 change only). Estimates with 95% confidence intervals not crossing 0 represent significant changes. $^{*}P < 0.05$. *LS* least squares. Reproduced from Pak et al. (2015)

et al. 1999, 2003; El-Solh et al. 2002; Chin et al. 2000; Zamarron et al. 2011; Zamarron-Sanz et al. 2006). Positive airway pressure (PAP) therapy may reduce ICAM-1 levels in OSA patients (Chin et al. 2000; Ohga et al. 2003; Zamarron et al. 2011). One prior study has examined VCAM-1, finding no PAP treatment effect (Chin et al. 2000). However, these studies had small samples and relatively short duration, and did not directly address the role of obesity on these relationships. See Fig. 8.3 for an illustration of how in a moderate-to-severe OSA population, adequate PAP usage limits significant increases in both ICAM-1 and VCAM-1 levels observed in PAP nonusers after 2 years (Pak et al. 2015). As obesity and OSA often coexist, limiting these increases with PAP usage may help to decrease the rate of progression of OSA-related cardiovascular disease. For ICAM-1, full usage decreased levels, with the largest effect occurring in the most obese subjects (Pak et al. 2015). For VCAM-1, increased levels over 2 years were observed for all PAP groups, but nonusers had much larger increases than full users. Although the VCAM-1 association appeared independent of obesity, larger increases in nonusers were again seen in the most obese. Obesity is an important risk factor for OSA (Young et al. 1993), and their shared pathways of oxidative stress and inflammation make discerning independent roles of obesity and OSA in cardiovascular disease difficult (Arnardottir et al. 2009). Future studies should consider the role of obesity when exploring the relationship between sleepiness and cardiovascular disease risk and the effect of treatment.

The exploration of subgroups to clarify the genetic and biological profile that ultimately predicts cardiovascular disease risk and explore the effects of intervention on characterized subgroups of susceptibility to sleepiness will be crucial. The studies would target the question of whether the benefits of CPAP (reduced cardiovascular markers, i.e., ICAM-1) are only found to be reduced in those with genetic sleepiness susceptibility. Randomized trials will be needed in order to determine differences in sleepy genotype and nonsleepy genotype to determine the improvement in symptoms and cardiovascular risk with CPAP and the effect of obesity on these relationships. If the cardiovascular benefits of CPAP are reduced in those with genetic sleepiness susceptibility, then treatment strategies may target those molecules [i.e., anti-ICAM-1 antibodies and antioxidants (Pak et al. 2014)].

8.4 Summary and Future Research Implications

Overall, the preliminary research findings suggest that biological and genetic variation is involved in the etiology of inflammation and oxidative stress may potentially impact sleepiness symptoms and cardiovascular disease risk. Replication of these findings, in combination with exploring how interventions targeting specific molecules within the oxidative stress and inflammatory pathway modulates an individual's susceptibility, will be important to guide treatment and management of symptoms and the prevention of cardiovascular disease. Replication of current genetic findings remains a challenge, however, with consistent control of confounders, consistent phenotype definitions, larger sample sizes, and consideration of population ethnicity, replication of findings will become more attainable.

References

Arnardottir ES, Mackiewicz M, Gislason T, Teff KL, Pack AI. Molecular signatures of obstructive sleep apnea in adults: a review and perspective. Sleep. 2009;32(4):447–70.

Arnaud C, Beguin PC, Lantuejoul S, Pepin JL, Guillermet C, Pelli G, et al. The inflammatory preatherosclerotic remodeling induced by intermittent hypoxia is attenuated by RANTES/CCL5 inhibition. Am J Respir Crit Care Med. 2011;184(6):724–31.

Ballantyne CM, Entman ML. Soluble adhesion molecules and the search for biomarkers for atherosclerosis. Circulation. 2002;106(7):766–7.

Bast A, Haenen GR, Doelman CJ. Oxidants and antioxidants: state of the art. Am J Med. 1991;91 (3C):2S–13S.

Bedard K, Attar H, Bonnefont J, Jaquet V, Borel C, Plastre O, et al. Three common polymorphisms in the CYBA gene form a haplotype associated with decreased ROS generation. Hum Mutat. 2009;30(7):1123–33.

Blankenberg S, Rupprecht HJ, Bickel C, Peetz D, Hafner G, Tiret L, et al. Circulating cell adhesion molecules and death in patients with coronary artery disease. Circulation. 2001;104(12): 1336–42.

Blankenberg S, Barbaux S, Tiret L. Adhesion molecules and atherosclerosis. Atherosclerosis. 2003;170(2):191–203.

Carpagnano GE, Spanevello A, Sabato R, Depalo A, Palladino GP, Bergantino L, et al. Systemic and airway inflammation in sleep apnea and obesity: the role of ICAM-1 and IL-8. Transl Res. 2010;155(1):35–43.

Chin K, Nakamura T, Shimizu K, Mishima M, Nakamura T, Miyasaka M, et al. Effects of nasal continuous positive airway pressure on soluble cell adhesion molecules in patients with obstructive sleep apnea syndrome. Am J Med. 2000;109(7):562–7.

Choi JB, Nelesen R, Loredo JS, Mills PJ, Ancoli-Israel S, Ziegler MG, et al. Sleepiness in obstructive sleep apnea: a harbinger of impaired cardiac function? Sleep. 2006;29(12):1531–6.

Das UN. Is obesity an inflammatory condition? Nutrition. 2001;17(11–12):953–66.

Dematteis M, Godin-Ribuot D, Arnaud C, Ribuot C, Stanke-Labesque F, Pepin JL, et al. Cardiovascular consequences of sleep-disordered breathing: contribution of animal models to understanding the human disease. ILAR J. 2009;50(3):262–81.

Dinges DF, Powell JW. Microcomputer analyses of performance on a portable, simple visual Rt task during sustained operations. Behav Res Methods Instrum Comput. 1985;17(6):652–5.

Dinges DF, Douglas SD, Zaugg L, Campbell DE, McMann JM, Whitehouse WG, et al. Leukocytosis and natural killer cell function parallel neurobehavioral fatigue induced by 64 hours of sleep deprivation. J Clin Invest. 1994;93(5):1930–9.

El-Solh AA, Mador MJ, Sikka P, Dhillon RS, Amsterdam D, Grant BJ. Adhesion molecules in patients with coronary artery disease and moderate-to-severe obstructive sleep apnea. Chest. 2002;121(5):1541–7.

Empana JP, Dauvilliers Y, Dartigues JF, Ritchie K, Gariepy J, Jouven X, et al. Excessive daytime sleepiness is an independent risk indicator for cardiovascular mortality in community-dwelling elderly: the three city study. Stroke. 2009;40(4):1219–24.

Engleman HM, Hirst WS, Douglas NJ. Under reporting of sleepiness and driving impairment in patients with sleep apnoea/hypopnoea syndrome. J Sleep Res. 1997;6(4):272–5.

Findley LJ, Barth JT, Powers DC, Wilhoit SC, Boyd DG, Suratt PM. Cognitive impairment in patients with obstructive sleep apnea and associated hypoxemia. Chest. 1986;90(5):686–90.

Gottlieb DJ, O'Connor GT, Wilk JB. Genome-wide association of sleep and circadian phenotypes. BMC Med Genet. 2007;8(Suppl 1(Journal Article)):S9.

Gozal D, Serpero LD, Kheirandish-Gozal L, Capdevila OS, Khalyfa A, Tauman R. Sleep measures and morning plasma TNF-alpha levels in children with sleep-disordered breathing. Sleep. 2010;33(3):319–25.

Gozal D, Khalyfa A, Capdevila OS, Kheirandish-Gozal L, Khalyfa AA, Kim J. Cognitive function in prepubertal children with obstructive sleep apnea: a modifying role for NADPH oxidase p22 subunit gene polymorphisms? Antioxid Redox Signal. 2012;16(2):171–7.

Gray SL, Hanlon JT, Landerman LR, Artz M, Schmader KE, Fillenbaum GG. Is antioxidant use protective of cognitive function in the community-dwelling elderly? Am J Geriatr Pharmacother. 2003;1(1):3–10.

Halliwell B, Whiteman M. Measuring reactive species and oxidative damage in vivo and in cell culture: how should you do it and what do the results mean? Br J Pharmacol. 2004;142(2):231–55.

Khalyfa A, Serpero LD, Kheirandish-Gozal L, Capdevila OS, Gozal D. TNF-alpha gene polymorphisms and excessive daytime sleepiness in pediatric obstructive sleep apnea. J Pediatr. 2011;158(1):77–82.

Kim CD, Kim YK, Lee SH, Hong KW. Rebamipide inhibits neutrophil adhesion to hypoxia/reoxygenation-stimulated endothelial cells via nuclear factor-kappaB-dependent pathway. J Pharmacol Exp Ther. 2000;294(3):864–9.

Kohler M, Stoewhas AC, Ayers L, Senn O, Bloch KE, Russi EW, et al. Effects of continuous positive airway pressure therapy withdrawal in patients with obstructive sleep apnea: a randomized controlled trial. Am J Respir Crit Care Med. 2011;184(10):1192–9.

Krueger JM. The role of cytokines in sleep regulation. Curr Pharm Des. 2008;14(32):3408–16.

Lavie L, Vishnevsky A, Lavie P. Evidence for lipid peroxidation in obstructive sleep apnea. Sleep. 2004;27(1):123–8.

Morrow JD, Roberts LJ. The isoprostanes: their role as an index of oxidant stress status in human pulmonary disease. Am J Respir Crit Care Med. 2002;166(12 Pt 2):S25–30.

Newman AB, Spiekerman CF, Enright P, Lefkowitz D, Manolio T, Reynolds CF, et al. Daytime sleepiness predicts mortality and cardiovascular disease in older adults. The Cardiovascular Health Study Research Group. J Am Geriatr Soc. 2000;48(2):115–23.

Ohga E, Nagase T, Tomita T, Teramoto S, Matsuse T, Katayama H, et al. Increased levels of circulating ICAM-1, VCAM-1, and L-selectin in obstructive sleep apnea syndrome. J Appl Physiol (1985). 1999;87(1):10–4.

Ohga E, Tomita T, Wada H, Yamamoto H, Nagase T, Ouchi Y. Effects of obstructive sleep apnea on circulating ICAM-1, IL-8, and MCP-1. J Appl Physiol (1985). 2003;94(1):179–84.

Pagel JF. Excessive daytime sleepiness. Am Fam Physician. 2009;79(5):391–6.

Pak VM, Grandner MA, Pack AI. Circulating adhesion molecules in obstructive sleep apnea and cardiovascular disease. Sleep Med Rev. 2014;18(1):25–34.

Pak VM, Keenan BT, Jackson N, Grandner MA, Maislin G, Teff K, et al. Adhesion molecule increases in sleep apnea: beneficial effect of positive airway pressure and moderation by obesity. Int J Obes. 2015;39(3):472–9.

Pak VM, Mazzotti DR, Keenan BT, Hirotsu C, Gehrman P, Bittencourt L, et al. Candidate gene analysis in the Sao Paulo Epidemiologic Sleep Study (EPISONO) shows an association of variant in PDE4D and sleepiness. Sleep Med. 2018a;47:106–12.

Pak VM, Dai F, Keenan BT, Gooneratne NS, Pack AI. Lower plasma choline levels are associated with sleepiness symptoms. Sleep Med. 2018b;44:89–96.

Patel SR, Zhu X, Storfer-Isser A, Mehra R, Jenny NS, Tracy R, et al. Sleep duration and biomarkers of inflammation. Sleep. 2009;32(2):200–4.

Pierola J, Alemany A, Yanez A, de-la-Pena M, Sanchez-de-la-Torre M, Esquinas C, et al. NADPH oxidase p22phox polymorphisms and oxidative stress in patients with obstructive sleep apnoea. Respir Med. 2011;105(11):1748–54.

Robinson GV, Smith DM, Langford BA, Davies RJO, Stradling JR. CPAP does not reduce 24 hour blood pressure in hypertensive obstructive sleep apnoea patients without daytime sleepiness. Thorax. 2004;59(1):16.

Sawa Y, Sugimoto Y, Ueki T, Ishikawa H, Sato A, Nagato T, et al. Effects of TNF-alpha on leukocyte adhesion molecule expressions in cultured human lymphatic endothelium. J Histochem Cytochem. 2007;55(7):721–33.

Sekut L, Yarnall D, Stimpson SA, Noel LS, Bateman-Fite R, Clark RL, et al. Anti-inflammatory activity of phosphodiesterase (PDE) IV inhibitors in acute and chronic models of inflammation. Clin Exp Immunol. 1995;100(1):126–32.

Selemidis S, Sobey CG, Wingler K, Schmidt HH, Drummond GR. NADPH oxidases in the vasculature: molecular features, roles in disease and pharmacological inhibition. Pharmacol Ther. 2008;120(3):254–91.

Singh TD, Patial K, Vijayan VK, Ravi K. Oxidative stress and obstructive sleep apnoea syndrome. Indian J Chest Dis Allied Sci. 2009;51(4):217–24.

Solfrizzi V, Panza F, Capurso A. The role of diet in cognitive decline. J Neural Transm (Vienna). 2003;110(1):95–110.

Tabner BJ, Turnbull S, Fullwood NJ, German M, Allsop D. The production of hydrogen peroxide during early-stage protein aggregation: a common pathological mechanism in different neurodegenerative diseases? Biochem Soc Trans. 2005;33(Pt 4):548–50.

Tsaluchidu S, Cocchi M, Tonello L, Puri BK. Fatty acids and oxidative stress in psychiatric disorders. BMC Psychiatry. 2008;8(Suppl 1(Journal Article)):S5.

Ursavas A, Karadag M, Rodoplu E, Yilmaztepe A, Oral HB, Gozu RO. Circulating ICAM-1 and VCAM-1 levels in patients with obstructive sleep apnea syndrome. Respiration. 2007;74(5):525–32.

Verdecchia P, Angeli F, Cavallini C. Ambulatory blood pressure for cardiovascular risk stratification. Circulation. 2007;115(16):2091–3.

Violi F, Sanguigni V, Loffredo L, Carnevale R, Buchetti B, Finocchi A, et al. Nox2 is determinant for ischemia-induced oxidative stress and arterial vasodilatation: a pilot study in patients with hereditary Nox2 deficiency. Arterioscler Thromb Vasc Biol. 2006;26(8):e131–2.

Wang Y, Zhang SX, Gozal D. Reactive oxygen species and the brain in sleep apnea. Respir Physiol Neurobiol. 2010;174(3):307–16.

Xu W, Chi L, Row BW, Xu R, Ke Y, Xu B, et al. Increased oxidative stress is associated with chronic intermittent hypoxia-mediated brain cortical neuronal cell apoptosis in a mouse model of sleep apnea. Neuroscience. 2004;126(2):313–23.

Xu Y, Zhang HT, O'Donnell JM. Phosphodiesterases in the central nervous system: implications in mood and cognitive disorders. Handb Exp Pharmacol. 2011;204:447–85.

Yamauchi M, Kimura H. Oxidative stress in obstructive sleep apnea: putative pathways to the cardiovascular complications. Antioxid Redox Signal. 2008;10(4):755–68.

Young T, Palta M, Dempsey J, Skatrud J, Weber S, Badr S. The occurrence of sleep-disordered breathing among middle-aged adults. N Engl J Med. 1993;328(17):1230–5.

Young T, Peppard PE, Gottlieb DJ. Epidemiology of obstructive sleep apnea: a population health perspective. Am J Respir Crit Care Med. 2002;165(9):1217–39.

Zamarron C, Riveiro A, Gude F. Circulating levels of vascular endothelial markers in obstructive sleep apnoea syndrome. Effects of nasal continuous positive airway pressure. Arch Med Sci. 2011;7(6):1023–8.

Zamarron-Sanz C, Ricoy-Galbaldon J, Gude-Sampedro F, Riveiro-Riveiro A. Plasma levels of vascular endothelial markers in obstructive sleep apnea. Arch Med Res. 2006;37(4):552–5.

Zhang HT, Crissman AM, Dorairaj NR, Chandler LJ, O'Donnell JM. Inhibition of cyclic AMP phosphodiesterase (PDE4) reverses memory deficits associated with NMDA receptor antagonism. Neuropsychopharmacology. 2000;23(2):198–204.

Zhang HT, Huang Y, Jin SL, Frith SA, Suvarna N, Conti M, et al. Antidepressant-like profile and reduced sensitivity to rolipram in mice deficient in the PDE4D phosphodiesterase enzyme. Neuropsychopharmacology. 2002;27(4):587–95.

Chapter 9
Diaphragm EMG Recording and Its Application in Sleep Medicine

Ying-Mei Luo and Yuan-Ming Luo

Abstract Pathophysiological changes in obstructive sleep apnea (OSA) related to neural respiratory drive can be assessed by diaphragm EMG recorded from surface electrodes, in particular, esophageal electrode. Although esophageal pressure was considered to be the gold standard in assessment of respiratory effort, it can be influenced by changes in lung volume and airflow. Diaphragm EMG recorded from esophageal electrode has an advantage over esophageal pressure in assessment of neural respiratory drive in patients with obstructive sleep apnea whose airflow and lung volume are not stable during overnight sleep. In this chapter, the recording of diaphragm EMG from an esophageal electrode catheter is discussed. Application of diaphragm EMG has been used to further understand the mechanism of pathophysiological changes in patients with OSA including those with both OSA and chronic obstructive pulmonary disease (COPD), overlap syndrome. Assessment of diaphragm EMG can also be used to differentiate central from obstructive sleep apneas.

Keywords Neural respiratory drive · Diaphragm EMG · Sleep apnea · Arousal · COPD

9.1 Recording of Diaphragm EMG

The diaphragm is the most important respiratory muscle and the diaphragm electromyogram (EMG) is useful to assess neural respiratory drive. However, the usefulness of the diaphragm EMG is dependent on the accurate recording of the signal

Y.-M. Luo
National Heart and Lung Institute, Imperial College, London, UK

Y.-M. Luo (✉)
Chinese National Researcher Center for Respiratory Disease, State Key Laboratory of Respiratory Disease, The First Affiliated Hospital of Guangzhou Medical University, Guangzhou, China

Sleep Center, The First Affiliated Hospital of Guangzhou Medical University, Guangzhou, China
e-mail: y.m.luo@vip.163.com

A. I. Pack, Q. Y. Li (eds.), *Sleep and its Disorders*, Translational Medicine Research,
https://doi.org/10.1007/978-94-024-2168-2_9

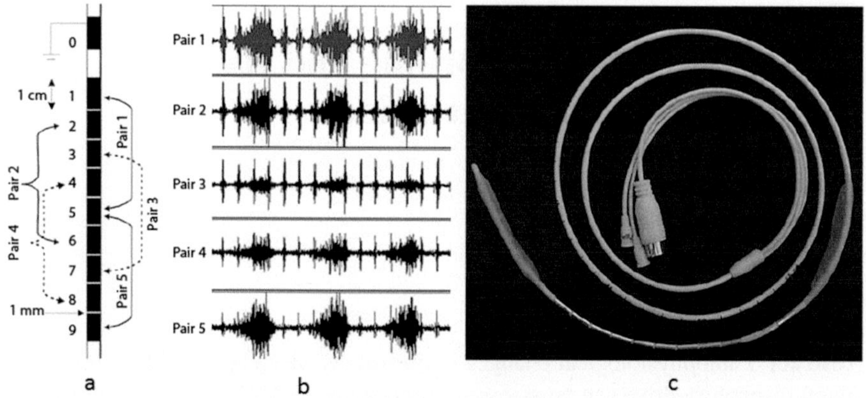

Fig. 9.1 Combined esophageal electrode and its positioning. (**a**) Configuration of electrode. (**b**) Diaphragmatic EMG recorded from multi-pair esophageal electrode after electrode catheter was optimally positioned, characterized by large EMG signals from pairs 1 and 5, the smallest EMG was recorded from pair 3. (**c**) Photograph of combined balloon electrode catheter [Figure from Luo et al. (2011)]

without artifact (Laveneziana et al. 2019). Although needle electrodes have been used in humans in some physiological studies, they are impractical for most clinical practice, particularly during sleep. Surface electrodes could be an alternative method for recording the diaphragm EMG, but this technique has disadvantages because of signal contamination, artifacts, and difficulty in standardization in positioning (Luo et al. 1998). In contrast, the diaphragm EMG recorded from an esophageal electrode is less affected by obesity and crosstalk signals (Luo et al. 1998). Consequently, esophageal diaphragm EMG has become popular in research and clinical practice (Luo et al. 2008a). One or two balloons are usually attached to an electrode catheter to simultaneously record esophageal pressure or transdiaphragmatic pressure (Pdi) while recording diaphragm EMG (Luo et al. 2008a). Although diaphragm EMG is recorded from esophageal electrodes, mainly from the crus, it is usually considered to be able to accurately reflect the electric activity of the entire diaphragm (American Thoracic Society/European Respiratory Society 2002).

For better recording of the diaphragm EMG, the esophageal electrode should be positioned close to the diaphragm. Luo and co-workers developed a technique to accurately position an esophageal electrode based on the amplitude and polarity of the diaphragm compound muscle action potential (CMAP) elicited by bilateral phrenic nerve stimulation (Luo et al. 1999, 2008a). Esophageal electrodes can also be positioned based on the spontaneous EMG signals recorded simultaneously from five pairs of electrodes (Luo et al. 2008b). The optimal position was characterized by a large EMG from two electrode pairs, which shared the middle electrode, and a small EMG from the pair straddling the middle electrode (Luo et al. 2011) (Fig. 9.1). When a catheter is positioned properly, the esophageal balloon records a negative pressure and the gastric balloon a positive pressure during inspiration for a subject with normal diaphragm function.

9.2 Assessment of Neural Respiratory Drive with Diaphragm EMG

It is useful to assess neural respiratory drive in patients with respiratory diseases including OSA and COPD because underlying physiological consequences of the diseases are related to changes in neural respiratory drive. The diaphragm EMG has long been considered to be a good tool in the assessment of neural respiratory drive. For example, it was shown that the diaphragm EMG increases gradually during CO_2 rebreathing and there is a linear relationship between root mean square of the diaphragm EMG and ventilation in normal subjects and patients with COPD (Luo and Moxham 2005) (Fig. 9.2). The observation that pressure support ventilation reduces both Pdi and diaphragm EMG equally in normal subjects suggests that two measures reflect neural respiratory drive. However, inspiratory pressure could underestimate neural respiratory drive in patients with COPD and sleep-disordered breathing because of changes in airflow and lung volume. We and others have shown that diaphragm EMG increases progressively during incremental exercise in COPD whereas Pdi reaches a plateau (Luo et al. 2011; Sinderby et al. 2001), indicating that diaphragm EMG is a better index in assessment of neural respiratory drive.

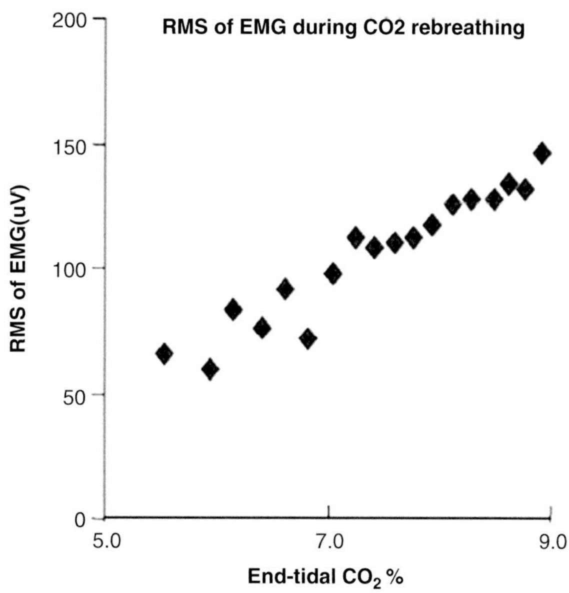

Fig. 9.2 Peak of root mean square (RMS) increases during CO_2 rebreathing. There is a good relationship between end-tidal CO_2 and the amplitude of the RMS. No plateau of EMG is observed [Figure from Luo and Moxham (2005)]

9.3 Neural Drive During Apneic Events in Patients with OSA

Clinically it has been hypothesized that episodes of increased neural respiratory drive occur during subtotal obstruction and the arousals associated with these obstructive events contribute to daytime sleepiness (Luo et al. 2008b). Measurement of esophageal pressure (Pes) could be useful in understanding the underlying physiological mechanism of OSA (Luo et al. 2008b). However, Pes during apneic episodes may be larger than that when airflow occurs even if neural respiratory drive is the same because inspiratory airflow and high lung volume both reduce the generation of Pes (Luo et al. 2009; Xiao et al. 2015). Consequently, Pes is actually not the "gold standard" to assess neural respiratory drive in patients with OSA, whose breathing by definition is associated with variable airflow and lung volume. Diaphragm EMG could be an alternative tool to accurately assess neural respiratory drive in OSA patients. Stoohs et al. (2005) reported that diaphragm EMG recorded from surface electrodes was able to measure respiratory effort. We recorded the diaphragm EMG and Pes during overnight polysomnography in patients with OSA and found that Pes increased gradually during apneic events and reached maximal at the end of the event. In contrast to the data of Pes, the highest neural respiratory drive assessed by diaphragm EMG is observed during the arousal phase (Luo et al. 2008b) (Fig. 9.3).

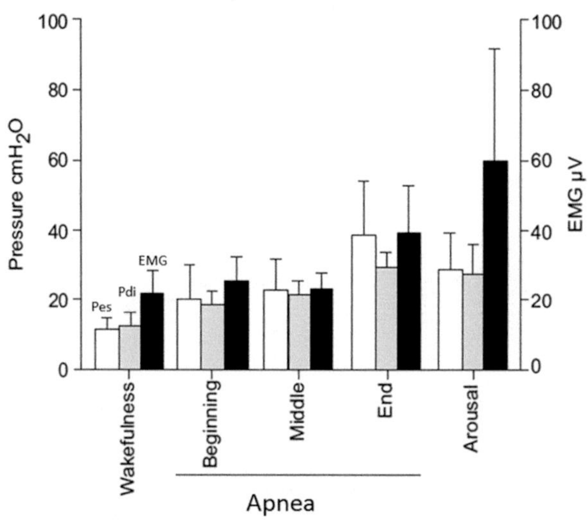

Fig. 9.3 Esophageal pressure (Pes; white bar), transdiaphragmatic pressure (Pdi; gray bar), and diaphragm electromyography (EMG; black bar) signal recorded from the esophageal electrode during obstructive sleep apnea. Data are presented as mean ± SD. Pes and Pdi increased gradually over the course of an apnea, reaching a maximum at the end of the apnea, and decreased significantly at the beginning of arousal. However, the diaphragm EMG signal was similar at the beginning and middle of the apnea, increased significantly at the end of the apnea, and increased further at the beginning of arousal [Figure from Luo et al. (2008b)]

9.4 The Mechanism of Arousal in Patients with OSA

One of the major pathophysiological changes in OSA is frequent arousals, contributing to excessive daytime sleepiness (Luo et al. 2008b). Some studies have argued that there is a threshold of respiratory effort or neural respiratory drive triggering arousal in patients with OSA based on recordings of Pes during overnight polysomnography (Kimoff et al. 1994; Gleeson et al. 1990). However, as described before, Pes is affected by changes in lung volume and airflow (Luo et al. 2008b; Luo and Moxham 2005; Sinderby et al. 2001; Xiao et al. 2012), and changes in these variables preclude Pes from accurately evaluating neural respiratory drive in patients with OSA. Although the severity of upper airway obstruction during apnea differs from that during hypopnea, pathophysiological changes for both events are similar (Luo et al. 2009; Kay et al. 1995) and a similar level of diaphragm EMG activity would be expected immediately preceding arousal in both apneic and hypopneic events if respiratory effort is responsible for arousal. We measured diaphragm EMG during both apnea and hypopneas in patients with OSA of varying severity and found that, when judged by diaphragm EMG, the variability of neural drive associated with arousal is large even when the examined arousals were confined to stage II supine sleep; diaphragm EMG at the end of hypopneas was larger than that at the end of apneas (Xiao et al. 2015) (Fig. 9.4). Moreover, diaphragm EMG could be similar at the end of both apneas and hypopneas with and without arousal (Xiao et al. 2015) (Fig. 9.5). In addition, although diaphragm EMG at the end of respiratory events was usually larger than the mean of diaphragm EMG in the middle of events, diaphragm EMG from some breathing cycles during the middle of apnea or hypopnea events was larger than those at the end of respiratory events associated with arousal (Xiao et al. 2015) (Fig. 9.6). The above data argue against the traditional concept that the magnitude of neural drive observed in apnea or hypopnea causes arousal and suggest that something else other than respiratory effort is responsible for arousal.

9.5 Distinguishing Central from Obstructive Sleep Apnea Events

Sleep apnea includes central sleep apnea and obstructive sleep apnea events. Because the mechanism responsible for central sleep apnea differs from that for obstructive sleep apnea and the treatment for obstructive apnea also differs from that for central sleep apnea, it is important for both clinical practice and research to accurately distinguish central from obstructive sleep apnea. Chest abdominal wall movement recorded by respiratory inductance plethysmography is usually taken as respiratory effort or neural respiratory drive for clinical diagnostic purposes. However, neural respiratory drive may not be reliably reflected by respiratory inductance plethysmography (RIP) because chest and abdominal wall motion could be influenced by lung volume and posture, leading to an overestimation of the

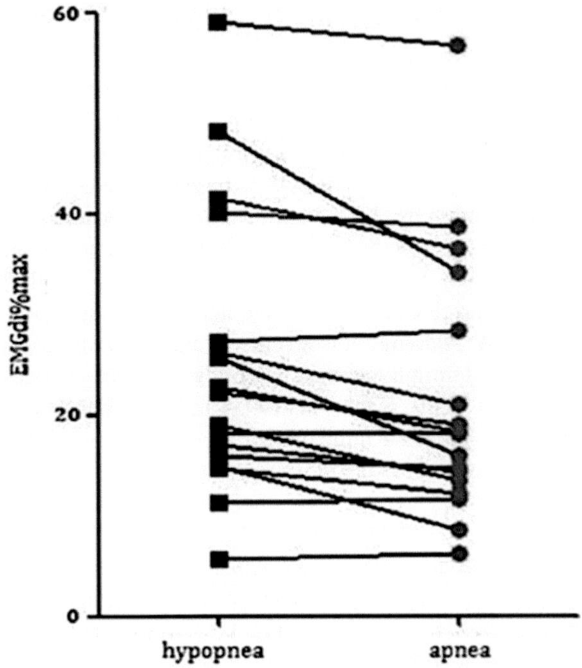

Fig. 9.4 Comparison of the diaphragm EMG at the end of respiratory events (apnea and hypopnea). Diaphragm EMG at the end of the hypopnea (25.3% ± 14.2% max, mean ± SD) is significantly larger than that observed during the apnea 21.7% ± 13.2%max ($p < 0.05$). Each dot represents the mean for one subject [Figure from Xiao et al. (2015)]

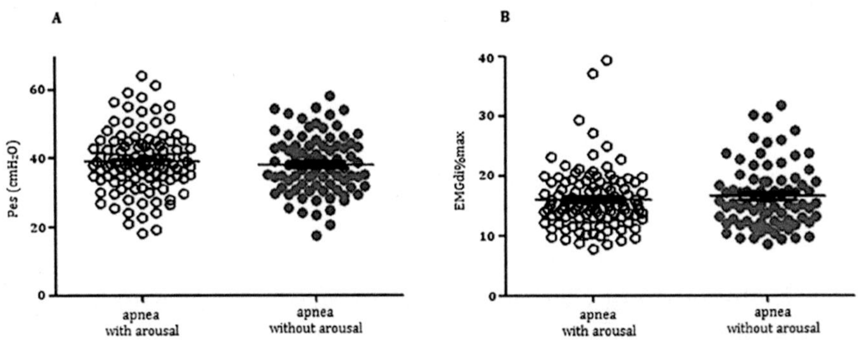

Fig. 9.5 The mean of the esophageal pressure (**a**) and diaphragm EMG (**b**) at the end of apneas that were associated with arousal from sleep are similar to those without arousal. They are not significantly different [Figure from Xiao et al. (2015)]

frequency of central apnea events (Luo et al. 2009) (Fig. 9.7). In contrast, Pes is considered to be an accurate method to assess neural respiratory drive and to distinguish obstructive from central apneic events. However, it has been documented that Pes can also be affected by variation of flow and lung volume, which occurs during apnea, especially during hypopnea. Because central apnea by definition, is due to cessation of neural respiratory drive, diaphragm EMG which is independent of changes in lung volume and airflow may be superior to other methods in

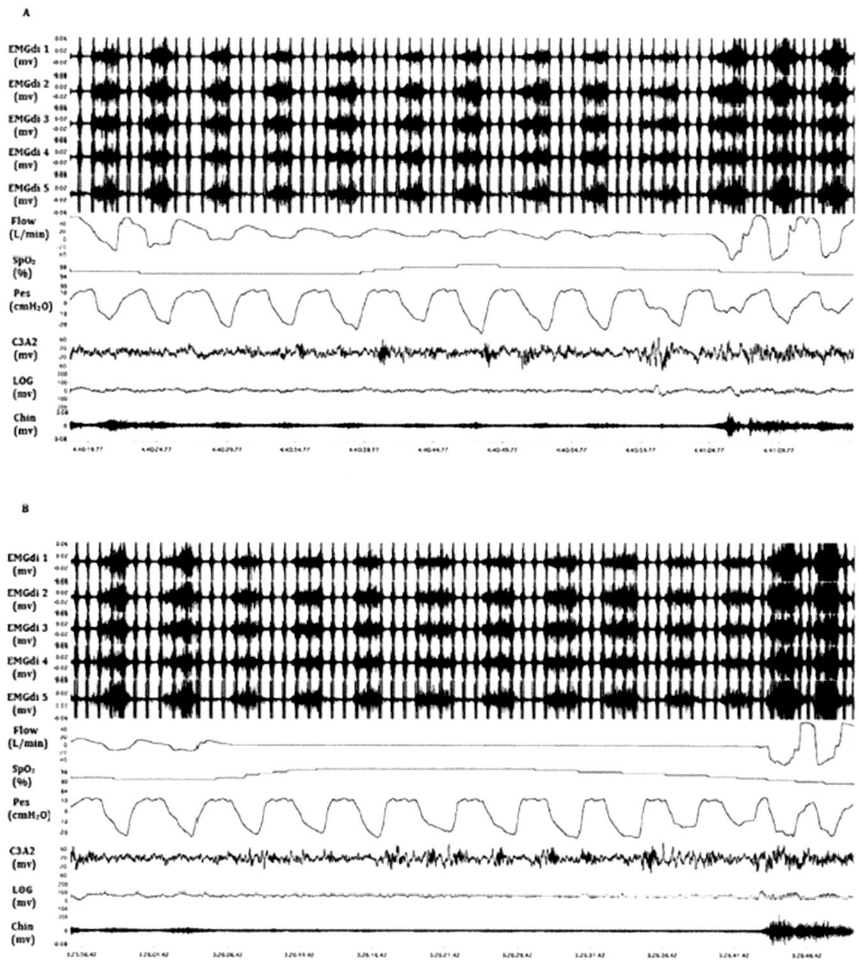

Fig. 9.6 Esophageal pressure (Pes) and diaphragm EMG from multiple electrodes during respiratory events and before respiratory events are sometimes larger than those at the end of the events, although arousal occurs only at the end of events for hypopnea (**a**) and apnea (**b**) [Figure from Xiao et al. (2015)]. Traces from top to bottom are diaphragm electromyography from five pairs of electrodes (EMGdi 1–5), airflow, Oxygen saturation (SaO_2), esophageal pressure (Pes), electroencephalography EEG recorded from C3A2 (C3A2), electrooculography recorded from left side (LOG), and electromyography recorded from chin (Chin)

differentiating central from obstructive apnea. Although recording the diaphragm EMG with a catheter could be theoretically uncomfortable and interfere with patients' sleep, the unpleasant sensation is similar to that caused by balloon catheter for measurement of esophageal pressure. The mean sleep time (7.0 h) in our study suggests that a thin esophageal catheter can be tolerated by most patients (Luo et al. 2009). It has been reported that up to 45% of central apnea events diagnosed by RIP could not be proved by diaphragm EMG (Luo et al. 2009). Therefore, a diagnosis of

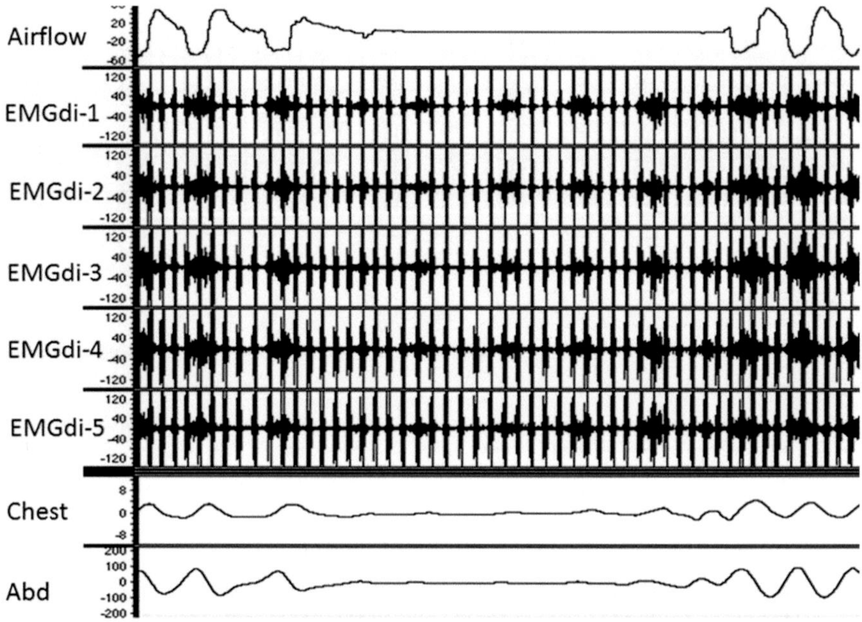

Fig. 9.7 An OSA episode is incorrectly diagnosed as CSA based on RIP. Signals (from top to bottom) are airflow, EMGdi 1-EMGdi 5, chest movement, and abdomen movement. This episode would have been scored as CSA if the judgment was based on the chest and abdominal movement recorded from RIP alone. However, this episode is scored as OSA based on EMGdi over the course of an apneic episode (Luo et al. 2009)

central sleep apnea should be further confirmed by diaphragm EMG when the diagnosis is in doubt. Although diaphragm EMG has traditionally been unwieldy, recent technical advances have resolved this and could allow the technique to potentially be the "gold standard" to differentiate central from obstructive apnea events.

9.6 Neural Respiratory Drive in Patients with COPD Alone During Sleep

It has been recognized that patients with COPD are subject to hypoxemia or even respiratory failure during sleep because of hypoventilation (Luo et al. 2014). However, it is not clear whether hypoventilation in patients with COPD during sleep is due to increases in upper airway resistance or reductions in neural drive. It is obvious that COPD patients with OSA (overlap syndrome) will have a sleep-related increase in upper airway resistance, which will contribute to the reduction of their ventilation during sleep. It has been shown that the reduction in ventilation from wakefulness to non-rapid eye movement (NREM) sleep in laryngectomized patients with constant upper airway resistance (breathing through a tracheal stoma) is similar to that when breathing through an intact upper airway, indicating that changes in upper airway resistance are not always responsible for reduction of ventilation during sleep (Morrell et al. 1996). We recently have performed a study to determine whether neural respiratory drive is the main factor contributing to sleep-related hypoventilation in patients with COPD (Luo et al. 2014). A study was done on 14 patients with COPD, who were free from obstructive sleep apnea (AHI < 5.0 events/h), confirmed by overnight polysomnography, showed that ventilation decreased during NREM and further decreased during REM when compared with wakefulness in patients with COPD. With a decrease in ventilation, there was almost proportional decrease in neural respiratory drive as assessed by diaphragm EMG (Luo et al. 2014) (Fig. 9.8). Although there was a reduction of the diaphragm EMG from wakefulness to NREM sleep in normal subjects, the reduction of neural drive in patients with COPD was much larger than that in normal subjects (Luo et al. 2014), probably because there is an additional increase in neural respiratory drive from the

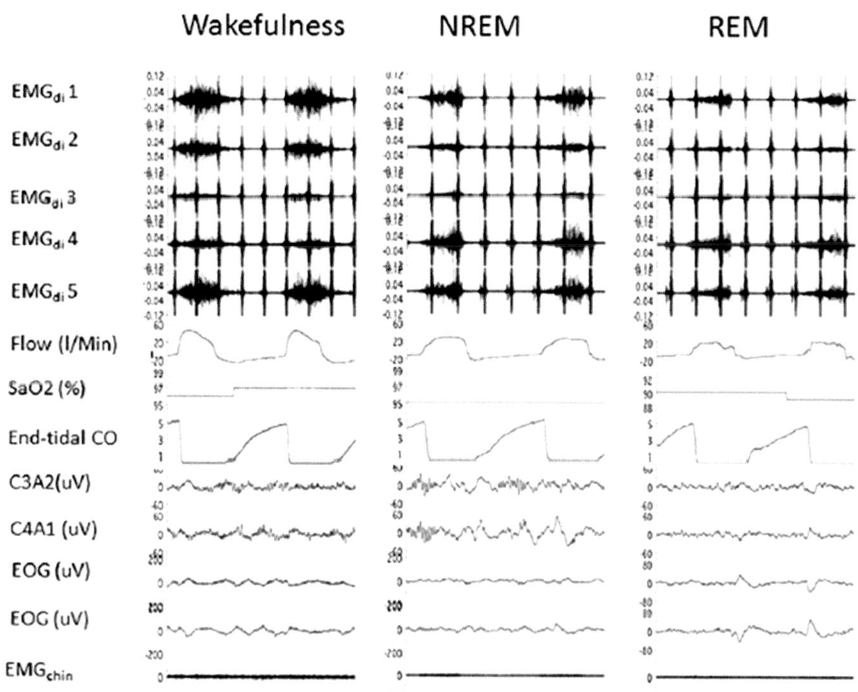

Fig. 9.8 Polysomnography including five-channel diaphragm EMG (EMGdi 1–5) from a multi-pair esophageal electrode, airflow from pneumotachograph (Flow), oxygen saturation (SaO_2), end-tidal CO_2, electroencephalogram (EEG; C3A2 and C4A1), and left and right electrooculograms (EOGs). Compared with wakefulness, EMGdi and airflow decrease in non-rapid eye movement (NREM), and further decrease in REM. Data are from a patient with chronic obstructive pulmonary disease (COPD) [Note, SaO_2 scale on REM panel differs from the others, figure from Luo et al. (2014)]

cortex in patients with COPD to compensate for hypoventilation during wakefulness (Luo et al. 2014).

9.7 Neural Respiratory Drive in Patients with Both COPD and OSA During Sleep

It has been previously reported that nocturnal oxygen desaturation is more severe in patients with both COPD and OSA, a phsenotype termed the "overlap syndrome," than in those with COPD alone (Marin et al. 2010; Sanders et al. 2003; Chaouat et al. 1995). However, this view is mainly derived from studies of patients who had predominantly mild or moderate COPD or who were recruited from OSA patients with obesity at a sleep center (Marin et al. 2010; Sanders et al. 2003; Chaouat et al. 1995), and thus may not represent a clinical cohort of patients with severe COPD (He et al. 2017). In contrast to hypoventilation in patients with COPD, OSA is characterized by increased upper airway resistance associated with an increase in neural respiratory drive (Luo et al. 2009). If patients with severe COPD develop OSA, the sleep-related reduction in neural respiratory drive associated with COPD could be offset by the increase in neural respiratory drive in OSA. Consequently, ventilation in patients with severe COPD may not further decrease when COPD and mild or modest OSA occur together (He et al. 2017) (Fig. 9.9). Indeed, a recent

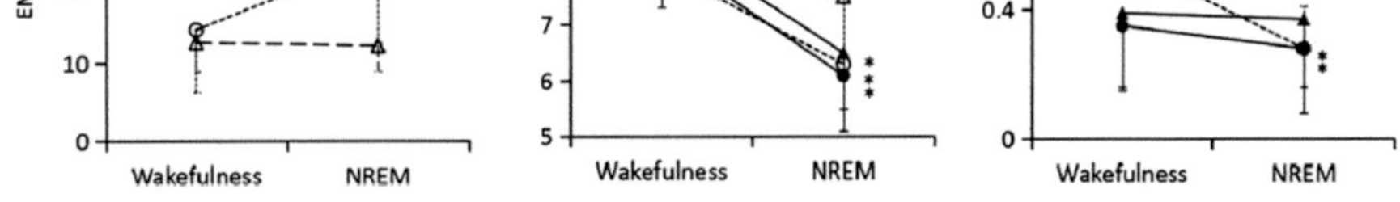

Fig. 9.9 Diaphragm EMG (EMGdi)% (left panel), ventilation (middle panel) and the VT/EMGdi (right panel) in patients with COPD alone, overlap syndrome, normal subjects and patients with obstructive sleep apnea (OSA). Ventilation decreases from wakefulness to sleep in all four groups but only in patients with COPD, overlap syndrome and OSA is the reduction statistically significant. EMGdi decreases significantly in patients with COPD alone but increases significantly in patients with OSA from wakefulness to non-rapid eye movement (NREM) sleep, whereas it remains unchanged in normal subjects and patients with overlap syndrome. VT/EMGdi decreases significantly from wakefulness to sleep in patients with overlap syndrome and those with OSA but it changes little in normal subjects and patients with COPD alone. The decrease in ventilation is associated with a reduction of EMGdi in patients with COPD alone whereas reduction in ventilation is associated with decreased VT/EMGdi in patients with overlap syndrome and those with OSA [Figure from Patout et al. (2015)]

cohort study on nonobese patients with severe COPD showed that the number of patients who required oxygen supplementation in patients with COPD alone was similar to that in those with overlap syndrome. This suggests that the prevalence of oxygen desaturation may be similar between patients with severe COPD alone and those with overlap syndrome providing that the impairment of lung function is similar (Soler et al. 2015). Our recent study also found that mean oxygen saturation and minimal oxygen saturations during overnight sleep were similar in COPD patients with or without OSA (He et al. 2017). Moreover, although patients with coexistent OSA and severe COPD usually have brief periods of desaturation, prolonged desaturation ($SaO_2 < 90$ for longer than 5 min) occurred actually more often in patients with severe COPD than in those with overlap syndrome (He et al. 2017). These findings suggest that if patients with severe COPD develop mild or moderate OSA, oxygen desaturation may not necessarily worsen. This view was supported by a recent study which showed that the clinical outcome of end-stage patients with overlap syndrome is not worse than those with COPD alone (Patout et al. 2015; Du et al. 2018). Inconsistent results in this important area indicate more research is required.

9.8 Conclusion

Diaphragm EMG recorded from a multi-pair esophageal electrode can be used to assess neural respiratory drive. Respiratory muscle dysfunction contributes to sleep-disordered breathing and sleep-related hypoventilation. Measurement of diaphragm EMG is useful to diagnose neural muscular disease when respiratory muscle function was affected. Diaphragm EMG can accurately distinguish central from obstructive sleep apnea and hypopnea. Although OSA-related arousal is usually considered to be triggered by neural respiratory drive, this concept has not been conclusively proven. Patients with both OSA and COPD, i.e., overlap syndrome, are not necessarily more severe than those with COPD alone in terms of hypoventilation and oxygen desaturation during sleep because reduction in neural respiratory drive inherent to COPD could be offset by an increase in neural respiratory drive associated with OSA.

References

American Thoracic Society/European Respiratory Society. ATS/ERS statement on respiratory muscle testing. Am J Respir Crit Care Med. 2002;166(4):518–624.

Chaouat A, Weitzenblum E, Krieger J, Ifoundza T, Oswald M, Kessler R. Association of chronic obstructive pulmonary disease and sleep apnea syndrome. Am J Respir Crit Care Med. 1995;151(1):82–6.

Du W, Liu J, Zhou J, Ye D, OuYang Y, Deng Q. Obstructive sleep apnea, COPD, the overlap syndrome, and mortality: results from the 2005–2008 National Health and Nutrition Examination Survey. Int J Chron Obstruct Pulmon Dis. 2018;13:665–74.

Gleeson K, Zwillich CW, White DP. The influence of increasing ventilatory effort on arousal from sleep. Am Rev Respir Dis. 1990;142(2):295–300.

He BT, Lu G, Xiao SC, Chen R, Steier J, Moxham J, et al. Coexistence of OSA may compensate for sleep related reduction in neural respiratory drive in patients with COPD. Thorax. 2017;72(3): 256–62.

Kay A, Trinder J, Kim Y. Individual differences in relationship between upper airway resistance and ventilation during sleep onset. J Appl Physiol (1985). 1995;79(2):411–9.

Kimoff RJ, Cheong TH, Olha AE, Charbonneau M, Levy RD, Cosio MG, et al. Mechanisms of apnea termination in obstructive sleep apnea. Role of chemoreceptor and mechanoreceptor stimuli. Am J Respir Crit Care Med. 1994;149(3 Pt 1):707–14.

Laveneziana P, Albuquerque A, Aliverti A, Babb T, Barreiro E, Dres M, et al. ERS statement on respiratory muscle testing at rest and during exercise. Eur Respir J. 2019;53(6):1801214.

Luo YM, Moxham J. Measurement of neural respiratory drive in patients with COPD. Respir Physiol Neurobiol. 2005;146(2–3):165–74.

Luo YM, Polkey MI, Johnson LC, Lyall RA, Harris ML, Green M, et al. Diaphragm EMG measured by cervical magnetic and electrical phrenic nerve stimulation. J Appl Physiol (1985). 1998;85(6):2089–99.

Luo YM, Lyall RA, Lou Harris M, Rafferty GF, Polkey MI, Moxham J. Quantification of the esophageal diaphragm electromyogram with magnetic phrenic nerve stimulation. Am J Respir Crit Care Med. 1999;160(5 Pt 1):1629–34.

Luo YM, Moxham J, Polkey MI. Diaphragm electromyography using an oesophageal catheter: current concepts. Clin Sci. 2008a;115(8):233–44.

Luo YM, Wu HD, Tang J, Jolley C, Steier J, Moxham J, et al. Neural respiratory drive during apnoeic events in obstructive sleep apnoea. Eur Respir J. 2008b;31(3):650–7.

Luo YM, Tang J, Jolley C, Steier J, Zhong NS, Moxham J, et al. Distinguishing obstructive from central sleep apnea events: diaphragm electromyogram and esophageal pressure compared. Chest. 2009;135(5):1133–41.

Luo YM, Li RF, Jolley C, Wu HD, Steier J, Moxham J, et al. Neural respiratory drive in patients with COPD during exercise tests. Respiration. 2011;81(4):294–301.

Luo YM, He BT, Wu YX, Yuan H, Xu J, Moxham J, et al. Neural respiratory drive and ventilation in patients with chronic obstructive pulmonary disease during sleep. Am J Respir Crit Care Med. 2014;190(2):227–9.

Marin JM, Soriano JB, Carrizo SJ, Boldova A, Celli BR. Outcomes in patients with chronic obstructive pulmonary disease and obstructive sleep apnea: the overlap syndrome. Am J Respir Crit Care Med. 2010;182(3):325–31.

Morrell MJ, Harty HR, Adams L, Guz A. Breathing during wakefulness and NREM sleep in humans without an upper airway. J Appl Physiol (1985). 1996;81(1):274–81.

Patout M, Ramsay M, Mackie M, Lhuillier E, Grey N, Arbane G, et al. Home mechanical ventilation (HMV): setup and outcome in Europe. Eur Respir J. 2015;46:OA4780.

Sanders MH, Newman AB, Haggerty CL, Redline S, Lebowitz M, Samet J, et al. Sleep and sleep-disordered breathing in adults with predominantly mild obstructive airway disease. Am J Respir Crit Care Med. 2003;167(1):7–14.

Sinderby C, Spahija J, Beck J, Kaminski D, Yan S, Comtois N, et al. Diaphragm activation during exercise in chronic obstructive pulmonary disease. Am J Respir Crit Care Med. 2001;163(7): 1637–41.

Soler X, Gaio E, Powell FL, Ramsdell JW, Loredo JS, Malhotra A, et al. High prevalence of obstructive sleep apnea in patients with moderate to severe chronic obstructive pulmonary disease. Ann Am Thorac Soc. 2015;12(8):1219–25.

Stoohs RA, Blum HC, Knaack L, Butsch-von-der-Heydt B, Guilleminault C. Comparison of pleural pressure and transcutaneous diaphragmatic electromyogram in obstructive sleep apnea syndrome. Sleep. 2005;28(3):321–9.

Xiao SC, Lu YR, Guo HX, Qiu ZH, Luo YM. Effect of expiratory load on neural inspiratory drive. Chin Med J. 2012;125(20):3629–34.

Xiao SC, He BT, Steier J, Moxham J, Polkey MI, Luo YM. Neural respiratory drive and arousal in patients with obstructive sleep apnea hypopnea. Sleep. 2015;38(6):941–9.

Chapter 10
Chronic Intermittent Hypoxia in Patients with OSA

Qing Yun Li, Chen Juan Gu, Ying Ni Lin, and Qiong Wang

Abstract Obstructive sleep apnea (OSA) is closely related to the increasing cardiovascular, metabolic, and cancer morbidities. Chronic intermittent hypoxia (CIH), which is marked by cyclic episodes of short duration of oxygen desaturation followed by resaturation during sleep, is a hallmark feature of OSA, and is regarded as the main mechanism contributing to the clinical consequences of OSA. The chapter provides an overview of the association between OSA and its comorbidities including cardiovascular diseases, metabolic diseases, cancer, and cognitive dysfunction, and the possible underlying mechanisms with an emphasis on the role of CIH.

Keywords Chronic intermittent hypoxia · Obstructive sleep apnea · Mortality · Morbidity

Abbreviations

AF	Atrial fibrillation
AHI	Apnea hypopnea index
ANS	Autonomic nervous system
AP-1	Activator protein-1
BMI	Body mass index
CAD	Coronary artery disease
CH	Continuous hypoxia
CIH	Chronic intermittent hypoxia
CPAP	Continuous positive airway pressure
CSC	Cancer stem cell
DHF	Diastolic heart failure
DNA	Deoxyribonucleic acid

Q. Y. Li (✉) · C. J. Gu · Y. N. Lin · Q. Wang
Department of Respiratory and Critical Care Medicine, Ruijin Hospital, Shanghai Jiao Tong University School of Medicine, Shanghai, China

A. I. Pack, Q. Y. Li (eds.), *Sleep and its Disorders*, Translational Medicine Research,
https://doi.org/10.1007/978-94-024-2168-2_10

FFA	Free fatty acid
FiO_2	Inspired O_2 fraction
Glut4	Glucose transporter type 4
HbA1c	Glycosylated hemoglobin
HDL	High-density lipoprotein
HF	Heart failure
HIF-1	Hypoxia-inducible factor-1
hs-TnT	High-sensitivity troponin T
IFG	Impaired fasting glucose
IGT	Impaired glucose tolerance
IH	Intermittent hypoxia
IR	Insulin resistance
LDL	Low-density lipoprotein
LTF	Long-term facilitation
LVEF	Left ventricular ejection fraction
MMR	Mismatch repair
mTOR	Mammalian target of rapamycin
NAFLD	Non-alcoholic fatty liver disease
NASH	Nonalcoholic steatohepatitis
NF-κB	Nuclear factor κB
NFAT	Nuclear factor of activated T-cells
nNOS	Neuronal nitric oxide synthase
NO	Nitric oxide
ODI	Oxygen desaturation index
OSA	Obstructive sleep apnea
PH	Pulmonary hypertension
PSG	Polysomnography
$PtiO_2$	Tissue oxygen partial pressure
RDI	Respiratory disturbance index
REM	Rapid eye movement
RHF	Right heart failure
RHTN	Resistant Hypertension
ROS	Reactive oxygen species
SaO_2	Arterial oxygen saturation
SCD-1	Stearoyl coenzyme A desaturase 1
SDB	Sleep-disordered breathing
SREBP-1c	Sterol regulatory element-binding protein 1c
T2DM	Type 2 diabetes mellitus
TAM	Tumor-associated macrophage
TC	Total cholesterol
TG	Triglycerides
Tregs	T regulatory lymphocytes
VEGF	Vascular endothelial growth factor
VLDL	Very low-density lipoprotein

10.1 Introduction

Obstructive sleep apnea (OSA) is a common sleep disorder characterized by repetitive episodes of upper airway obstruction during sleep. OSA is associated with significant morbidity, including cardiovascular diseases (Drager et al. 2011; Kasai et al. 2012; Somers et al. 2008), metabolic dysfunction (Shaw et al. 2008; Pamidi and Tasali 2012; Kent et al. 2014), neurocognitive impairment (Beebe et al. 2003), and cancer (Campos-Rodriguez et al. 2013; Christensen et al. 2013; Martinez-Garcia et al. 2014a; Nieto et al. 2012). OSA patients manifest a typical pattern of chronic intermittent hypoxia (CIH) marked by cyclic episodes of short duration of oxygen desaturation followed by resaturation during sleep. The condition is chronic and can last for weeks to months or longer (Dewan et al. 2015).

As a hallmark of OSA, CIH is regarded as the main mechanism contributing to the clinical consequences of OSA. The Molecular Signatures of Obstructive Sleep Apnea (MSOSA) study investigated the cyclical IH characteristics in OSA patients. Analysis of these data revealed that those oxygen desaturation/resaturation cycles are nonsinusoidal. Desaturation time increases in an almost linear fashion as desaturation amplitude increases and in contrast, resaturation time stays relatively constant (Fig. 10.1a) (Lim et al. 2015). The authors also detected within-patient variation in the severity of oxygen desaturation across the night (Fig. 10.1b) and observed that patients with a higher number of desaturation events are more likely to experience greater variation in desaturation nadirs (Lim et al. 2015).

Cyclical changes of short duration of desaturation followed by reoxygenation in organs and tissues, are similar to repeated ischemia and reperfusion events, which induce the production of reactive oxygen species (ROS) and thereby cause oxidative stress (Lavie 2015). Of note, a recurrent, shorter, and faster resaturation accelerates ROS production and release from the mitochondria compared with a longer resaturation schedule (Lim et al. 2015). IH-related ROS production and oxidative stress activate redox-sensitive signaling pathways and transcription factors, including the hypoxia-inducible factor-1 (HIF-1), c-fos, nuclear factor of activated T-cells (NFAT), nuclear factor kB (NF-κB), and activator protein 1 (AP1), and affect the expression of downstream genes encoding inflammatory cytokines and adhesion molecules. Consequently, leukocytes, platelets, and endothelial cells are activated, which in turn facilitates the production of ROS, inflammatory cytokines, and adhesion molecules. This oxidative-inflammatory cycle causes damage to tissues and organs, and likely contributes to OSA-associated multisystem comorbidity (Lavie 2015; Nanduri et al. 2008).

In this chapter, we reviewed the association between OSA and its comorbidities, and the possible underlying mechanisms with an emphasis on the role of CIH.

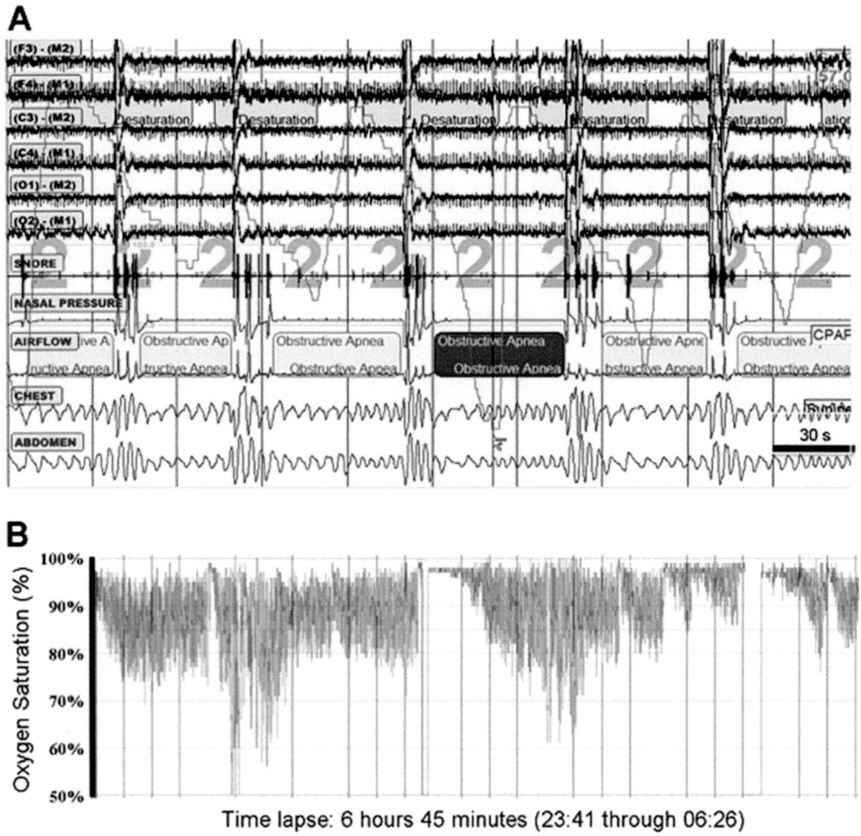

Fig. 10.1 Patient with severe OSA. (**A**) oxygen desaturation/resaturation cycle is not sinusoidal. (**B**) oxygen desaturation/resaturation has considerable variability across the sleep period in patients with OSA, including different nadirs and periods of normoxia. [Reproduced with permission from APS 2015: Lim et al. (2015)]

10.2 CIH and Cardiovascular Diseases

OSA is regarded as an independent risk factor for cardiovascular morbidity, including systemic hypertension, pulmonary hypertension, cardiac arrhythmias, coronary artery disease, and heart failure (Pack and Gislason 2009; Bradley and Floras 2009). The available evidence strongly implicates CIH as a major perpetuating factor of cardiovascular diseases and dysfunction, although it is likely that negative intrathoracic pressure swings and sleep fragmentation also contribute to OSA-related cardiovascular pathophysiology (Dewan et al. 2015).

10.2.1 *Clinical Evidence*

10.2.1.1 Hypertension

Population-based studies have revealed an independent relationship between OSA and hypertension. The adjusted odds ratio (OR) for hypertension increases with increasing OSA severity over long-term follow-up (Peppard et al. 2000; Nieto et al. 2000). The cross-sectional analyses of 6120 participants in the Sleep Heart Health Study (SHHS) found that among patients aged 40–59 years, the OR of systolic/diastolic hypertension increased significantly with more hypoxic sleep time (Haas et al. 2005). In European Sleep Apnoea Database cohort study, multiple regression analysis illustrated that oxygen desaturation index (ODI) independently correlated with prevalent hypertension, but not apnea hypopnea index (AHI) (Tkacova et al. 2014). Consistently, another retrospective cohort study also showed that indices of hypoxia during sleep and daytime mean oxygen saturation (SaO_2), rather than AHI, were included in the most precise predictive factors for hypertension, implying that CIH plays an essential role in OSA-related hypertension. Continuous positive airway pressure (CPAP), which abolishes airway obstructions and arterial oxygenation, has been shown to prevent and treat hypertension in OSA patients (Logan et al. 2003).

10.2.1.2 Pulmonary Hypertension

OSA is associated with pulmonary hypertension (PH). Vascular remodeling and hypertension were found in rodent models of CIH (Nisbet et al. 2009; Campen et al. 2005). Clinical studies showed that PH could occur in 20–41% of OSA patients in the absence of cardiac and lung diseases, mostly mild-to-moderate pulmonary hypertension (Sajkov et al. 1994, 1999; Sanner et al. 1997). OSA-related PH may be the consequence of pulmonary vascular remodeling induced by CIH and further result in persistent hypoxemia during wakefulness (Sajkov et al. 1994, 1999). Those with PH are more likely to suffer from daytime hypoxemia and have an increased pulmonary vascular response to hypoxia than non-PH subjects matched for BMI, lung function, and OSA severity (Sajkov et al. 1994, 1999). This may cause further pulmonary vascular remodeling and progressive PH (Sajkov et al. 1999). Response to CPAP in OSA with PH remains controversial, possibly due to small sample size and lack of detailed characterization of the etiology of PH in OSA (Alchanatis et al. 2001; Sforza et al. 1990; Sajkov et al. 2002; Arias et al. 2006; Nahmias et al. 1996).

10.2.1.3 Cardiac Arrhythmias

Cardiac arrhythmias, including bradycardia/tachycardia, ventricular ectopy, atrial premature contractions, and atrial fibrillation (AF) occur commonly in OSA patients (Rossi et al. 2013). AF, nonsustained ventricular tachycardia, and complex ventricular ectopy are more prevalent in patients with OSA than in non-OSA subjects after adjustment for potential confounders (Mehra et al. 2006). OSA patients with nadir nocturnal SaO_2 lower than 60% are at increased risk of developing ventricular arrhythmias (Shepard et al. 1985). Untreated OSA patients with AF recurrence show a greater fall in nocturnal SaO_2 (Kanagala et al. 2003). Gami et al. found that the decrease in nocturnal SaO_2 was more important than AHI in predicting the development of AF in OSA patients <65 years old (Gami et al. 2007). Cadby et al. showed that both AHI and TS90 (time spent with SaO_2 below 90%) were the independent predictors of AF in OSA patients (Cadby et al. 2015). Neither of these two studies detected an association between arousal index and AF, indicating that OSA-related CIH rather than sleep fragmentation contributes to the interaction between OSA and AF (Gami et al. 2007; Cadby et al. 2015). CPAP is effective in preventing OSA-associated arrhythmias (Abe et al. 2010), lowering the likelihood of recurrence of AF after cardioversion (Kanagala et al. 2003), and reducing ventricular premature beats during sleep in OSA patients with heart failure (HF) (Ryan et al. 2005). CPAP prevents the occurrence rather than the recurrence of AF after cavotricuspid isthmus radiofrequency ablation, indicating a better efficacy of CPAP in patients postablation without preexisting AF (Bazan et al. 2013).

10.2.1.4 Coronary Artery Disease

OSA constitutes a major treatable risk factor for coronary artery disease (CAD). The prevalence of OSA in patients with CAD is about 30% (Peker et al. 1999), while among hospitalized male patients with acute myocardial infarction (AMI), the prevalence rises to nearly 70% (Konecny et al. 2010). In a case control study that recruited men undergoing coronary angiography because of angina pectoris, patients with angina pectoris presented a significantly higher ODI or AHI and also had a lower mean value of the lowest SaO_2 than controls. Multiple logistic regression analysis showed that the risk of CAD increased with an increase of ODI or AHI after adjustment for age, hypertension, diabetes, smoking habits, and BMI, indicating that sleep-disordered breathing (SDB) with nocturnal desaturations was an independent predictor of symptomatic CAD (Mooe et al. 1996). It should also be noted that obesity was associated with more severe SDB and could confound the association between SDB and CAD in the study. An ODI or AHI in the highest quartile (ODI $\geq$ 7 events/h or AHI $\geq$ 12 events/h), a history of hypertension, and a 5-U increase in BMI were related to comparable ORs for CAD (3.6, 4.5, 4.2, and 4.8, respectively) (Mooe et al. 1996). In another study, an ODI of $\geq$5 events/h and an AHI of $\geq$10 events/h have been shown to independently correlate with cerebrovascular events in CAD patients (Mooe et al. 2001). Marin et al. (2005) reported a higher incidence of fatal cardiovascular events (1.06 per 100 person-years) and nonfatal cardiovascular events (2.13 per 100 person-years) in patients with severe OSA than simple snorers, patients with untreated mild-to-moderate OSA, patients treated with CPAP, and healthy participants over a follow-up period of 10 years. Multivariate analysis, adjusted for potential confounders, showed that untreated severe OSA significantly increased the risk of fatal (OR 2.87) and nonfatal (OR 3.17) cardiovascular events compared with healthy participants. Episodes of nocturnal myocardial ischemia, marked by ST-segment depression, are commonly concomitant with apnea hypopnea or desaturation events and/or rapid eye movement (REM) sleep in patients with OSA and CAD (Schafer et al. 1997; Mooe et al. 2000). Oxygen desaturation together with age, sleep efficiency, and severity of ischemic heart disease, but not AHI, are the main factors associated with nocturnal myocardial ischemia (Peled et al. 1999). CPAP modestly reduces carotid intima-media thickness and arterial pulse-wave velocity, the early signs of atherosclerosis, in severe OSA patients (Drager et al. 2007). A 3-month CPAP treatment in severe OSA patients with CAD effectively improves left ventricular function (Liu et al. 2014). Importantly, for CAD patients with OSA, treatment for OSA significantly decreases the risk of cardiovascular death, recurrent myocardial infarction, hospitalization for heart failure, and coronary revascularization (Milleron et al. 2004; Garcia-Rio et al. 2013). The role of OSA in leading to cardiovascular events was evaluated in a randomized trial. The Sleep Apnea Cardiovascular Endpoints (SAVE) trial enrolled patients with moderate-to-severe OSA and a history of cardiovascular or cerebrovascular disease, who were randomly assigned to therapeutic CPAP or usual care and followed for an average of 3.7 years. The primary analysis gave negative results that CPAP, with a mean duration of only 3.3 h treatment per night, did not lower the rate of primary end point (death from cardiovascular causes, myocardial infarction, stroke, or hospitalization for unstable angina, heart failure, or transient ischemic attack) (hazard ratio with CPAP, 1.10; 95% CI, 0.91 to 1.32; $P = 0.34$) (McEvoy et al. 2016). In contrast, the RICCADSA study involving OSA patients with established CAD showed a significant reduction in cardiovascular risk in those who used CPAP for $\geq$4 h/night compared with those who used CPAP <4 h/night or did not receive CPAP treatment after a median follow-up of 57 months. This indicates that good CPAP adherence is required to achieve cardiovascular benefits in OSA patients (Peker et al. 2016).

10.2.1.5 Heart Failure

The prevalence of OSA in heart failure (HF) ranges from 12 to 53% (Vazir et al. 2007; Yumino et al. 2009). Cross-sectional data from 6424 men and women showed a 2.20-fold increased odds of having HF associated with OSA after adjustment for confounders including age, race, sex, smoking status, number of cigarettes smoked per day, self-reported diabetes, self-reported hypertension, use of antihypertension medications, systolic blood pressure, BMI, total cholesterol, and high-density lipoprotein cholesterol (Shahar et al. 2001). SHHS demonstrated that OSA was a predictor for incident HF in men (adjusted hazard ratio 1.13 per 10-unit increase in AHI) but not in women. The reason why the authors had less power to detect the association of OSA with HF in women could be the low prevalence of severe OSA in women (Gottlieb et al. 2010). Moreover, there is a high prevalence of SDB, including both OSA and CSA, in patients with heart failure with preserved left ventricular ejection fraction (HFpEF) (Bitter et al. 2009).

CIH is the main contributor to HF in OSA patients. Mean nocturnal SaO_2 differentiates between OSA patients with and without right heart failure (RHF). Additionally, persistent hypoxemia and/or hypercapnia over a 24-h period is a novel mediator of RHF in OSA patients (Bradley et al. 1985). In a small cohort study with symptomatic diastolic heart failure (DHF), overnight minimum percentage SaO_2, but not AHI, was associated with more severe diastolic dysfunction (Chan et al. 1997). Similar results were obtained in a clinic-based study of patients without known heart diseases, which also identified worsening nocturnal hypoxemia as an independent indicator for isolated septal growth as well as decreased nitric oxide-mediated dilation in large arteries (Kraiczi et al. 2001).

Several randomized controlled trials have reported that CPAP treatment significantly reverses the decline of left ventricular ejection fraction (LVEF) in HF patients combined with OSA (Usui et al. 2005; Mansfield et al. 2004). The efficacy of CPAP has been further confirmed by another study that showed an improvement in stroke volume and cardiac output after 1-month of CPAP therapy (Kasai et al. 2015). Additionally, adaptive servo-ventilation (ASV) improves the prognosis of HFpEF patients with SDB with favorable effects such as improvement of cardiac diastolic function, and arterial stiffness after a 6-month follow-up (Yoshihisa et al. 2013). Positive airway pressure (PAP), including both ASV and CPAP, also improves right heart and pulmonary function, and may reduce all-cause mortality in HFpEF patients with SDB (Yoshihisa et al. 2015). However, in the Treatment of Sleep-Disordered Breathing with Predominant Central Sleep Apnea by Adaptive Servo-Ventilation in Patients with Heart Failure (SERVE-HF) trial, the incidence of the primary end point [the first event of death from any cause, lifesaving cardiovascular intervention (cardiac transplantation, implantation of a ventricular assist device, resuscitation after sudden cardiac arrest, or appropriate lifesaving shock), or unplanned hospitalization for worsening heart failure] did not differ significantly between the ASV group, with a low adherence of average 3.4 h per night, and the control group. However, all-cause and cardiovascular mortality were both increased with the use of ASV (Cowie et al. 2015). The explanation of the negative results may be that attenuating CSA, which is a compensatory mechanism in HF patients, with ASV may be detrimental. But compared with CSA, OSA causes more adverse cardiac loading by increasing the left ventricular afterload, which can be reversed by PAP. Therefore, the SERVE-HF results cannot be simply extrapolated to HF patients with OSA.

10.2.1.6 Stroke

OSA prevalence in stroke patients ranges from 50 to 70% (Hermann and Bassetti 2009). Cross-sectional analysis revealed that patients with AHI $\geq$ 20 events/h had an increased risk for stroke (OR $=$ 4.33) compared with those without OSA after adjustment for known confounding factors (Arzt et al. 2005). In a prospective study of patients with CAD over a 10-year follow-up, sleep apnea was presented in 54% of these patients. Patients with an ODI $\geq$ 5 events/h were at greater risk for stroke (Valham et al. 2008). Wessendorf et al. observed higher plasma levels of fibrinogen, and average minimal SaO_2 was identified as an independent predictor of fibrinogen levels in stroke patients (Wessendorf et al. 2000). This indicates that OSA-related hypoxia may mediate the interaction between fibrinogen and OSA in promoting stroke. Regarding the impact of CPAP on stroke, most studies focus on CPAP treatment for OSA patients after a stroke. In outpatients with OSA, 2–4 weeks after a stroke, CPAP treatment resulted in a greater improvement in the depression score, but not in cognitive or physical function over 4 weeks (Sandberg et al. 2001). As opposed to the controversial effects of CPAP on neurocognitive outcomes in stroke patients with OSA (Hsu et al. 2006), several long-term follow-up studies have shown that CPAP reduces the incidence of cardiovascular events (Martinez-Garcia et al. 2012), and more importantly, improves the long-term survival in stroke patients with moderate-to-severe OSA (Parra et al. 2015; Martinez-Garcia et al. 2009).

10.2.2 Mechanisms

The intermediary pathways linking OSA to cardiovascular disease have been elucidated over the last two decades. The main trigger is CIH, which leads to an array of injurious effects on the heart and vessels through several maladaptive mechanisms, including oxidative stress, inflammation, vascular endothelial dysfunction, and IH-induced sympathetic surges.

10.2.2.1 Dysregulation of Autonomic Nervous System

One major mechanism of cardiovascular disease, especially hypertension in OSA is sympathetic overactivation (Somers et al. 1995). OSA-related CIH sensitizes the arterial chemoreflex, leading to tonic activation of sympathetic outflow even during normoxic daytime wakefulness. Studies in OSA patients and animal models show that acute hypoxia exaggerates ventilatory and pressor responses and increases muscle sympathetic nerve activity (Hedner et al. 1992; Leuenberger et al. 1995; Peng et al. 2006). The underlying mechanism for IH-induced chemoreflex sensitization includes elevated reactive oxygen species (ROS) production in the carotid body, ROS-dependent signaling, and angiotensin II (Ang-II)-related upregulation of type I Ang-II receptors and NADPH oxidase activation (Nanduri et al. 2008; Prabhakar and Kumar 2010). Additionally, CIH directly affects central sites of sympathetic regulation, possibly through upregulation of noradrenergic terminal density in neurons, decreased expression of neuronal nitric oxide synthase (nNOS) in neurons in the paraventricular nucleus of the hypothalamus, and ROS-related activation of brain renin–Ang-II system (Nanduri et al. 2008; Weiss et al. 2007). Moreover, derangements in parasympathetic and sympathetic tone during and after episodes of intermittent hypoxia provide a substrate that increases the potential for cardiac arrhythmogenesis. Apneic episodes concomitant with hypoxia stimulate the carotid body and increase vagal tone, which can lead to bradyarrhythmias and heart block (Zwillich et al. 1982). The following resumption of breathing with or without arousals increases sympathetic tone characterized by hyperpnea and may cause tachyarrhythmias in OSA patients (Rossi et al. 2013).

10.2.2.2 Oxidative Stress and Inflammation

Another trigger for cardiovascular injury in OSA is intermittent hypoxia-related oxidative stress and proinflammatory state, characterized by the elevation of biomarkers of oxidative stress and inflammation in OSA patients (Shamsuzzaman et al. 2002; Lavie et al. 2008; Ye et al. 2010; Thunstrom et al. 2015). Rodent models have demonstrated that intermittent hypoxia leads to a state of oxidative stress through either suppression of antioxidant capacity and/or overproduction of reactive oxygen and nitrogen species (Badran et al. 2014). The increased production of ROS and oxidative stress, on one hand, directly cause cardiovascular damage, and on the other, they also promote systemic inflammation, via mitochondrial dysfunction, activation of hypoxia-inducible transcription factors, and reduction in antioxidants, to exaggerate cardiovascular injury (Rossi et al. 2013; Prabhakar and Kumar 2004).

Oxidative stress-related myocardial cell injury, as exhibited by increased troponin levels, as well as myocyte hypertrophy and fibrosis, eventually culminate in left ventricular dysfunction in rodent models of intermittent hypoxia (Liu et al. 2010; Chen et al. 2005; Hayashi et al. 2008). Augmentation of systemic inflammation in response to CIH exposure fosters the early development and growth of atherosclerotic lesions and promotes plaque rupture, leading to increased risk of CAD, stroke, and worse clinical outcomes (Levy et al. 2009; Capone et al. 2012; Jackman et al. 2014; Jagadapillai et al. 2014). Furthermore, chronic intermittent hypoxia-induced cellular inflammation, cardiac myocyte dysfunction, and changes in cardiac structure create heterogeneous regions of myocyte excitability and increase the risk for re-entrant arrhythmias (Rossi et al. 2013). PH in intermittent hypoxia-treated mice is associated with increased levels of the NADPH oxidase subunits NOX4 and p22phox, indicating that NADPH oxidase-derived ROS contributes to the development of PH (Nisbet et al. 2009).

10.2.2.3 Endothelial Dysfunction

Diminished endothelial function is an important consequence of CIH, with several potential mechanisms involved, including endothelin release and attenuated production of nitric oxide (NO). Rats exposed to intermittent hypoxia showed an elevated plasma endothelin level (Kanagy et al. 2001), which is associated with endothelin-induced vascular contraction and is an important precursor of atherosclerosis (Allahdadi et al. 2005; Lefebvre et al. 2006). Consistently, CPAP attenuates the elevations of endothelin and BP in acute untreated OSA patients (Phillips et al. 1999), and reverses the decrease of circulating NO in OSA patients (Ip et al. 2000). The hypoxemia-driven effects on endothelin and NO likely contribute to the endothelial dysfunction in OSA patients (Kato et al. 2000).

10.3 CIH and Metabolic Dysfunction

10.3.1 CIH and Impaired Glucose Metabolism: Clinical Evidence

OSA increases the risk of type 2 diabetes mellitus (T2DM) and a great proportion of T2DM patients suffer from concomitant OSA (Shaw et al. 2008; Tahrani et al. 2012). In a meta-analysis of six prospective cohort studies including 5953 participants with follow-up periods of 2.7–16 years, moderate to severe OSA was associated with an increased risk of T2DM (Wang et al. 2013a). An ODI > 5 events/h was a predictor of developing diabetes (OR = 4.4) during a mean period of 11-year follow-up (Lindberg et al. 2012). OSA exacerbates the progression of T2DM, as manifested by difficulty in controlling blood glucose and increased occurrence of diabetic complications. The adjusted mean glycosylated hemoglobin (HbA_1c) was increased by 1.49%, 1.93%, and 3.69% in patients with mild, moderate, and severe OSA, respectively (Aronsohn et al. 2010). Concomitant OSA was independently associated with diabetic peripheral neuropathy and nephropathy (OR = 2.64), and baseline AHI was an independent predictor of estimated glomerular filtration rate (eGFR) (Tahrani et al. 2012, 2013).

In addition to T2DM, OSA is reported to be associated with prediabetic state, including impaired fasting glucose (IFG) and impaired glucose tolerance (IGT). The prevalence of IFG and IGT is higher in OSA patients (20–67%) (Pamidi and Tasali 2012). Data from the SHHS revealed that in 2588 participants without known diabetes, OSA subjects had significantly higher adjusted prevalence and adjusted odds of IFG and IFG plus IGT (Seicean et al. 2008). Insulin resistance (IR), another important marker of prediabetes, is also found to be independently associated with OSA. In 118 subjects without diabetes, those with mild, moderate, and severe OSA displayed a 26.7%, 36.5%, and 43.7% reduction in insulin sensitivity, respectively, compared with normal subjects, independent of age, sex, race, and percent body fat (Punjabi and Beamer 2009). In young, lean, and healthy men, who were free of cardio-metabolic diseases, the presence of mild OSA was associated with a 27% decrease in insulin sensitivity (Pamidi et al. 2012).

Studies have examined the efficacy of CPAP on glucose metabolism in OSA. Dawson et al. (2008) reported that an average 41-day CPAP treatment decreased and stabilized sleeping glucose levels, when they used a continuous glucose monitoring system to measure interstitial glucose every 5 min during polysomnography (PSG) in 20 T2DM patients with newly diagnosed OSA. Babu et al. (2005) showed that

CPAP treatment (83 ± 50 days) significantly reduced the mean 1-h postprandial glucose values and HbA_1c level. A parallel RCT enrolling OSA patients with T2DM with HbA1c levels ≥6.5% showed a decrease in HbA1c level and an improvement of insulin resistance in the CPAP group compared with those without CPAP. In CPAP-treated patients, the 6-month change in HbA1c levels was associated with mean nocturnal oxygen saturation (Martinez-Ceron et al. 2016). Moreover, CPAP improved insulin sensitivity in severe OSA as assessed by IGT (Weinstock et al. 2012) and nondiabetic patients with moderate-to-severe OSA without changing BMI (Yang et al. 2013). These findings suggest that OSA is related to impaired glucose homeostasis independent of obesity, and that CPAP can be an important therapeutic approach for patients with OSA and impaired glucose metabolism.

However, two RCTs showed that PAP did not influence glycemic control, including the HbA1c level, fasting plasma glucose, and insulin resistance, but improved blood pressure (Shaw et al. 2016; Myhill et al. 2012). One of the explanations could be that the enrolled patients had a mean baseline HbA1c level of about 7%, which means that the T2DM patients were already relatively well controlled, and thus, there was limited scope for further improvement with CPAP.

10.3.2 CIH and Impaired Glucose Metabolism: Mechanisms

Insulin resistance (IR) and impaired pancreatic β-cell function are the two main features involved in the pathogenesis of T2DM. Evidence from human and animal models showed that CIH causes IR in the absence of obesity, while data regarding the effects of CIH on pancreatic β-cell function is relatively limited.

10.3.2.1 CIH and Insulin Resistance

Several human and animal studies have shown that CIH induces IR (Iiyori et al. 2007; Chen et al. 2010; Louis and Punjabi 2009; Carreras et al. 2012; Polak et al. 2013). However, the potential molecular mechanisms underlying CIH-induced IR are not fully elucidated. CIH-related activation of sympathetic nerve system, possibly through increased release of catecholamine in adrenal medulla and dysregulation of insulin pathway in liver, may be involved (Shin et al. 2014a; Mesarwi et al. 2015). Some studies have shown, however, that CIH decreases the whole-body insulin sensitivity independent of sympathetic activation (Iiyori et al. 2007; Shin et al. 2014b). Further, CIH may also activate the hypothalamic–pituitary–adrenal axis and facilitate the release of corticosteroids. Yokoe et al. (2008) revealed that intermittent hypoxia reversed the normal diurnal blood glucose rhythm and exacerbated diurnal peak corticosterone, which was temporally associated with the peak in blood glucose. Moreover, CIH-induced oxidative stress and inflammation also partially contribute to IR in OSA patients (Tasali and Ip 2008).

CIH-induced IR through altering the production of adipokines. Adiponectin functions as an insulin sensitizer by decreasing hepatic glucose output, thereby contributing to the regulation of the whole-body glucose homeostasis. Magalang et al. (2009) reported that 48-h exposure to cyclic intermittent hypoxia significantly decreased the secretion of total and high-molecular weight adiponectin by 3T3-L1 adipocytes. Clinical studies have shown that hypoadiponectinemia is related to sympathetic activation, IR and severity of OSA (Lam et al. 2008). Thus, hypoadiponectinemia may contribute to alterations in metabolic processes leading to IR under intermittent hypoxia. Further, CIH increases the gene expression and circulating protein levels of leptin, which is produced primarily by adipose tissue and acts both centrally and peripherally to regulate insulin sensitivity. Thus, changes in leptin in CIH may also contribute in IR (Reinke et al. 2011).

10.3.2.2 CIH and β-Cell Dysfunction

The effect of CIH on pancreatic β-cells is not well known. Current evidence suggests the coexistence of protective and injurious pathways in pancreas as a result of intermittent hypoxia. Intermittent hypoxia promotes both apoptosis and proliferation of β-cells in mice. The net effect of exposure is increased turnover or increased replication of pancreatic β-cells (Yokoe et al. 2008; Xu et al. 2009). Similarly, our group also found that 8-week intermittent hypoxia exposure increased β-cell mass in lean C57BL/6J mice (Gu et al. 2013).

Regarding the effects of CIH on the function of pancreatic β-cells, a rodent model of CIH demonstrated that 6-week exposure to intermittent hypoxia impaired the function of pancreatic β-cells, marked by augmented basal insulin secretion, defective proinsulin processing, and impaired glucose-stimulated insulin secretion (Shin et al. 2014a). Mitochondrial ROS levels increase in pancreatic β-cells with intermittent hypoxia, and administration of ROS scavenger reversed the basal insulin secretion and proinsulin processing (Wang et al. 2013b). Thus, oxidative stress in CIH plays a role in pancreatic β-cell dysfunction (Wang et al. 2013b). Moreover, in a mouse model of diabetes mellitus, 14-day exposure to intermittent hypoxia-induced pancreatic apoptosis and exacerbated dysfunction of pancreatic β-cells, possibly mediated by the intermittent hypoxia-induced increase in free fatty acids and a shift in composition of fatty acids toward long-chain saturated fatty acid species (Sherwani et al. 2013).

10.3.3 CIH and Impaired Lipid Metabolism: Clinical Evidence

Several studies have demonstrated that OSA is independently associated with impaired lipid metabolism. Data from the SHHS showed that in men <65 years, fasting levels of total cholesterol (TC) and triglycerides (TG) directly correlated with the severity of OSA (Newman et al. 2001). Another cross-sectional study revealed that nocturnal hypoxia and OSA severity were independent indicators for higher TG and lower high-density lipoprotein (HDL) levels after adjustment for confounding factors (Trzepizur et al. 2013). Furthermore, there is a relationship between OSA and the progression of non-alcoholic fatty liver disease (NAFLD). In obese adult patients with NAFLD, OSA is related to elevated alanine aminotransferase (ALT) levels and a trend toward histologic evidence of progressive liver diseases (Kallwitz et al. 2007). In pediatric NAFLD, OSA is also associated with biochemical, immunohistochemical, and histological features of nonalcoholic steatohepatitis (NASH) and fibrosis (Nobili et al. 2014). CPAP may be beneficial to improve lipid profile in OSA patients. A randomized controlled trial including 220 OSA patients demonstrated that 1-month nasal CPAP produced a decrease in plasma TC by 10.8 mg/dl (Nobili et al. 2014). However, another study showed that CPAP decreased serum TG levels only when it was combined with weight loss (Chirinos et al. 2014). A study examined the effect of CPAP on postprandial lipids and reported a beneficial effect of CPAP on decreasing TG and TC, which consequently reduced the risk for cardiovascular events (Phillips et al. 2011). More recently, a meta-regression analysis of 29 studies including a total of 1958 subjects revealed that CPAP treatment for OSA seems to improve dyslipidemia, manifested by the decrease in the levels of TC and low-density lipoprotein (LDL), and the increase in the levels of HDL, without affecting TG levels (Nadeem et al. 2014).

10.3.4 CIH and Impaired Lipid Metabolism: Mechanisms

Animal studies unambiguously showed that CIH is a direct cause of hyperlipidemia. Increased TC and TG levels are correlated with the degree of hypoxemia and are more marked in lean than obese mice (Li et al. 2007a). In C57BL/6J mice on a high-cholesterol diet, 12-week exposure to intermittent hypoxia increased serum levels of very low-density lipoprotein (VLDL) and LDL (Li et al. 2007a). Similar changes in response to CIH occurred in atherosclerosis-prone apolipoprotein E-deficient mice (Jun et al. 2010).

CIH induces hyperlipidemia through consistent upregulation of hepatic genes, which play an essential role in regulation of lipid biosynthesis (Li et al. 2005, 2007a, b). In particular, CIH significantly enhances expressions of sterol regulatory element-binding protein 1 (SREBP-1), a key regulator of lipid biosynthesis, and stearoyl-coenzyme A desaturase 1 (SCD-1), an important gene for TG and phospholipids biosynthesis (Li et al. 2007b), possibly through HIF-1 signaling (Li et al. 2006). Consistently, interruption of SREBP-1 signaling in transgenic mice (Li et al. 2007b) and depletion of SCD-1 with antisense oligonucleotides in C57BL/6J mice prevent intermittent hypoxia-induced hyperlipidemia (Li et al. 2007b; Savransky et al. 2008). In addition to enhanced lipid biosynthesis, lipolysis may be another putative mechanism of dyslipidemia during CIH. Intermittent hypoxia increases hepatic TG and facilitates hepatic VLDL secretion without affecting de novo fatty acid synthesis, suggesting that peripheral lipolysis is the main source of free fatty acids (FFA) in TG and VLDL (Li et al. 2005). A study in apolipoprotein E-deficient mice showed an increase in FFA levels, indicating that intermittent hypoxia induces adipose tissue lipolysis (Jun et al. 2010). The activation of sympathetic nervous system in response to intermittent hypoxia exposure could potentially induce lipolysis (Lam et al. 2008; Lafontan and Langin 2009; Zechner et al. 2009). The confluence of increased FFA delivery and impaired β-oxidation may also underlie the association between OSA and accumulation of fat in the liver and liver injury (Tanne et al. 2005; Polotsky et al. 2009, Savransky et al. 2007). Thus, CIH may disrupt lipid metabolism through the interactions of upregulated hepatic lipids biosynthesis, increased adipose tissue lipolysis, and FFA flux to the liver.

Furthermore, CIH exposure in mice activates NADPH oxidase in liver and induces oxidative stress. Lipid peroxidation and inflammation may play a role in intermittent hypoxia-induced progression of NAFLD (Jun et al. 2008). In a mouse model of diet-induced fatty liver, intermittent hypoxia-induced lobular inflammation and fibrosis in the liver, converting hepatic steatosis to steatohepatitis. Significant increases in lipid peroxidation and myeloperoxidase have been observed in liver with significant increased hepatic levels of pro-inflammatory cytokines IL-1β, IL-6, and CXC chemokine MIP-2 (Li et al. 2007b).

10.4 CIH and Neurocognitive Dysfunction

10.4.1 Clinical Evidence

Hypoxemia and sleep fragmentation can independently and even synergistically mediate neurocognitive dysfunction in OSA patients and contribute to different aspects of cognitive impairment. Specifically, vigilance is more related to sleep fragmentation, whereas hypoxemia accounts for a wider range of impairment including changes in global cognitive function, executive function, attention, and visuo-constructive abilities (Quan et al. 2011; Shpirer et al. 2012; Findley et al. 1986; Ferini-Strambi et al. 2003; Bucks et al. 2013). Compared with OSA patients without hypoxemia, hypoxemic patients suffer from more severe cognitive impairment (Findley et al. 1986). Severity of nocturnal hypoxemia, but not the frequency of apneic events, is related to a higher risk of cognitive impairment in OSA patients (Kotterba et al. 1998). Furthermore, neuroimaging studies have demonstrated that the severity of hypoxemia is associated with decreased gray matter volumes in the parietal and prefrontal cortices, hippocampal atrophy, reduced frontal activation, and cortical metabolic changes in OSA patients (Canessa et al. 2011; Gale and Hopkins 2004; Zhang et al. 2011; Tonon et al. 2007).

The efficacy of CPAP treatment on cognitive function in OSA patients remains uncertain, possibly due to varied duration of CPAP usage, assessments of different cognitive domains, different sample characteristics and designs across studies. Ferini-Strambi et al. (2003) observed that a 15-day CPAP treatment was sufficient to restore attentive, visuospatial learning, and motor performances in severe OSA patients, and increasing therapy duration to 4 months did not further improve cognitive tests. Studies with a relatively small sample size showed that CPAP treatment for 3–6 months significantly reversed deficits in several cognitive domains in OSA patients (Dalmases et al. 2015; Naegele et al. 1998; Bedard et al. 1993), while a large, randomized sham-controlled trial only detected mild and transient improvement in executive and frontal lobe function in severe OSA patients (Kushida et al. 2012). In contrast, a multicenter study showed that a substantial proportion of moderate-to-severe OSA patients still suffered from residual sleepiness and neurobehavioral abnormalities despite adequate CPAP use (Antic et al. 2011). Thus, it is crucial to adequately assess patients after CPAP therapy and seek alternate etiologies and treatments for residual abnormalities.

10.4.2 Mechanisms

Animal studies showed that intermittent hypoxia-induced cognitive deficits may be partially attributed to death and structural changes of neuronal cells, possibly through oxidative stress and inflammation-related pathways. In adult rats, IH exposure is associated with increases in neuronal apoptosis and cytoarchitectural disorganization in hippocampal CA1 region and the frontoparietal cortex, which are involved in learning and memory (Gozal et al. 2001). Oxidative tissue injury and low-grade neuro-inflammation, consequently causing neuronal cell damage and resulting in cognitive deficits, have been found in mice hippocampus in the presence of CIH (Zhu et al. 2007; Sapin et al. 2015).

Alterations in the cellular and molecular substrates of synaptic plasticity within the cortex and hippocampus also mediate intermittent hypoxia-induced neurocognitive dysfunction. Intermittent hypoxia can disrupt the N-methyl-D-aspartate (NMDA)-dependent pathway, which is implicated in memory formation via diminishing the ability of hippocampal neurons to sustain long-term potentiation (Payne et al. 2004). Additionally, intermittent hypoxia reduces NMDA receptor-binding sites and the density of NMDA NR1 (NMDA receptors 1)-expressing cells in the CA1 field of hippocampus, suggesting the involvement of excitotoxic processes that may underlie the unique vulnerability of NMDA NR1-expressing cells to intermittent hypoxia (Gozal et al. 2001; Pichiule et al. 1996).

Disruption of blood–brain barrier also plays a role in intermittent hypoxia-related cognitive impairment. It has been demonstrated that in susceptible individuals, altered microvessel permeability changes the concentration of solutes, cells, and water, thereby altering neuronal morphology and synaptic plasticity and causing cognitive impairment (Lim and Pack 2014).

10.5 CIH and Tumor

10.5.1 Clinical Evidence

The relationship between OSA and cancer has been established by several large cohort studies (Campos-Rodriguez et al. 2013; Martinez-Garcia et al. 2014a; Nieto et al. 2012; Kendzerska et al. 2014). Data from the Wisconsin Sleep Cohort showed that increased cancer mortality correlated with percent nighttime with oxygen saturation below 90% ($TSat_{90}$) (Nieto et al. 2012). Two Spanish cohort studies further confirmed the association between OSA and cancer mortality, and consistently identified $TSat_{90}$, rather than AHI, as an independent predictor for increased cancer incident, particularly in patients younger than 65 years (Campos-Rodriguez et al. 2013; Martinez-Garcia et al. 2014a). In the Canadian cohort study of more than 10,000 patients who had suspected OSA, Kendzerska et al. (2014) found that oxygen desaturation, but not AHI, was associated with smoking-related cancers, although they failed to detect a significant relationship between OSA severity and the overall prevalent or incident cancer in the whole cohort. Another Denmark cohort study also showed no association between symptoms of SDB and incident cancer, but only found higher cancer incidence in patients younger than 50 years with high daytime sleepiness (Christensen et al. 2013). With regard to the cancer locations, studies from Spain and Canada showed that colorectal, prostate, lung, and breast cancers are most common in OSA patients (Campos-Rodriguez et al. 2013; Kendzerska et al. 2014). The American insurance database, however, in nearly 5.6 million individuals showed the adjusted risks of pancreatic and kidney cancer and melanoma were significantly higher in patients with OSA, while the risks of colorectal, breast, and prostate cancers appeared to be lower (Gozal et al. 2016). OSA patients, especially with insomnia, have been shown to have higher risk of primary brain cancers (Chen and Hwang 2014). In patients with cutaneous malignant melanoma, both AHI and ODI are independently associated with an increased melanoma growth rate and other aggressiveness factors including increased maximum tumor thickness in millimeters (Breslow index), presence of ulceration and mitotic index (Martinez-Garcia et al. 2014b). Of note, a recent study reported that OSA increased expression of a disproportionate number of genes mapping to neoplastic pathways in circulating leukocytes, and more importantly, expression of these genes could be modestly reduced by effective CPAP treatment (Gharib et al. 2014).

10.5.2 Mechanisms

Proof-of-concept animal studies have explored the effect of intermittent hypoxia on tumor malignancy. Using a murine melanoma model, Almendros et al. (Almendros et al. 2012a, b, 2013) have lent support to the notion that intermittent hypoxia-enhanced tumor proliferation and metastasis in a murine melanoma model. Several studies have been conducted to explore the underlying mechanisms of how OSA-like intermittent hypoxia pattern affects tumor behavior. The proposed hypotheses include intermittent hypoxia-induced oxidative stress, genomic instability, angiogenesis, and immunological microenvironment alterations (Kukwa et al. 2015).

Rapid proliferation of cancer cells and abnormal vasculature network results in heterogeneous hypoxic microenvironments within tumors, which may be responsible for tumor aggressive behavior and resistance to therapeutic intervention. Cycles of hypoxia and reoxygenation leads to ROS production and hence may directly cause DNA damage. On the other hand, hypoxia inhibits multiple DNA repair pathways, consequently resulting in incomplete or inaccurate DNA replication (Klein and Glazer 2010). Additionally, increased ROS modifies proteins or lipids and regulates critical transcription factors in redox-sensitive signaling pathways, such as HIF-1, NF-κB, and AP-1 (Lavie 2015), leading to self-renewal and apoptotic imbalance, angiogenesis, and platelet aggregation in tumors. The pattern of OSA-like intermittent hypoxia in tumor is generally different from that in OSA. In particular, cycles of hypoxia and reoxygenation in tumors vary from minutes to hours (Toffoli and Michiels 2008), while intermittent hypoxia in OSA is high-frequency and could result in one or more hypoxic event per minute. Despite the difference in the pattern of intermittent hypoxia, nocturnal repetitive blood oxygen desaturation in OSA could result in relapsing swings in tumor oxygen supply and exaggerate ROS-related changes in tumors, thereby leading to poor clinical prognosis.

Studies have shown that OSA-like intermittent hypoxia promotes tumor angiogenesis in rodent models (Almendros et al. 2012b; Vilaseca et al. 2017; Zhang et al. 2018), which alters hypoxic microenvironment in tumors. Serum levels of vascular endothelial growth factor (VEGF), a potent angiogenic cytokine, have been found to be elevated in OSA patients and are strongly associated with the degree of nocturnal hypoxemia (Schulz et al. 2002; Teramoto et al. 2003). Consistently, increased VEGF levels were observed in intermittent hypoxia-exposed mice (Almendros et al. 2012b; Vilaseca et al. 2017; Zhang et al. 2018). In an OSA mouse model bearing kidney cancer, exposure to intermittent hypoxia increased the endothelial cell contents, which was positively correlated with serum VEGF levels (Vilaseca et al. 2017). Additionally, intermittent hypoxia promoted VEGF expression in macrophages, but not in the kidney adenocarcinoma cells (RENCA cells) or endothelial cells. This indicates that increased tumor angiogenesis upon exposure to intermittent hypoxia was more likely due to an increased expression of VEGF by cell populations such as macrophages rather than directly in tumor cells or endothelial cells (Vilaseca et al. 2017). VEGF expression is regulated by HIF-1, which is a heterodimer composed of an alpha subunit (HIF-1α) and a beta subunit (HIF-1β). Under hypoxic conditions, HIF-1α rapidly transfers to the nucleus and binds to HIF-1β, and then the complex binds to hypoxia response elements, which induces transcription of HIF-1 target genes. Monocytes from OSA patients have higher levels of HIF-1α and VEGF compared with those of control subjects and CPAP-treated patients. The mRNA levels of HIF-1α and VEGF are positively correlated with nighttime oxygen saturation levels $<90\%$ (CT90) (Cubillos-Zapata et al. 2018). Knockdown of HIF-1α reduced VEGF levels in intermittent hypoxia-exposed healthy monocytes, suggesting that intermittent hypoxia induces VEGF expression via activation of HIF-1α. Application of monocyte supernatants from OSA patients, but not from the control or CPAP-treated groups, increased the tumor sphere sizes and tumor viability in human pancreas (BxPC3) and colon (LoVo) tumor cells. This was reversed by addition of anti-VEGF antibody, indicating that intermittent hypoxia may promote tumor progress through activation of HIF-1α/VEGF pathway in monocytes (Cubillos-Zapata et al. 2018).

The immune system is involved in multiple cancer-related processes. Much attention has been paid to tumor-associated macrophages (TAMs), which are subdivided into two major populations, namely tumor-inhibitory (M1) and tumor-promoting (M2) phenotypes (Almendros et al. 2014). Compelling evidence have shown that TAMs migration to tumor and polarization toward M2 promote cancer growth and development, are accomplished by the involvement of multiple regulators, such as NF-κB, STAT 3, STAT6, Notch, PPAR-γ, and c-Myc (Tang et al. 2013; Guo et al. 2013). Almendros et al. (2014) have demonstrated that OSA-like intermittent hypoxia exposure induced a shift of TAMs polarity toward M2 pro-tumoral phenotype, which promoted tumors invasiveness and metastasis. They also reported that intermittent hypoxia-induced phenotypic alterations in adipose tissue macrophages surrounding the tumor and their increased infiltration within the tumor contributed to the accelerated tumor progression associated with intermittent hypoxia in OSA (Almendros et al. 2015). Additionally, intermittent hypoxia exposure promoted the recruitment of other immune cells including T-regulated lymphocytes (Tregs) and bone marrow-derived inhibitory cells (MDSCs) (Almendros et al. 2015; Campillo et al. 2017), and reduced intra-tumoral CD8+ T cells function as effector cytotoxic T lymphocytes (CTLs) (Akbarpour et al. 2017), indicating an impaired immunosurveillance within tumor tissues produced by intermittent hypoxia. Activation of cycloxygenase-2 (COX-2)/prostaglandin E_2 (PGE_2) pathway contributes to the initiation and maintenance of M2 polarized TAMs, dysfunction of CTLs and natural killer cells (NK cells), and recruitment of Tregs and MDSCs (Chen and Smyth 2011). Intermittent hypoxia increased intra-tumoral levels of COX-2 and PGE_2 in a Lewis lung cancer mouse model. Administration of celecoxib, which is a specific inhibitor for COX-2, decreased COX-2 and PGE_2 levels, inhibited the process of TAMs polarization toward M2 and recruitment of Tregs and MDSCs, and thereby prevented intermittent hypoxia-induced tumor progression (Campillo et al. 2017). This suggests that intermittent hypoxia may alter the host immune response to cancer and accelerate tumor progression, at least partially, through activation of COX-2/PGE_2 pathway. However, more animal and human studies are still needed to confirm the role of abnormal immune responses in OSA-related cancer development and to investigate whether intervention targeting the immune system might improve cancer prognosis in OSA.

Exosomes are small vesicles that contain proteins, lipids, mRNAs, and miRNAs, and represent an important mode of intercellular communication (Raposo and Stoorvogel 2013). Studies have shown that exosomes affect tumor-related pathways such as cancer stemness, angiogenesis, and metastasis within the tumor microenvironment (Azmi et al. 2013). Plasma exosomes from intermittent hypoxia-exposed mice increased cell proliferation, migration, and invasion of epithelial lung tumor cells, and disrupted endothelial cell barrier integrity and tight junctions. Analysis of exosomal miRNA expression profiling and mRNA expression profiles derived from lung tumor cells identified 11 differentially expressed miRNAs and their tumor cell targets including AMP-activated protein kinase (AMPK) signaling and Hippo signaling (Almendros et al. 2016). Therefore, exosomes released upon intermittent hypoxia may serve as vehicles of intercellular communication that alter the connections between tumor cells and surrounding stroma and underlie adverse cancer prognosis.

In addition to the evidence showing a promoting effect of intermittent hypoxia on tumor progression, Gallego-Martin et al. (2017) reported that 3-month exposure to intermittent hypoxia increased the spontaneous tumorigenesis associated with normal aging in 15-month-old male outbred Swiss CD1 mice. In particular, the percentage of animals exposed to severe intermittent hypoxia exhibiting tumors in at least one organ was almost twice that of the group subjected to room air or mild intermittent hypoxia. Lung tumors showed a significantly higher prevalence in the group exposed to severe intermittent hypoxia compared with the normoxic control, while skin tumorigenesis did not differ among the groups (Gallego-Martin et al. 2017). However, further studies are required to explore how intermittent hypoxia promotes tumorigenesis.

In conclusion, the past several decades have brought major advances in understanding OSA and CIH. Data from both epidemiologic and animal studies suggest a dominant role of OSA-associated CIH as a major contributor to multiple organ comorbidity and mortality. However, studies are still needed to address the underlying mechanisms and the effectiveness of CPAP treatment.

References

Abe H, Takahashi M, Yaegashi H, Eda S, Tsunemoto H, Kamikozawa M, Koyama J, Yamazaki K, Ikeda U. Efficacy of continuous positive airway pressure on arrhythmias in obstructive sleep apnea patients. Heart Vessel. 2010;25(1):63–9.

Akbarpour M, Khalyfa A, Qiao Z, Gileles-Hillel A, Almendros I, Farre R, Gozal D. Altered CD8+ T-cell lymphocyte function and TC1 cell stemness contribute to enhanced malignant tumor properties in murine models of sleep apnea. Sleep. 2017;40(2) https://doi.org/10.1093/sleep/zsw040.

Alchanatis M, Tourkohoriti G, Kakouros S, Kosmas E, Podaras S, Jordanoglou JB. Daytime pulmonary hypertension in patients with obstructive sleep apnea: the effect of continuous positive airway pressure on pulmonary hemodynamics. Respiration. 2001;68(6):566–72.

Allahdadi KJ, Walker BR, Kanagy NL. Augmented endothelin vasoconstriction in intermittent hypoxia-induced hypertension. Hypertension. 2005;45(4):705–9.

Almendros I, Montserrat JM, Ramirez J, Torres M, Duran-Cantolla J, Navajas D, Farre R. Intermittent hypoxia enhances cancer progression in a mouse model of sleep apnoea. Eur Respir J. 2012a;39(1):215–7.

Almendros I, Montserrat JM, Torres M, Bonsignore MR, Chimenti L, Navajas D, Farre R. Obesity and intermittent hypoxia increase tumor growth in a mouse model of sleep apnea. Sleep Med. 2012b;13(10):1254–60.

Almendros I, Montserrat JM, Torres M, Dalmases M, Cabanas ML, Campos-Rodriguez F, Navajas D, Farre R. Intermittent hypoxia increases melanoma metastasis to the lung in a mouse model of sleep apnea. Respir Physiol Neurobiol. 2013;186(3):303–7.

Almendros I, Wang Y, Becker L, Lennon FE, Zheng J, Coats BR, Schoenfelt KS, Carreras A, Hakim F, Zhang SX, et al. Intermittent hypoxia-induced changes in tumor-associated macrophages and tumor malignancy in a mouse model of sleep apnea. Am J Respir Crit Care Med. 2014;189(5):593–601.

Almendros I, Gileles-Hillel A, Khalyfa A, Wang Y, Zhang SX, Carreras A, Farre R, Gozal D. Adipose tissue macrophage polarization by intermittent hypoxia in a mouse model of OSA: effect of tumor microenvironment. Cancer Lett. 2015;361(2):233–9.

Almendros I, Khalyfa A, Trzepizur W, Gileles-Hillel A, Huang L, Akbarpour M, Andrade J, Farre R, Gozal D. Tumor cell malignant properties are enhanced by circulating exosomes in sleep apnea. Chest. 2016;150(5):1030–41.

Antic NA, Catcheside P, Buchan C, Hensley M, Naughton MT, Rowland S, Williamson B, Windler S, McEvoy RD. The effect of CPAP in normalizing daytime sleepiness, quality of life, and neurocognitive function in patients with moderate to severe OSA. Sleep. 2011;34(1): 111–9.

Arias MA, Garcia-Rio F, Alonso-Fernandez A, Martinez I, Villamor J. Pulmonary hypertension in obstructive sleep apnoea: effects of continuous positive airway pressure: a randomized, controlled cross-over study. Eur Heart J. 2006;27(9):1106–13.

Aronsohn RS, Whitmore H, Van Cauter E, Tasali E. Impact of untreated obstructive sleep apnea on glucose control in type 2 diabetes. Am J Respir Crit Care Med. 2010;181(5):507–13.

Arzt M, Young T, Finn L, Skatrud JB, Bradley TD. Association of sleep-disordered breathing and the occurrence of stroke. Am J Respir Crit Care Med. 2005;172(11):1447–51.

Azmi AS, Bao B, Sarkar FH. Exosomes in cancer development, metastasis, and drug resistance: a comprehensive review. Cancer Metastasis Rev. 2013;32(3–4):623–42.

Babu AR, Herdegen J, Fogelfeld L, Shott S, Mazzone T. Type 2 diabetes, glycemic control, and continuous positive airway pressure in obstructive sleep apnea. Arch Intern Med. 2005;165(4): 447–52.

Badran M, Ayas N, Laher I. Cardiovascular complications of sleep apnea: role of oxidative stress. Oxidative Med Cell Longev. 2014;2014:985258.

Bazan V, Grau N, Valles E, Felez M, Sanjuas C, Cainzos-Achirica M, Benito B, Jauregui-Abularach M, Gea J, Bruguera-Cortada J, et al. Obstructive sleep apnea in patients with typical atrial flutter: prevalence and impact on arrhythmia control outcome. Chest. 2013;143(5): 1277–83.

Bedard MA, Montplaisir J, Malo J, Richer F, Rouleau I. Persistent neuropsychological deficits and vigilance impairment in sleep apnea syndrome after treatment with continuous positive airways pressure (CPAP). J Clin Exp Neuropsychol. 1993;15(2):330–41.

Beebe DW, Groesz L, Wells C, Nichols A, McGee K. The neuropsychological effects of obstructive sleep apnea: a meta-analysis of norm-referenced and case-controlled data. Sleep. 2003;26(3): 298–307.

Bitter T, Faber L, Hering D, Langer C, Horstkotte D, Oldenburg O. Sleep-disordered breathing in heart failure with normal left ventricular ejection fraction. Eur J Heart Fail. 2009;11(6):602–8.

Bradley TD, Floras JS. Obstructive sleep apnoea and its cardiovascular consequences. Lancet. 2009;373(9657):82–93.

Bradley TD, Rutherford R, Grossman RF, Lue F, Zamel N, Moldofsky H, Phillipson EA. Role of daytime hypoxemia in the pathogenesis of right heart failure in the obstructive sleep apnea syndrome. Am Rev Respir Dis. 1985;131(6):835–9.

Bucks RS, Olaithe M, Eastwood P. Neurocognitive function in obstructive sleep apnoea: a meta-review. Respirology. 2013;18(1):61–70.

Cadby G, McArdle N, Briffa T, Hillman DR, Simpson L, Knuiman M, Hung J. Severity of OSA is an independent predictor of incident atrial fibrillation hospitalization in a large sleep-clinic cohort. Chest. 2015;148(4):945–52.

Campen MJ, Shimoda LA, O'Donnell CP. Acute and chronic cardiovascular effects of intermittent hypoxia in C57BL/6J mice. J Appl Physiol (1985). 2005;99(5):2028–35.

Campillo N, Torres M, Vilaseca A, Nonaka PN, Gozal D, Roca-Ferrer J, Picado C, Montserrat JM, Farre R, Navajas D, et al. Role of Cyclooxygenase-2 on intermittent hypoxia-induced lung tumor malignancy in a mouse model of sleep apnea. Sci Rep. 2017;7(44693):44693.

Campos-Rodriguez F, Martinez-Garcia MA, Martinez M, Duran-Cantolla J, Pena Mde L, Masdeu MJ, Gonzalez M, Campo F, Gallego I, Marin JM, et al. Association between obstructive sleep apnea and cancer incidence in a large multicenter Spanish cohort. Am J Respir Crit Care Med. 2013;187(1):99–105.

Canessa N, Castronovo V, Cappa SF, Aloia MS, Marelli S, Falini A, Alemanno F, Ferini-Strambi L. Obstructive sleep apnea: brain structural changes and neurocognitive function before and after treatment. Am J Respir Crit Care Med. 2011;183(10):1419–26.

Capone C, Faraco G, Coleman C, Young CN, Pickel VM, Anrather J, Davisson RL, Iadecola C. Endothelin 1-dependent neurovascular dysfunction in chronic intermittent hypoxia. Hypertension. 2012;60(1):106–13.

Carreras A, Kayali F, Zhang J, Hirotsu C, Wang Y, Gozal D. Metabolic effects of intermittent hypoxia in mice: steady versus high-frequency applied hypoxia daily during the rest period. Am J Physiol Regul Integr Comp Physiol. 2012;303(7):R700–9.

Chan J, Sanderson J, Chan W, Lai C, Choy D, Ho A, Leung R. Prevalence of sleep-disordered breathing in diastolic heart failure. Chest. 1997;111(6):1488–93.

Chen JC, Hwang JH. Sleep apnea increased incidence of primary central nervous system cancers: a nationwide cohort study. Sleep Med. 2014;15(7):749–54.

Chen EP, Smyth EM. COX-2 and PGE2-dependent immunomodulation in breast cancer. Prostaglandins Other Lipid Mediat. 2011;96(1–4):14–20.

Chen L, Einbinder E, Zhang Q, Hasday J, Balke CW, Scharf SM. Oxidative stress and left ventricular function with chronic intermittent hypoxia in rats. Am J Respir Crit Care Med. 2005;172(7):915–20.

Chen L, Cao ZL, Han F, Gao ZC, He QY. Chronic intermittent hypoxia from pedo-stage decreases glucose transporter 4 expression in adipose tissue and causes insulin resistance. Chin Med J. 2010;123(4):463–70.

Chirinos JA, Gurubhagavatula I, Teff K, Rader DJ, Wadden TA, Townsend R, Foster GD, Maislin G, Saif H, Broderick P, et al. CPAP, weight loss, or both for obstructive sleep apnea. N Engl J Med. 2014;370(24):2265–75.

Christensen AS, Clark A, Salo P, Nymann P, Lange P, Prescott E, Rod NH. Symptoms of sleep disordered breathing and risk of cancer: a prospective cohort study. Sleep. 2013;36(10): 1429–35.

Cowie MR, Woehrle H, Wegscheider K, Angermann C, d'Ortho MP, Erdmann E, Levy P, Simonds AK, Somers VK, Zannad F, et al. Adaptive servo-ventilation for central sleep apnea in systolic heart failure. N Engl J Med. 2015;373(12):1095–105.

Cubillos-Zapata C, Hernandez-Jimenez E, Avendano-Ortiz J, Toledano V, Varela-Serrano A, Fernandez-Navarro I, Casitas R, Carpio C, Aguirre LA, Garcia-Rio F, et al. Obstructive sleep apnea monocytes exhibit high levels of vascular endothelial growth factor secretion, augmenting tumor progression. Mediat Inflamm. 2018;2018(7373921):7373921.

Dalmases M, Sole-Padulles C, Torres M, Embid C, Nunez MD, Martinez-Garcia MA, Farre R, Bargallo N, Bartres-Faz D, Montserrat JM. Effect of CPAP on cognition, brain function, and structure among elderly patients with OSA: a randomized pilot study. Chest. 2015;148(5): 1214–23.

Dawson A, Abel SL, Loving RT, Dailey G, Shadan FF, Cronin JW, Kripke DF, Kline LE. CPAP therapy of obstructive sleep apnea in type 2 diabetics improves glycemic control during sleep. J Clin Sleep Med. 2008;4(6):538–42.

Dewan NA, Nieto FJ, Somers VK. Intermittent hypoxemia and OSA: implications for comorbidities. Chest. 2015;147(1):266–74.
Drager LF, Bortolotto LA, Figueiredo AC, Krieger EM, Lorenzi GF. Effects of continuous positive airway pressure on early signs of atherosclerosis in obstructive sleep apnea. Am J Respir Crit Care Med. 2007;176(7):706–12.
Drager LF, Polotsky VY, Lorenzi-Filho G. Obstructive sleep apnea: an emerging risk factor for atherosclerosis. Chest. 2011;140(2):534–42.
Ferini-Strambi L, Baietto C, Di Gioia MR, Castaldi P, Castronovo C, Zucconi M, Cappa SF. Cognitive dysfunction in patients with obstructive sleep apnea (OSA): partial reversibility after continuous positive airway pressure (CPAP). Brain Res Bull. 2003;61(1):87–92.
Findley LJ, Barth JT, Powers DC, Wilhoit SC, Boyd DG, Suratt PM. Cognitive impairment in patients with obstructive sleep apnea and associated hypoxemia. Chest. 1986;90(5):686–90.
Gale SD, Hopkins RO. Effects of hypoxia on the brain: neuroimaging and neuropsychological findings following carbon monoxide poisoning and obstructive sleep apnea. J Int Neuropsychol Soc. 2004;10(1):60–71.
Gallego-Martin T, Farre R, Almendros I, Gonzalez-Obeso E, Obeso A. Chronic intermittent hypoxia mimicking sleep apnoea increases spontaneous tumorigenesis in mice. Eur Respir J. 2017;49:1602111.
Gami AS, Hodge DO, Herges RM, Olson EJ, Nykodym J, Kara T, Somers VK. Obstructive sleep apnea, obesity, and the risk of incident atrial fibrillation. J Am Coll Cardiol. 2007;49(5):565–71.
Garcia-Rio F, Alonso-Fernandez A, Armada E, Mediano O, Lores V, Rojo B, Fernandez-Lahera J, Fernandez-Navarro I, Carpio C, Ramirez T. CPAP effect on recurrent episodes in patients with sleep apnea and myocardial infarction. Int J Cardiol. 2013;168(2):1328–35.
Gharib SA, Seiger AN, Hayes AL, Mehra R, Patel SR. Treatment of obstructive sleep apnea alters cancer-associated transcriptional signatures in circulating leukocytes. Sleep. 2014;37(4): 709–714, 714A–T.
Gottlieb DJ, Yenokyan G, Newman AB, O'Connor GT, Punjabi NM, Quan SF, Redline S, Resnick HE, Tong EK, Diener-West M, et al. Prospective study of obstructive sleep apnea and incident coronary heart disease and heart failure: the sleep heart health study. Circulation. 2010;122(4): 352–60.
Gozal D, Daniel JM, Dohanich GP. Behavioral and anatomical correlates of chronic episodic hypoxia during sleep in the rat. J Neurosci. 2001;21(7):2442–50.
Gozal D, Ham SA, Mokhlesi B. Sleep apnea and cancer: analysis of a nationwide population sample. Sleep. 2016;39(8):1493–500.
Gu CJ, Li M, Li QY, Li N. Chronic intermittent hypoxia increases beta cell mass and activates the mammalian target of rapamycin/hypoxia inducible factor 1/vascular endothelial growth factor A pathway in mice pancreatic islet. Chin Med J. 2013;126(12):2368–73.
Guo C, Buranych A, Sarkar D, Fisher PB, Wang XY. The role of tumor-associated macrophages in tumor vascularization. Vasc Cell. 2013;5(1):20.
Haas DC, Foster GL, Nieto FJ, Redline S, Resnick HE, Robbins JA, Young T, Pickering TG. Age-dependent associations between sleep-disordered breathing and hypertension: importance of discriminating between systolic/diastolic hypertension and isolated systolic hypertension in the Sleep Heart Health Study. Circulation. 2005;111(5):614–21.
Hayashi T, Yamashita C, Matsumoto C, Kwak CJ, Fujii K, Hirata T, Miyamura M, Mori T, Ukimura A, Okada Y, et al. Role of gp91phox-containing NADPH oxidase in left ventricular remodeling induced by intermittent hypoxic stress. Am J Phys Heart Circ Phys. 2008;294(5): H2197–203.
Hedner JA, Wilcox I, Laks L, Grunstein RR, Sullivan CE. A specific and potent pressor effect of hypoxia in patients with sleep apnea. Am Rev Respir Dis. 1992;146(5 Pt 1):1240–5.
Hermann DM, Bassetti CL. Sleep-related breathing and sleep-wake disturbances in ischemic stroke. Neurology. 2009;73(16):1313–22.

Hsu CY, Vennelle M, Li HY, Engleman HM, Dennis MS, Douglas NJ. Sleep-disordered breathing after stroke: a randomised controlled trial of continuous positive airway pressure. J Neurol Neurosurg Psychiatry. 2006;77(10):1143–9.

Iiyori N, Alonso LC, Li J, Sanders MH, Garcia-Ocana A, O'Doherty RM, Polotsky VY, O'Donnell CP. Intermittent hypoxia causes insulin resistance in lean mice independent of autonomic activity. Am J Respir Crit Care Med. 2007;175(8):851–7.

Ip MS, Lam B, Chan LY, Zheng L, Tsang KW, Fung PC, Lam WK. Circulating nitric oxide is suppressed in obstructive sleep apnea and is reversed by nasal continuous positive airway pressure. Am J Respir Crit Care Med. 2000;162(6):2166–71.

Jackman KA, Zhou P, Faraco G, Peixoto PM, Coleman C, Voss HU, Pickel V, Manfredi G, Iadecola C. Dichotomous effects of chronic intermittent hypoxia on focal cerebral ischemic injury. Stroke. 2014;45(5):1460–7.

Jagadapillai R, Mellen NM, Sachleben LR Jr, Gozal E. Ceftriaxone preserves glutamate transporters and prevents intermittent hypoxia-induced vulnerability to brain excitotoxic injury. PLoS One. 2014;9(7):e100230.

Jun J, Savransky V, Nanayakkara A, Bevans S, Li J, Smith PL, Polotsky VY. Intermittent hypoxia has organ-specific effects on oxidative stress. Am J Physiol Regul Integr Comp Physiol. 2008;295(4):R1274–81.

Jun J, Reinke C, Bedja D, Berkowitz D, Bevans-Fonti S, Li J, Barouch LA, Gabrielson K, Polotsky VY. Effect of intermittent hypoxia on atherosclerosis in apolipoprotein E-deficient mice. Atherosclerosis. 2010;209(2):381–6.

Kallwitz ER, Herdegen J, Madura J, Jakate S, Cotler SJ. Liver enzymes and histology in obese patients with obstructive sleep apnea. J Clin Gastroenterol. 2007;41(10):918–21.

Kanagala R, Murali NS, Friedman PA, Ammash NM, Gersh BJ, Ballman KV, Shamsuzzaman AS, Somers VK. Obstructive sleep apnea and the recurrence of atrial fibrillation. Circulation. 2003;107(20):2589–94.

Kanagy NL, Walker BR, Nelin LD. Role of endothelin in intermittent hypoxia-induced hypertension. Hypertension. 2001;37(2 Pt 2):511–5.

Kasai T, Floras JS, Bradley TD. Sleep apnea and cardiovascular disease: a bidirectional relationship. Circulation. 2012;126(12):1495–510.

Kasai T, Yumino D, Redolfi S, Su MC, Ruttanaumpawan P, Mak S, Newton GE, Floras JS, Bradley TD. Overnight effects of obstructive sleep apnea and its treatment on stroke volume in patients with heart failure. Can J Cardiol. 2015;31(7):832–8.

Kato M, Roberts-Thomson P, Phillips BG, Haynes WG, Winnicki M, Accurso V, Somers VK. Impairment of endothelium-dependent vasodilation of resistance vessels in patients with obstructive sleep apnea. Circulation. 2000;102(21):2607–10.

Kendzerska T, Leung RS, Hawker G, Tomlinson G, Gershon AS. Obstructive sleep apnea and the prevalence and incidence of cancer. CMAJ. 2014;186(13):985–92.

Kent BD, Grote L, Ryan S, Pepin JL, Bonsignore MR, Tkacova R, Saaresranta T, Verbraecken J, Levy P, Hedner J, et al. Diabetes mellitus prevalence and control in sleep-disordered breathing: the European Sleep Apnea Cohort (ESADA) study. Chest. 2014;146(4):982–90.

Klein TJ, Glazer PM. The tumor microenvironment and DNA repair. Semin Radiat Oncol. 2010;20 (4):282–7.

Konecny T, Kuniyoshi FH, Orban M, Pressman GS, Kara T, Gami A, Caples SM, Lopez-Jimenez F, Somers VK. Under-diagnosis of sleep apnea in patients after acute myocardial infarction. J Am Coll Cardiol. 2010;56(9):742–3.

Kotterba S, Rasche K, Widdig W, Duscha C, Blombach S, Schultze-Werninghaus G, Malin JP. Neuropsychological investigations and event-related potentials in obstructive sleep apnea syndrome before and during CPAP-therapy. J Neurol Sci. 1998;159(1):45–50.

Kraiczi H, Caidahl K, Samuelsson A, Peker Y, Hedner J. Impairment of vascular endothelial function and left ventricular filling: association with the severity of apnea-induced hypoxemia during sleep. Chest. 2001;119(4):1085–91.

Kukwa W, Migacz E, Druc K, Grzesiuk E, Czarnecka AM. Obstructive sleep apnea and cancer: effects of intermittent hypoxia? Future Oncol. 2015;11(24):3285–98.

Kushida CA, Nichols DA, Holmes TH, Quan SF, Walsh JK, Gottlieb DJ, Simon RD Jr, Guilleminault C, White DP, Goodwin JL, et al. Effects of continuous positive airway pressure on neurocognitive function in obstructive sleep apnea patients: the Apnea Positive Pressure Long-term Efficacy Study (APPLES). Sleep. 2012;35(12):1593–602.

Lafontan M, Langin D. Lipolysis and lipid mobilization in human adipose tissue. Prog Lipid Res. 2009;48(5):275–97.

Lam JC, Xu A, Tam S, Khong PI, Yao TJ, Lam DC, Lai AY, Lam B, Lam KS, Mary SM. Hypoadiponectinemia is related to sympathetic activation and severity of obstructive sleep apnea. Sleep. 2008;31(12):1721–7.

Lavie L. Oxidative stress in obstructive sleep apnea and intermittent hypoxia—revisited—the bad ugly and good: implications to the heart and brain. Sleep Med Rev. 2015;20:27–45.

Lavie L, Dyugovskaya L, Polyakov A. Biology of peripheral blood cells in obstructive sleep apnea—the tip of the iceberg. Arch Physiol Biochem. 2008;114(4):244–54.

Lefebvre B, Godin-Ribuot D, Joyeux-Faure M, Caron F, Bessard G, Levy P, Stanke-Labesque F. Functional assessment of vascular reactivity after chronic intermittent hypoxia in the rat. Respir Physiol Neurobiol. 2006;150(2–3):278–86.

Leuenberger U, Jacob E, Sweer L, Waravdekar N, Zwillich C, Sinoway L. Surges of muscle sympathetic nerve activity during obstructive apnea are linked to hypoxemia. J Appl Physiol (1985). 1995;79(2):581–8.

Levy P, Pepin JL, Arnaud C, Baguet JP, Dematteis M, Mach F. Obstructive sleep apnea and atherosclerosis. Prog Cardiovasc Dis. 2009;51(5):400–10.

Li J, Thorne LN, Punjabi NM, Sun CK, Schwartz AR, Smith PL, Marino RL, Rodriguez A, Hubbard WC, O'Donnell CP, et al. Intermittent hypoxia induces hyperlipidemia in lean mice. Circ Res. 2005;97(7):698–706.

Li J, Bosch-Marce M, Nanayakkara A, Savransky V, Fried SK, Semenza GL, Polotsky VY. Altered metabolic responses to intermittent hypoxia in mice with partial deficiency of hypoxia-inducible factor-1alpha. Physiol Genomics. 2006;25(3):450–7.

Li J, Savransky V, Nanayakkara A, Smith PL, O'Donnell CP, Polotsky VY. Hyperlipidemia and lipid peroxidation are dependent on the severity of chronic intermittent hypoxia. J Appl Physiol (1985). 2007a;102(2):557–63.

Li J, Nanayakkara A, Jun J, Savransky V, Polotsky VY. Effect of deficiency in SREBP cleavage-activating protein on lipid metabolism during intermittent hypoxia. Physiol Genomics. 2007b;31(2):273–80.

Lim DC, Pack AI. Obstructive sleep apnea and cognitive impairment: addressing the blood-brain barrier. Sleep Med Rev. 2014;18(1):35–48.

Lim DC, Brady DC, Po P, Chuang LP, Marcondes L, Kim EY, Keenan BT, Guo X, Maislin G, Galante RJ, et al. Simulating obstructive sleep apnea patients' oxygenation characteristics into a mouse model of cyclical intermittent hypoxia. J Appl Physiol (1985). 2015;118(5):544–57.

Lindberg E, Theorell-Haglow J, Svensson M, Gislason T, Berne C, Janson C. Sleep apnea and glucose metabolism: a long-term follow-up in a community-based sample. Chest. 2012;142(4): 935–42.

Liu JN, Zhang JX, Lu G, Qiu Y, Yang D, Yin GY, Zhang XL. The effect of oxidative stress in myocardial cell injury in mice exposed to chronic intermittent hypoxia. Chin Med J. 2010;123 (1):74–8.

Liu X, Feng L, Cao G, Huang H, Xu Q, Yu J, Zhang S, Zhou M. Cardiac structure and function improvements in coronary artery disease combined with severe obstructive sleep apnea/ hypopnea syndrome patients via noninvasive positive pressure ventilation therapy. Coron Artery Dis. 2014;25(6):516–20.

Logan AG, Tkacova R, Perlikowski SM, Leung RS, Tisler A, Floras JS, Bradley TD. Refractory hypertension and sleep apnoea: effect of CPAP on blood pressure and baroreflex. Eur Respir J. 2003;21(2):241–7.

Louis M, Punjabi NM. Effects of acute intermittent hypoxia on glucose metabolism in awake healthy volunteers. J Appl Physiol (1985). 2009;106(5):1538–44.

Magalang UJ, Cruff JP, Rajappan R, Hunter MG, Patel T, Marsh CB, Raman SV, Parinandi NL. Intermittent hypoxia suppresses adiponectin secretion by adipocytes. Experimental Clin Endocrinol Diabetes. 2009;117(3):129–34.

Mansfield DR, Gollogly NC, Kaye DM, Richardson M, Bergin P, Naughton MT. Controlled trial of continuous positive airway pressure in obstructive sleep apnea and heart failure. Am J Respir Crit Care Med. 2004;169(3):361–6.

Marin JM, Carrizo SJ, Vicente E, Agusti AG. Long-term cardiovascular outcomes in men with obstructive sleep apnoea-hypopnoea with or without treatment with continuous positive airway pressure: an observational study. Lancet. 2005;365(9464):1046–53.

Martinez-Ceron E, Barquiel B, Bezos AM, Casitas R, Galera R, Garcia-Benito C, Hernanz A, Alonso-Fernandez A, Garcia-Rio F. Effect of continuous positive airway pressure on glycemic control in patients with obstructive sleep apnea and type 2 diabetes. A Randomized Clinical Trial. Am J Respir Crit Care Med. 2016;194(4):476–85.

Martinez-Garcia MA, Soler-Cataluna JJ, Ejarque-Martinez L, Soriano Y, Roman-Sanchez P, Illa FB, Canal JM, Duran-Cantolla J. Continuous positive airway pressure treatment reduces mortality in patients with ischemic stroke and obstructive sleep apnea: a 5-year follow-up study. Am J Respir Crit Care Med. 2009;180(1):36–41.

Martinez-Garcia MA, Campos-Rodriguez F, Soler-Cataluna JJ, Catalan-Serra P, Roman-Sanchez P, Montserrat JM. Increased incidence of nonfatal cardiovascular events in stroke patients with sleep apnoea: effect of CPAP treatment. Eur Respir J. 2012;39(4):906–12.

Martinez-Garcia MA, Campos-Rodriguez F, Duran-Cantolla J, de la Pena M, Masdeu MJ, Gonzalez M, Del Campo F, Serra PC, Valero-Sanchez I, Ferrer MJ, et al. Obstructive sleep apnea is associated with cancer mortality in younger patients. Sleep Med. 2014a;15(7):742–8.

Martinez-Garcia MA, Martorell-Calatayud A, Nagore E, Valero I, Selma MJ, Chiner E, Landete P, Montserrat JM, Carrera C, Perez-Gil A, et al. Association between sleep disordered breathing and aggressiveness markers of malignant cutaneous melanoma. Eur Respir J. 2014b;43(6): 1661–8.

McEvoy RD, Antic NA, Heeley E, Luo Y, Ou Q, Zhang X, Mediano O, Chen R, Drager LF, Liu Z, et al. CPAP for prevention of cardiovascular events in obstructive sleep apnea. N Engl J Med. 2016;375(10):919–31.

Mehra R, Benjamin EJ, Shahar E, Gottlieb DJ, Nawabit R, Kirchner HL, Sahadevan J, Redline S. Association of nocturnal arrhythmias with sleep-disordered breathing: the Sleep Heart Health Study. Am J Respir Crit Care Med. 2006;173(8):910–6.

Mesarwi OA, Sharma EV, Jun JC, Polotsky VY. Metabolic dysfunction in obstructive sleep apnea: a critical examination of underlying mechanisms. Sleep Biol Rhythms. 2015;13(1):2–17.

Milleron O, Pilliere R, Foucher A, de Roquefeuil F, Aegerter P, Jondeau G, Raffestin BG, Dubourg O. Benefits of obstructive sleep apnoea treatment in coronary artery disease: a long-term follow-up study. Eur Heart J. 2004;25(9):728–34.

Mooe T, Rabben T, Wiklund U, Franklin KA, Eriksson P. Sleep-disordered breathing in men with coronary artery disease. Chest. 1996;109(3):659–63.

Mooe T, Franklin KA, Wiklund U, Rabben T, Holmstrom K. Sleep-disordered breathing and myocardial ischemia in patients with coronary artery disease. Chest. 2000;117(6):1597–602.

Mooe T, Franklin KA, Holmstrom K, Rabben T, Wiklund U. Sleep-disordered breathing and coronary artery disease: long-term prognosis. Am J Respir Crit Care Med. 2001;164(10 Pt 1): 1910–3.

Myhill PC, Davis WA, Peters KE, Chubb SA, Hillman D, Davis TM. Effect of continuous positive airway pressure therapy on cardiovascular risk factors in patients with type 2 diabetes and obstructive sleep apnea. J Clin Endocrinol Metab. 2012;97(11):4212–8.

Nadeem R, Singh M, Nida M, Kwon S, Sajid H, Witkowski J, Pahomov E, Shah K, Park W, Champeau D. Effect of CPAP treatment for obstructive sleep apnea hypopnea syndrome on lipid profile: a meta-regression analysis. J Clin Sleep Med. 2014;10(12):1295–302.

Naegele B, Pepin JL, Levy P, Bonnet C, Pellat J, Feuerstein C. Cognitive executive dysfunction in patients with obstructive sleep apnea syndrome (OSAS) after CPAP treatment. Sleep. 1998;21 (4):392–7.

Nahmias J, Lao R, Karetzky M. Right ventricular dysfunction in obstructive sleep apnoea: reversal with nasal continuous positive airway pressure. Eur Respir J. 1996;9(5):945–51.

Nanduri J, Yuan G, Kumar GK, Semenza GL, Prabhakar NR. Transcriptional responses to intermittent hypoxia. Respir Physiol Neurobiol. 2008;164(1–2):277–81.

Newman AB, Nieto FJ, Guidry U, Lind BK, Redline S, Pickering TG, Quan SF. Relation of sleep-disordered breathing to cardiovascular disease risk factors: the Sleep Heart Health Study. Am J Epidemiol. 2001;154(1):50–9.

Nieto FJ, Young TB, Lind BK, Shahar E, Samet JM, Redline S, D'Agostino RB, Newman AB, Lebowitz MD, Pickering TG. Association of sleep-disordered breathing, sleep apnea, and hypertension in a large community-based study. Sleep Heart Health Study. JAMA. 2000;283 (14):1829–36.

Nieto FJ, Peppard PE, Young T, Finn L, Hla KM, Farre R. Sleep-disordered breathing and cancer mortality: results from the Wisconsin Sleep Cohort Study. Am J Respir Crit Care Med. 2012;186(2):190–4.

Nisbet RE, Graves AS, Kleinhenz DJ, Rupnow HL, Reed AL, Fan TH, Mitchell PO, Sutliff RL, Hart CM. The role of NADPH oxidase in chronic intermittent hypoxia-induced pulmonary hypertension in mice. Am J Respir Cell Mol Biol. 2009;40(5):601–9.

Nobili V, Cutrera R, Liccardo D, Pavone M, Devito R, Giorgio V, Verrillo E, Baviera G, Musso G. Obstructive sleep apnea syndrome affects liver histology and inflammatory cell activation in pediatric nonalcoholic fatty liver disease, regardless of obesity/insulin resistance. Am J Respir Crit Care Med. 2014;189(1):66–76.

Pack AI, Gislason T. Obstructive sleep apnea and cardiovascular disease: a perspective and future directions. Prog Cardiovasc Dis. 2009;51(5):434–51.

Pamidi S, Tasali E. Obstructive sleep apnea and type 2 diabetes: is there a link? Front Neurol. 2012;3:126.

Pamidi S, Wroblewski K, Broussard J, Day A, Hanlon EC, Abraham V, Tasali E. Obstructive sleep apnea in young lean men: impact on insulin sensitivity and secretion. Diabetes Care. 2012;35 (11):2384–9.

Parra O, Sanchez-Armengol A, Capote F, Bonnin M, Arboix A, Campos-Rodriguez F, Perez-Ronchel J, Duran-Cantolla J, Martinez-Null C, de la Pena M, et al. Efficacy of continuous positive airway pressure treatment on 5 year survival in patients with ischaemic stroke and obstructive sleep apnea: a randomized controlled trial. J Sleep Res. 2015;24(1):47–53.

Payne RS, Goldbart A, Gozal D, Schurr A. Effect of intermittent hypoxia on long-term potentiation in rat hippocampal slices. Brain Res. 2004;1029(2):195–9.

Peker Y, Kraiczi H, Hedner J, Loth S, Johansson A, Bende M. An independent association between obstructive sleep apnoea and coronary artery disease. Eur Respir J. 1999;14(1):179–84.

Peker Y, Glantz H, Eulenburg C, Wegscheider K, Herlitz J, Thunstrom E. Effect of positive airway pressure on cardiovascular outcomes in coronary artery disease patients with nonsleepy obstructive sleep apnea. The RICCADSA Randomized Controlled Trial. Am J Respir Crit Care Med. 2016;194(5):613–20.

Peled N, Abinader EG, Pillar G, Sharif D, Lavie P. Nocturnal ischemic events in patients with obstructive sleep apnea syndrome and ischemic heart disease: effects of continuous positive air pressure treatment. J Am Coll Cardiol. 1999;34(6):1744–9.

Peng YJ, Yuan G, Ramakrishnan D, Sharma SD, Bosch-Marce M, Kumar GK, Semenza GL, Prabhakar NR. Heterozygous HIF-1alpha deficiency impairs carotid body-mediated systemic responses and reactive oxygen species generation in mice exposed to intermittent hypoxia. J Physiol. 2006;577(Pt 2):705–16.

Peppard PE, Young T, Palta M, Skatrud J. Prospective study of the association between sleep-disordered breathing and hypertension. N Engl J Med. 2000;342(19):1378–84.

Phillips BG, Narkiewicz K, Pesek CA, Haynes WG, Dyken ME, Somers VK. Effects of obstructive sleep apnea on endothelin-1 and blood pressure. J Hypertens. 1999;17(1):61–6.

Phillips CL, Yee BJ, Marshall NS, Liu PY, Sullivan DR, Grunstein RR. Continuous positive airway pressure reduces postprandial lipidemia in obstructive sleep apnea: a randomized, placebo-controlled crossover trial. Am J Respir Crit Care Med. 2011;184(3):355–61.

Pichiule P, Chavez JC, Boero J, Arregui A. Chronic hypoxia induces modification of the N-methyl-D-aspartate receptor in rat brain. Neurosci Lett. 1996;218(2):83–6.

Polak J, Shimoda LA, Drager LF, Undem C, McHugh H, Polotsky VY, Punjabi NM. Intermittent hypoxia impairs glucose homeostasis in C57BL6/J mice: partial improvement with cessation of the exposure. Sleep. 2013;36(10):1483–1490; 1490a–b.

Polotsky VY, Patil SP, Savransky V, Laffan A, Fonti S, Frame LA, Steele KE, Schweizter MA, Clark JM, Torbenson MS, et al. Obstructive sleep apnea, insulin resistance, and steatohepatitis in severe obesity. Am J Respir Crit Care Med. 2009;179(3):228–34.

Prabhakar NR, Kumar GK. Oxidative stress in the systemic and cellular responses to intermittent hypoxia. Biol Chem. 2004;385(3–4):217–21.

Prabhakar NR, Kumar GK. Mechanisms of sympathetic activation and blood pressure elevation by intermittent hypoxia. Respir Physiol Neurobiol. 2010;174(1–2):156–61.

Punjabi NM, Beamer BA. Alterations in glucose disposal in sleep-disordered breathing. Am J Respir Crit Care Med. 2009;179(3):235–40.

Quan SF, Chan CS, Dement WC, Gevins A, Goodwin JL, Gottlieb DJ, Green S, Guilleminault C, Hirshkowitz M, Hyde PR, et al. The association between obstructive sleep apnea and neurocognitive performance—the Apnea Positive Pressure Long-term Efficacy Study (APPLES). Sleep. 2011;34(3):303–314b.

Raposo G, Stoorvogel W. Extracellular vesicles: exosomes, microvesicles, and friends. J Cell Biol. 2013;200(4):373–83.

Reinke C, Bevans-Fonti S, Drager LF, Shin MK, Polotsky VY. Effects of different acute hypoxic regimens on tissue oxygen profiles and metabolic outcomes. J Appl Physiol (1985). 2011;111 (3):881–90.

Rossi VA, Stradling JR, Kohler M. Effects of obstructive sleep apnoea on heart rhythm. Eur Respir J. 2013;41(6):1439–51.

Ryan CM, Usui K, Floras JS, Bradley TD. Effect of continuous positive airway pressure on ventricular ectopy in heart failure patients with obstructive sleep apnoea. Thorax. 2005;60(9): 781–5.

Sajkov D, Cowie RJ, Thornton AT, Espinoza HA, McEvoy RD. Pulmonary hypertension and hypoxemia in obstructive sleep apnea syndrome. Am J Respir Crit Care Med. 1994;149(2 Pt 1): 416–22.

Sajkov D, Wang T, Saunders NA, Bune AJ, Neill AM, Douglas Mcevoy R. Daytime pulmonary hemodynamics in patients with obstructive sleep apnea without lung disease. Am J Respir Crit Care Med. 1999;159(5 Pt 1):1518–26.

Sajkov D, Wang T, Saunders NA, Bune AJ, McEvoy RD. Continuous positive airway pressure treatment improves pulmonary hemodynamics in patients with obstructive sleep apnea. Am J Respir Crit Care Med. 2002;165(2):152–8.

Sandberg O, Franklin KA, Bucht G, Eriksson S, Gustafson Y. Nasal continuous positive airway pressure in stroke patients with sleep apnoea: a randomized treatment study. Eur Respir J. 2001;18(4):630–4.

Sanner BM, Doberauer C, Konermann M, Sturm A, Zidek W. Pulmonary hypertension in patients with obstructive sleep apnea syndrome. Arch Intern Med. 1997;157(21):2483–7.

Sapin E, Peyron C, Roche F, Gay N, Carcenac C, Savasta M, Levy P, Dematteis M. Chronic intermittent hypoxia induces chronic low-grade neuroinflammation in the dorsal hippocampus of mice. Sleep. 2015;38(10):1537–46.

Savransky V, Nanayakkara A, Vivero A, Li J, Bevans S, Smith PL, Torbenson MS, Polotsky VY. Chronic intermittent hypoxia predisposes to liver injury. Hepatology. 2007;45(4):1007–13.

Savransky V, Jun J, Li J, Nanayakkara A, Fonti S, Moser AB, Steele KE, Schweitzer MA, Patil SP, Bhanot S, et al. Dyslipidemia and atherosclerosis induced by chronic intermittent hypoxia are attenuated by deficiency of stearoyl coenzyme A desaturase. Circ Res. 2008;103(10):1173–80.
Schafer H, Koehler U, Ploch T, Peter JH. Sleep-related myocardial ischemia and sleep structure in patients with obstructive sleep apnea and coronary heart disease. Chest. 1997;111(2):387–93.
Schulz R, Hummel C, Heinemann S, Seeger W, Grimminger F. Serum levels of vascular endothelial growth factor are elevated in patients with obstructive sleep apnea and severe nighttime hypoxia. Am J Respir Crit Care Med. 2002;165(1):67–70.
Seicean S, Kirchner HL, Gottlieb DJ, Punjabi NM, Resnick H, Sanders M, Budhiraja R, Singer M, Redline S. Sleep-disordered breathing and impaired glucose metabolism in normal-weight and overweight/obese individuals: the Sleep Heart Health Study. Diabetes Care. 2008;31(5): 1001–6.
Sforza E, Krieger J, Weitzenblum E, Apprill M, Lampert E, Ratamaharo J. Long-term effects of treatment with nasal continuous positive airway pressure on daytime lung function and pulmonary hemodynamics in patients with obstructive sleep apnea. Am Rev Respir Dis. 1990;141(4 Pt 1):866–70.
Shahar E, Whitney CW, Redline S, Lee ET, Newman AB, Nieto FJ, O'Connor GT, Boland LL, Schwartz JE, Samet JM. Sleep-disordered breathing and cardiovascular disease: cross-sectional results of the Sleep Heart Health Study. Am J Respir Crit Care Med. 2001;163(1):19–25.
Shamsuzzaman AS, Winnicki M, Lanfranchi P, Wolk R, Kara T, Accurso V, Somers VK. Elevated C-reactive protein in patients with obstructive sleep apnea. Circulation. 2002;105(21):2462–4.
Shaw JE, Punjabi NM, Wilding JP, Alberti KG, Zimmet PZ. Sleep-disordered breathing and type 2 diabetes: a report from the International Diabetes Federation Taskforce on Epidemiology and Prevention. Diabetes Res Clin Pract. 2008;81(1):2–12.
Shaw JE, Punjabi NM, Naughton MT, Willes L, Bergenstal RM, Cistulli PA, Fulcher GR, Richards GN, Zimmet PZ. The effect of treatment of obstructive sleep apnea on glycemic control in type 2 diabetes. Am J Respir Crit Care Med. 2016;194(4):486–92.
Shepard JW Jr, Garrison MW, Grither DA, Dolan GF. Relationship of ventricular ectopy to oxyhemoglobin desaturation in patients with obstructive sleep apnea. Chest. 1985;88(3): 335–40.
Sherwani SI, Aldana C, Usmani S, Adin C, Kotha S, Khan M, Eubank T, Scherer PE, Parinandi N, Magalang UJ. Intermittent hypoxia exacerbates pancreatic beta-cell dysfunction in a mouse model of diabetes mellitus. Sleep. 2013;36(12):1849–58.
Shin MK, Han W, Bevans-Fonti S, Jun JC, Punjabi NM, Polotsky VY. The effect of adrenal medullectomy on metabolic responses to chronic intermittent hypoxia. Respir Physiol Neurobiol. 2014a;203:60–7.
Shin MK, Yao Q, Jun JC, Bevans-Fonti S, Yoo DY, Han W, Mesarwi O, Richardson R, Fu YY, Pasricha PJ, et al. Carotid body denervation prevents fasting hyperglycemia during chronic intermittent hypoxia. J Appl Physiol (1985). 2014b;117(7):765–76.
Shpirer I, Elizur A, Shorer R, Peretz RB, Rabey JM, Khaigrekht M. Hypoxemia correlates with attentional dysfunction in patients with obstructive sleep apnea. Sleep Breath = Schlaf Atmung. 2012;16(3):821–7.
Somers VK, Dyken ME, Clary MP, Abboud FM. Sympathetic neural mechanisms in obstructive sleep apnea. J Clin Invest. 1995;96(4):1897–904.
Somers VK, White DP, Amin R, Abraham WT, Costa F, Culebras A, Daniels S, Floras JS, Hunt CE, Olson LJ, et al. Sleep apnea and cardiovascular disease: an American Heart Association/ American College of Cardiology Foundation Scientific Statement from the American Heart Association Council for High Blood Pressure Research Professional Education Committee, Council on Clinical Cardiology, Stroke Council, and Council on Cardiovascular Nursing. J Am Coll Cardiol. 2008;52(8):686–717.
Tahrani AA, Ali A, Raymond NT, Begum S, Dubb K, Mughal S, Jose B, Piya MK, Barnett AH, Stevens MJ. Obstructive sleep apnea and diabetic neuropathy: a novel association in patients with type 2 diabetes. Am J Respir Crit Care Med. 2012;186(5):434–41.

Tahrani AA, Ali A, Raymond NT, Begum S, Dubb K, Altaf QA, Piya MK, Barnett AH, Stevens MJ. Obstructive sleep apnea and diabetic nephropathy: a cohort study. Diabetes Care. 2013;36 (11):3718–25.

Tang X, Mo C, Wang Y, Wei D, Xiao H. Anti-tumour strategies aiming to target tumour-associated macrophages. Immunology. 2013;138(2):93–104.

Tanne F, Gagnadoux F, Chazouilleres O, Fleury B, Wendum D, Lasnier E, Lebeau B, Poupon R, Serfaty L. Chronic liver injury during obstructive sleep apnea. Hepatology. 2005;41(6):1290–6.

Tasali E, Ip MS. Obstructive sleep apnea and metabolic syndrome: alterations in glucose metabolism and inflammation. Proc Am Thorac Soc. 2008;5(2):207–17.

Teramoto S, Kume H, Yamamoto H, Ishii T, Miyashita A, Matsuse T, Akishita M, Toba K, Ouchi Y. Effects of oxygen administration on the circulating vascular endothelial growth factor (VEGF) levels in patients with obstructive sleep apnea syndrome. Int Med. 2003;42(8):681–5.

Thunstrom E, Glantz H, Fu M, Yucel-Lindberg T, Petzold M, Lindberg K, Peker Y. Increased inflammatory activity in nonobese patients with coronary artery disease and obstructive sleep apnea. Sleep. 2015;38(3):463–71.

Tkacova R, McNicholas WT, Javorsky M, Fietze I, Sliwinski P, Parati G, Grote L, Hedner J. Nocturnal intermittent hypoxia predicts prevalent hypertension in the European Sleep Apnoea Database cohort study. Eur Respir J. 2014;44(4):931–41.

Toffoli S, Michiels C. Intermittent hypoxia is a key regulator of cancer cell and endothelial cell interplay in tumours. FEBS J. 2008;275(12):2991–3002.

Tonon C, Vetrugno R, Lodi R, Gallassi R, Provini F, Iotti S, Plazzi G, Montagna P, Lugaresi E, Barbiroli B. Proton magnetic resonance spectroscopy study of brain metabolism in obstructive sleep apnoea syndrome before and after continuous positive airway pressure treatment. Sleep. 2007;30(3):305–11.

Trzepizur W, Le Vaillant M, Meslier N, Pigeanne T, Masson P, Humeau MP, Bizieux-Thaminy A, Goupil F, Chollet S, Ducluzeau PH, et al. Independent association between nocturnal intermittent hypoxemia and metabolic dyslipidemia. Chest. 2013;143(6):1584–9.

Usui K, Bradley TD, Spaak J, Ryan CM, Kubo T, Kaneko Y, Floras JS. Inhibition of awake sympathetic nerve activity of heart failure patients with obstructive sleep apnea by nocturnal continuous positive airway pressure. J Am Coll Cardiol. 2005;45(12):2008–11.

Valham F, Mooe T, Rabben T, Stenlund H, Wiklund U, Franklin KA. Increased risk of stroke in patients with coronary artery disease and sleep apnea: a 10-year follow-up. Circulation. 2008;118(9):955–60.

Vazir A, Hastings PC, Dayer M, McIntyre HF, Henein MY, Poole-Wilson PA, Cowie MR, Morrell MJ, Simonds AK. A high prevalence of sleep disordered breathing in men with mild symptomatic chronic heart failure due to left ventricular systolic dysfunction. Eur J Heart Fail. 2007;9(3): 243–50.

Vilaseca A, Campillo N, Torres M, Musquera M, Gozal D, Montserrat JM, Alcaraz A, Touijer KA, Farre R, Almendros I. Intermittent hypoxia increases kidney tumor vascularization in a murine model of sleep apnea. PLoS One. 2017;12(6):e0179444.

Wang X, Bi Y, Zhang Q, Pan F. Obstructive sleep apnoea and the risk of type 2 diabetes: a meta-analysis of prospective cohort studies. Respirology. 2013a;18(1):140–6.

Wang N, Khan SA, Prabhakar NR, Nanduri J. Impairment of pancreatic beta-cell function by chronic intermittent hypoxia. Exp Physiol. 2013b;98(9):1376–85.

Weinstock TG, Wang X, Rueschman M, Ismail-Beigi F, Aylor J, Babineau DC, Mehra R, Redline S. A controlled trial of CPAP therapy on metabolic control in individuals with impaired glucose tolerance and sleep apnea. Sleep. 2012;35(5):617–625b.

Weiss JW, Liu MD, Huang J. Physiological basis for a causal relationship of obstructive sleep apnoea to hypertension. Exp Physiol. 2007;92(1):21–6.

Wessendorf TE, Thilmann AF, Wang YM, Schreiber A, Konietzko N, Teschler H. Fibrinogen levels and obstructive sleep apnea in ischemic stroke. Am J Respir Crit Care Med. 2000;162(6): 2039–42.

Xu J, Long YS, Gozal D, Epstein PN. Beta-cell death and proliferation after intermittent hypoxia: role of oxidative stress. Free Radic Biol Med. 2009;46(6):783–90.
Yang D, Liu Z, Yang H, Luo Q. Effects of continuous positive airway pressure on glycemic control and insulin resistance in patients with obstructive sleep apnea: a meta-analysis. Sleep Breath = Schlaf Atmung. 2013;17(1):33–8.
Ye L, Ma GH, Chen L, Li M, Liu JL, Yang K, Li QY, Li N, Wan HY. Quantification of circulating cell-free DNA in the serum of patients with obstructive sleep apnea-hypopnea syndrome. Lung. 2010;188(6):469–74.
Yokoe T, Alonso LC, Romano LC, Rosa TC, O'Doherty RM, Garcia-Ocana A, Minoguchi K, O'Donnell CP. Intermittent hypoxia reverses the diurnal glucose rhythm and causes pancreatic beta-cell replication in mice. J Physiol. 2008;586(3):899–911.
Yoshihisa A, Suzuki S, Yamaki T, Sugimoto K, Kunii H, Nakazato K, Suzuki H, Saitoh S, Takeishi Y. Impact of adaptive servo-ventilation on cardiovascular function and prognosis in heart failure patients with preserved left ventricular ejection fraction and sleep-disordered breathing. Eur J Heart Fail. 2013;15(5):543–50.
Yoshihisa A, Suzuki S, Yamauchi H, Sato T, Oikawa M, Kobayashi A, Yamaki T, Sugimoto K, Kunii H, Nakazato K, et al. Beneficial effects of positive airway pressure therapy for sleep-disordered breathing in heart failure patients with preserved left ventricular ejection fraction. Clin Cardiol. 2015;38(7):413–21.
Yumino D, Wang H, Floras JS, Newton GE, Mak S, Ruttanaumpawan P, Parker JD, Bradley TD. Prevalence and physiological predictors of sleep apnea in patients with heart failure and systolic dysfunction. J Card Fail. 2009;15(4):279–85.
Zechner R, Kienesberger PC, Haemmerle G, Zimmermann R, Lass A. Adipose triglyceride lipase and the lipolytic catabolism of cellular fat stores. J Lipid Res. 2009;50(1):3–21.
Zhang X, Ma L, Li S, Wang Y, Wang L. A functional MRI evaluation of frontal dysfunction in patients with severe obstructive sleep apnea. Sleep Med. 2011;12(4):335–40.
Zhang XB, Yang YY, Zeng Y, Zeng HQ, Fu BB, Ko CY, Luo X, Du YP, Chen LD, Lai YT, et al. Anti-tumor effect of endostatin in a sleep-apnea mouse model with tumor. Clin Transl Oncol. 2018;6(10):018–1955.
Zhu Y, Fenik P, Zhan G, Mazza E, Kelz M, Aston-Jones G, Veasey SC. Selective loss of catecholaminergic wake active neurons in a murine sleep apnea model. J Neurosci. 2007;27(37):10060–71.
Zwillich C, Devlin T, White D, Douglas N, Weil J, Martin R. Bradycardia during sleep apnea. Characteristics and mechanism. J Clin Invest. 1982;69(6):1286–92.

Chapter 11
Neural Injury in Models of Intermittent Hypoxia

Sigrid C. Veasey

Abstract Intermittent fluctuation in oxyhemoglobin saturation in sleep is a hallmark feature of obstructive sleep apnea (OSA). Initially, because the desaturation events are so brief, there was a general belief that the events were of little consequence. Studies in animal models have highlighted the effects of brief episodic fluctuation in oxygen on neuronal function, and it is now clear that intermittent hypoxia (IH) can have lasting effects on brain health and function. Intriguing divergent effects are observed with mild short-term exposure compared with more severe, long-term exposure to intermittent hypoxia. Mild infrequent variations in oxyhemoglobin saturation can promote neuronal plasticity, axonal growth, and enhance ventilation, while more frequent and greater variations in oxyhemoglobin are associated with neuronal injury, neuron loss, and lasting neurobehavioral impairments and neurodegeneration. Intriguingly molecular mechanisms for the protective and injurious side of IH are in part shared. In this chapter, we review the full spectrum of IH in humans with OSA, relate these patterns of IH to neural consequences in animal models, discuss the molecular mechanisms of neuronal effects across the various IH patterns, and then discuss the implications of collective findings for clinical care of individuals with OSA.

Keywords Episodic hypoxia · Intermittent hypoxia · Hypoxia-inducible factor · Long-term facilitation · Phrenic · Hypoglossal

11.1 Intermittent Hypoxia from the Clinical Perspective

OSA manifests as frequent sleep state dependent reductions in ventilation occurring in large part from partial or complete upper airway obstruction. Thus, each obstructive event results, not only in oxyhemoglobin desaturation, but also hypercapnia, increased sympathetic drive, changes in cardiac preload, afterload, and output, as

S. C. Veasey (✉)
Division of Sleep Medicine, Department of Medicine, Perelman School of Medicine, University of Pennsylvania, Philadelphia, PA, USA
e-mail: veasey@mail.med.upenn.edu

A. I. Pack, Q. Y. Li (eds.), *Sleep and its Disorders*, Translational Medicine Research,
https://doi.org/10.1007/978-94-024-2168-2_11

well as arousal and sleep disruption (Remmers et al. 1978; Tolle et al. 1983; Shiomi et al. 1991). IH can have sustained effects on sympathetic drive (Katragadda et al. 1997). Specifically, sympathetic drive is lower in sleep overall, relative to wakefulness. With sufficiently frequent and severe oxyhemoglobin desaturations, sympathetic activity remains high across the nighttime sleep period, thereby preventing the normal "nocturnal dipping" of blood pressure, and with greater changes in oxyhemoglobin saturation, sympathetic drive will remain heightened even across the day (Somers et al. 1988; Gilmartin et al. 2010). Sustained increases in sympathetic drive, in turn, raise blood pressure, promote thrombosis, and may induce vascular remodeling, narrowing, and stiffening of arterial vessels [for review, see Austin et al. (2013)]. All these changes have the potential to negatively impact neural health, including the promotion of cerebral microvascular disease and stroke. As we consider OSA as typically a disease present for years before diagnosis and treatment, it is important to appreciate that the consequences of IH in OSA extend beyond acute direct neuronal changes to include the above-mentioned pathophysiological changes that, in turn, may also impact neural function.

Patterns and severity of hypoxemia in OSA are influenced by numerous factors. Within a given obstructive sleep-disordered breathing event, the oxyhemoglobin saturation nadir is determined by (1) the effect of the obstruction on ventilation (apnea or hypopnea), (2) the functional residual capacity of the lungs in the particular sleep stage in which an event occurs, and (3) central ventilatory control and responsiveness in that sleep stage for that individual. For example, patients with underlying impaired respiratory control at baseline may have a higher arousal threshold for carbon dioxide (CO_2) and/or hypoxemia severity and therefore longer events with lower oxygen and higher CO_2 arterial values. Progesterone, and potentially estrogen, have stimulatory effects on ventilation (Behan and Wenninger 2008), so that premenopausal females typically have higher oxygen values for a similar level of obstruction as males or postmenopausal females. Additionally, individuals with significant underlying restrictive lung disease or severe obesity, who have reduced functional residual capacity in the lungs in sleep, will have more rapid decline in oxygen values and thus may have more severe oxyhemoglobin desaturations across an obstructive sleep-disordered breathing event of a given length (Dempsey et al. 2010). The oxyhemoglobin patterns will also vary with stage of sleep. For example, in rapid eye movement (REM) sleep, most accessory muscles are paralyzed (further reducing the functional residual capacity) (Douglas et al. 1982). Obstructive sleep-disordered breathing events may be limited to REM sleep (when upper airway muscle tone is most reduced and ventilatory responsiveness is also reduced). In this case, IH occurs sparsely across the night but in 3–10 min periods. There are also individuals who have IH for reasons of OSA combined with a pulmonary or neuromuscular abnormality (e.g., severe chronic obstructive lung disease or unilateral diaphragmatic paralysis). These individuals may have not only IH but also sustained hypoxemia, particularly across REM sleep (Anderson et al. 1996).

At present, the risk of cardiovascular morbidities and mortality, and cognitive impairments in OSA have been largely related to the apnea/hypopnea index, which largely relates to oxygen desaturation frequency (Nieto et al. 2000; Young and Peppard 2000; Shahar et al. 2001; Stone et al. 2016). While clinical studies have not parceled out in humans the relative risk of the particular patterns described above, work in animal models (described below) suggests that very different outcomes are possible with the variations in oxyhemoglobin patterns. In clinical studies, it is quite difficult to distinguish effects of IH from the interconnected pathophysiological effects of obstructive sleep-disordered breathing events described above. Moreover, because obesity is a major risk factor for OSA, it is very difficult in clinical studies to delineate what the consequences of OSA are from the consequences of diabetes, hypertension, cardiovascular disease, etc. In light of these challenges, animal studies have been helpful in elucidating potential detrimental and beneficial effects of IH on the brain and the mechanisms by which IH influences neural function and injury.

11.2 Historical Perspective of IH Animal Studies and Various Patterns of IH Examined

There is a very intriguing, early body of research examining intervals of hypoxia lasting hours (h), alternating with hours of normoxia. While this pattern of chronic sustained IH is more consistent with the pattern of sleep-related hypoxia that might be observed in chronic lung or neuromuscular disease, these studies highlight several important observations shared with IH, while providing important distinctions in molecular pathways influenced by the temporal pattern of hypoxic exposure, as described below.

11.2.1 Chronic Sustained Intermittent Hypoxia

The first published account of IH exposures in animals dates back to 1948, well before the clinical recognition of OSA (Altland 1948). The work was presented in abstract form describing rats exposed to hypoxia for 4 h/day for 3 months. Remarkably, this particular pattern of IH exposure was shown to have effects on hematocrit, body growth and spermatogenesis that persisted for weeks into the recovery period (Altland 1948). Neuronal function and health, however, were not examined (Altland 1948). One of the first descriptions of IH effects on the brain came from Alberghina and Giuffrida in 1981 (Alberghina and Giuffrida 1981), with a demonstration that intermittent sustained hypoxia (hypoxia for 17 h/day for 6 days) reduces lipid biogenesis in the brain. Serra et al. (1981), using the same protocol, also in 1981, showed reduced labeled precursor uptake for deoxyribonucleic and ribonucleic acids and proteins, particularly in mitochondrial fractions. In both studies, effects were observed in the cortex and hippocampus without an effect observed in the striatum, suggesting regional or cell type differential susceptibility to IH. As with the first paradigm, effects lasted beyond exposure and in this case were evident for at least 12 h after the last exposure. In another model of sustained IH (10 h/day) for 10 days, Meyer and Doelle (1988) found that even 3 months after IH exposure, there were alterations in the endoplasmic reticulum and ribosomes, with more free polysomes, in the cortices. Hermans et al. (1992) found that sustained (4 h once daily for 5 days) IH in utero across the last third of gestation, resulted in enduring behavioral disturbances (Hermans et al. 1992). Specifically, the awake righting reflex was delayed on postnatal days 6 and 7. Open-field locomotor activity was reduced in females but not males at 19 days, supporting a gender effect of IH. Intriguingly, even later as young adults (postnatal days 60–65), mice exposed in utero to IH had less locomotor activity for the first half of the lights off (active) period.

The body has important adaptive responses to chronic sustained hypoxia. Adaptive responses include increasing red blood cells to carry more oxygen, expanding the vasculature also to deliver more oxygen, and a shift in metabolism toward glycolysis. The molecular response to these physiological changes includes increasing erythropoietin to increase red blood cell mass, increasing vascular growth factors, and activating specific transcriptional pathways to promote glycolysis over aerobic metabolism [for reviews, see Jelkmann (2007) and Prabhakar and Semenza (2015)]. Perhaps the most established molecular response to sustained hypoxia was discovered by Wang and Semenza, who discovered hypoxia-inducible factor-1 alpha (HIF1a) as a major transcriptional activator (Wang and Semenza 1993), essential for the erythropoietin response to hypoxia (Heinicke et al. 2003). For the past three decades, some athletes have taken advantage of brief intermittent sustained mild hypoxia (2–5 exposures of 3–5 min) exposures to increase erythropoietin and physical endurance (Heinicke et al. 2003; Piehl Aulin et al. 1998).

11.2.2 Early Studies of IH Studies Specifically Modeling OSA

As mentioned above, the more typical patterns of IH in OSA involve 10–30 s oxyhemoglobin desaturations occurring every 1–12 min. Some of the earliest identified studies of IH modeling OSA were performed to determine whether IH could result in increases in blood pressure that were sustained across long normoxic periods. Early studies led by Eugene Fletcher demonstrated lasting increases in blood pressure in rats exposed to 8 h/day of IH for 35 days (Fletcher et al. 1992, 1995; Fletcher 1995). Follow-up studies were designed to localize the neuronal responses to IH that might contribute to hypertension. C-fos is an immediate early gene that is used as a proxy for neuronal activation, particularly when the protein translocates to neuronal nuclei (Takemoto et al. 1995). Using immunohistochemistry for c-fos in the brainstem, Greenberg (Greenberg et al. 1999) examined c-fos response within the brainstem to this long-term IH (LTIH) and found that c-fos increased in neuronal nuclei in brain regions controlling sympathetic activity (including the nucleus tractus solitarius, caudal serotoninergic raphe obscurus, and the ventral lateral medulla) in response to LTIH. The regional pattern of c-fos expression was remarkably consistent across all rats exposed to LTIH. The brainstem c-fos activation induced by IH was evident 12–18 h after the last IH exposure. The persistence in c-fos activation many hours after the last LTIH exposure supports the concept that LTIH can have lasting effects on brain responses and function. Additionally, this work supports the concept that cardiovascular responses to OSA may at least in part be secondary to neurogenic changes in response to LTIH. In a follow-up study, the same researchers examined the cortical c-fos response to LTIH and found that here, too, only very specific neurons were activated in response to LTIH (Sica et al. 2000). These groups included layers II/III of the cortex, particularly the cingulate and piriform cortices (Sica et al. 2000), areas also implicated in sympathetic responses. Collectively, this early body of work provides evidence that the brain responds to LTIH; the response can last longer than the IH exposure, and that the response within the brain at least for this immediate early gene activation is regionally, and potentially neuronal group specific.

11.2.3 Chronic Versus Sustained IH Effects on the Brain

Despite the neuronal contribution to hypertension observed in animal models described above, IH in OSA was considered to be of little clinical concern in inducing neural injury given the rapid return to normoxia after each obstructive sleep-disordered breathing event. Yet more recent research has clearly demonstrated that although IH events are brief in OSA, injury can be significant and even more profound than constant hypoxia. Specifically, several groups of researchers have directly compared chronic sustained and IH for its effects on brain function and neuronal health. In neonatal pups with surgical ligation of one carotid artery that is then exposed to chronic hypoxia or CIH for the same total hypoxia exposure time and same level of hypoxia, it is the CIH group that has more profound central injuries, relative to constant hypoxia, including higher brain lactate, larger grade ischemic insult and a greater gliosis response (Nagata et al. 2000). The N-acetyl aspartate/creatine (NAA/Cr) ratio is a marker of neuronal integrity that can be measured with proton nuclear magnetic resonance spectroscopy. In comparing the effects of IH and constant hypoxia in the neonatal mouse, greater reductions in NAA/Cr are observed in IH than in constant hypoxia (Douglas et al. 2007). Collectively, these studies support the concept that IH not only causes neural injury but under some circumstances may cause greater injury than constant hypoxia. While the molecular basis for the worsened outcomes with IH than in sustained hypoxia has not been fully elucidated, it is known that the largely adaptive responses to chronic hypoxia (erythropoietin and HIF1a) are not typically present in models of brief IH and in most individuals with OSA who do not spend a significant portion of the night hypoxemic (Pokala et al. 1995).

11.3 Beneficial Effects of Acute Intermittent Hypoxia on Phrenic Nerve Function

One of the most remarkable IH findings is that even very brief exposures to IH (three 5 min exposures) can have lasting effects on a respiratory neuronal function beyond the termination of the stimulus. This prolonged effect on neuronal activity or function is termed plasticity. Respiratory plasticity was originally described by Millhorn et al. with repeated carotid sinus stimulation (Millhorn et al. 1980). Understanding that the carotid sinus can be stimulated by hypoxia, IH (using the same temporal pattern as carotid nerve stimulation) was tested for effects on phrenic nerve activity and found to promote phrenic nerve long-term facilitation in anesthetized rats (Hayashi et al. 1993). Similarly in anaesthetized rats, IH, administered as three bursts of 3 min of hypoxia (arterial oxygen 35–45 mmHg) while holding carbon dioxide constant (acute IH), results in a sustained (at least 60 min) increase in phrenic nerve activity (Dwinell et al. 1997). Intriguingly, phrenic plasticity was not observed in response to sustained hypoxia (Baker and Mitchell 2000). There is, at least in rats, a genetic basis for acute IH in that only specific strains and substrains of rats show evidence of the phrenic nerve long-term facilitation (LTF) response (Janssen and Fregosi 2000; Fuller et al. 2001). Genetics underlying the strain differences in phrenic LTF responses to acute IH have not been elucidated. LTF response to short-term IH is also age-dependent in males, in that it is only observed in very young adult male rats; in middle-aged male rats, the response is completely blunted (Zabka et al. 2001). There are gender differences in this age-dependency of effect in that while older male rats do not show acute IH phrenic LTF, older female rats do (Behan et al. 2002).

The molecular basis of the phrenic LTF response to acute IH has been extensively evaluated and involves several complex molecular signaling pathways. Central to phrenic LTF from acute IH is the activation of caudal serotoninergic raphe neurons (Ling et al. 2001). These activated neurons send increased serotonin (5-HT) to phrenic motoneurons, which is essential for acute IH plasticity (Baker-Herman and Mitchell 2002). Repeated activation of 5-HT receptors (subtypes 2A, 2C, and/or 7) initiate several cell signaling pathways that ultimately increase the production and activation of brain-derived neurotrophic factor (BDNF) (Leal et al. 2014). BDNF then activates the troponin receptor kinase B (Trk-B) receptor on the motoneurons to phosphorylate and activate an extracellular signal kinase (ERK) or mitogen-activated protein kinase (MAPK) (Wilkerson and Mitchell 2009; Dougherty et al. 2015). Each of these components is critical to acute IH phrenic LTF (Ling et al. 2001). A second distinct pathway has been identified that activates protein kinase A that in turn activates TRK to activate AKT which augments glutamatergic signaling, leading to LTF (Nichols et al. 2012). The system is not redundant in that the former PKC pathway is activated in moderate acute IH while the latter pathway is activated in severe hypoxia ($paO_2 < 35$ mmHg) (Nichols et al. 2012). Terada and Mitchell examined the role of sleep in the phrenic LTF response to acute IH (Terada and Mitchell 2011). Acute IH increases diaphragmatic LTF in both wakefulness and

NREM sleep but does not affect phrenic activity in REM sleep. Daily acute IH does not influence either baseline diaphragmatic activity or induce LTF lasting hours and, therefore, cannot induce a metaplasticity of the phrenic response that would last across longer periods of sleep to protect sleep-disordered breathing. Nonetheless, now understanding the molecular mechanisms of acute IH, pharmacologic targets along the acute IH LTF pathways may be tested for effectiveness in improving ventilation during sleep.

11.4 The "More Is Not Better" Side of Intermittent Hypoxia

In light of the above responses, it would seem that IH is beneficial and should help prevent patients with OSA from having apneic events in sleep, at least across portions of the night. In this section below, research is summarized to support the concept that the above-described effects with acute IH are not always observed in chronic IH (CIH). Indeed, acute IH to mild levels of hypoxemia can augment respiratory nerve activity, while longer more severe CIH has detrimental effects on neural function.

11.4.1 Effects of Chronic Intermittent Hypoxia on Carotid Body Activation

Peng and Prabhakar examined whether moderate 1-week CIH, modeling OSA, induced phrenic LTF (Peng and Prabhakar 2003). Importantly, the investigators found that CIH for 1 week prior to acute IH enhanced phrenic LTF, while sustained hypoxia actually prevented the LTF, and the CIH-enhanced LTF effect could be blunted by giving a reactive oxygen species scavenger (Peng and Prabhakar 2003). Thus, CIH can influence the above acute IH phrenic LTF and this effect appears to involve reactive oxygen species.

Appreciating that the carotid body is the gatekeeper for cardiorespiratory responses to hypoxia of all forms, including IH, mechanisms whereby CIH activates carotid body glomus cells were recently addressed. One of the critical steps toward glomus cell activation is an increase in intracellular calcium (Kumar and Prabhakar 2012). A rise in intracellular calcium may emanate from endoplasmic reticulum or mitochondrial stores within or through influx via voltage-gated calcium channels. However, Makarenko et al., found that blocking T-type voltage-gated calcium channels (VGCCs) prevented the CIH effect on intracellular calcium in glomus cells (Makarenko et al. 2012). A reactive oxygen species scavenger prevented the CIH-induced increase in calcium as well, suggesting that ROS activates the Type 3.2 VGCC to increase intracellular calcium (Makarenko et al. 2012). Mechanisms by which calcium influx into the glomus cells leads to long-term facilitation of ventilatory responses remain to be elucidated. Importantly CIH, but not chronic hypoxia, increases phosphorylation of CREB (a transcriptional regulator for cAMP-responsive element) in the carotid body glomus cells (Wang et al. 2000), which could then activate a transcriptional and translational response to increase activity. Additionally, CIH increases glutamate responses within the carotid body (Liu et al. 2009). This activation manifests clinically as heightened sympathetic drive as described below with resultant hypertension in OSA.

11.4.1.1 Oxygen Sensing at the Carotid Body Across IH

One of the most significant advances in IH neurobiology has been the incredible detailing of oxygen sensing mechanisms in the carotid body, and while it is quite complicated, it is worthwhile considering, as this is certainly one of the first chains of events in IH neural cardiopulmonary responses. The overall picture is that fluctuations in oxygen in IH increase the availability of reactive oxygen species that sets up a complex signaling pathway leading to sympathetic activity through gaseous transmitters in the carotid body. In greater detail, seated just at the bifurcation of the carotid artery into internal and external carotid arteries, carotid bodies are well-poised to almost immediately detect fluctuations in oxygen delivery to the brain. The actual oxygen sensing cells are the glomus cells described above. But just how do glomus cells translate low oxygen tension into calcium influx? The reoxygenation phase in IH increases reactive oxygen species within the carotid body, which then oxidatively modify and inactivate hemoxygenase-2 (Yuan et al. 2004). In normoxia, hemoxygenase-2 is constitutively active, catalyzing the synthesis of carbon monoxide. Carbon monoxide then, in normoxia, activates protein kinase G, which phosphorylates and inactivates cystathionine g-ligase (CSE) an enzyme critical for hydrogen sulfide (H2S) production (Yuan et al. 2015a). In CIH with hemoxygenase-2 inactivated carbon monoxide is not present to suppress ultimately CSE from making H2S. H2S excites carotid glomus cells by inhibiting background (TASK) potassium channels, and increasing intracellular calcium (Buckler 2012; Li et al. 2010; Telezhkin et al. 2010). Inhibition of CSE and transgenic absence of CSE both prevent IH activation of sympathetic drive (Yuan et al. 2016). It is exciting to consider that drugs targeting carotid body CSE might provide an important therapeutic avenue to reduce sympathetic drive in OSA.

11.4.1.2 Chronic IH Activation of Sympathetic Activity

As described above, CIH results in chronic activation of carotid sinus neurons. How this translates into increased blood pressure has been carefully examined and recently reviewed (Kumar et al. 2015). The adrenal medulla is essential for CIH-induced hypertension in that rats subjected to bilateral adrenal medullectomy confer resistance to hypertension produced by CIH (Bao et al. 1997). It is quite interesting that several of the same mediators in CIH responses in adrenal medullary chromaffin cells are the same players in the carotid glomus cellular response, including increased intracellular calcium and increased reactive oxygen species. CIH seems to disturb the balance of hypoxia-inducible factors (HIFs) 1 and 2. HIF-1α promotes glycolysis over oxidative phosphorylation and a pro-oxidant state (increased NADPH oxidase, which is critical to the CIH-increased ROS, even in glomus cells), while HIF-2α promotes the transcription of many antioxidant enzymes (superoxide dismutases 1 and 2 and catalase) (Semenza and Prabhakar 2018). Overall, CIH-induced carotid sinus nerve activation leads to sympathetic nerve activation that in turn somehow alters the balance of HIF-1α and -2α to favor a pro-oxidant HIF-1α state (Peng et al. 2006, 2014; Nanduri et al. 2009).

Overall, these well-delineated pathways provide several promising targets for the prevention of OSA-related hypertension, including targeting NADPH oxidase inhibitors and drugs that influence H2S production.

11.4.2 Chronic Intermittent Hypoxia Impact on Hippocampal Neurons and Function

The hippocampus is particularly sensitive to hypoxia (Kirino and Sano 1984), and within the hippocampus neurons in the CA1 region are the most vulnerable to constant hypoxia (Schmidt-Kastner and Freund 1991). David Gozal and colleagues began examining the mechanisms of this differential vulnerability of CA1 compared to CA3 neurons to longer-term severe CIH, finding increased hypoxic depolarization in CA1 vs. CA3 pyramidal neurons (Kreisman et al. 2000). Then, in considering OSA, his group utilized a longer and more frequent exposure of IH (40 events/h to FIO_2 concentrations around 10% continuously for 1–14 days) in young adult rats (2 months old) (Gozal et al. 2001). This long-term IH (LTIH) did not alter total hourly amounts of wakefulness, NREM or REM sleep, but markedly impaired performance in spatial memory (hippocampal-dependent) task, the Morris water maze. Not only was performance acutely impaired but even after 14 days into recovery performance remained impaired. Histological examination of the hippocampus revealed apoptosis in the CA1, supporting heightened vulnerability for the CA1 also with LTIH. Additionally, 14 days of IH (LTIH) resulted in an astrocytosis within the hippocampus. This landmark study provided the first evidence that LTIH could impart lasting functional impairments and neural injury. A similar immediate effect of LTIH on hippocampal-dependent memory was observed in developing rats (age 15–30 days) (Row et al. 2002). Here, the effect was more pronounced in male rats than in females. Shortly thereafter, Michael Decker with David Rye confirmed spatial memory impairments in developing rats exposed to LTIH and found that impairments in performance persisted at least until the age of young adults (2mos) (Decker et al. 2003). Additionally, these rats had sustained reductions in wakefulness and increases in REM sleep (Decker et al. 2003). In an effort to begin to elucidate major molecular pathways involved in a relatively non-biased manner,

Evelyn Gozal and colleagues analyzed proteomic differences within the CA1 (LTIH vulnerable hippocampus) and CA3 (relatively LTIH resistant) regions of the hippocampus (Gozal et al. 2002). Overall, the proteomic changes in CA1 not evident in CA3 included alterations in cytoskeletal, metabolic/energetic, and chaperone proteins. Intriguingly, there is a strong age-dependency to the vulnerability to IH, in that rats pups exposed at very early stages (postnatal day 2–5) develop less hippocampal neuronal apoptosis relative to older pups. The most vulnerable group spanned rat pups of 10–25 days, so that rats older at the time of exposure (up to 120 days of age studied) had less apoptosis. It is important to recognize that the duration of LTIH may also be important as 2 vs. 4 or more weeks may also have very different effects on hippocampal responses to LTIH. Specifically, apoptosis of CA1 pyramidal neurons peaks at day 3 of LTIH exposure, and phosphorylation of CREB peaks at day 14 and then declines gradually to normoxic levels by day 30 of LTIH (Goldbart et al. 2003a). Similarly, phosphorylated protein kinase B (AKT) and phosphorylated glycogen synthase kinase B (GSK-B) both decline across the first day of exposure and then gradually return to baseline levels over 2 week (Goldbart et al. 2003b). A temporal pattern in hippocampal function was also observed in that long-term potentiation in hippocampal brain slices was markedly reduced (34% of baseline) at day 3 IH and then improved to 54% of baseline by day 7 IH (Payne et al. 2004).

Clinical imaging studies of the hippocampus in patients with OSA demonstrate reduced volume, less gray matter, and potentially some reversal with treatment. Clearly, understanding the molecular mechanisms by which OSA and IH can disturb hippocampal function is of utmost importance. It is quite interesting then that some of the same molecular pathways as described above for acute IH phrenic LTF and for carotid body and adrenal medullary responses to LTIH, are highlighted here as well. Specifically, LTIH increases oxidative stress in the hippocampus, increasing peroxynitrite and reducing nitric oxide (NO) availability. In animals exposed to LTIH, this reduction in NO availability impairs calcium-activated potassium channels on CA1 pyramidal neurons (Tjong et al. 2008a). Melatonin supplementation can, interestingly prevent the LTIH-induced impaired potassium channel responses (Tjong et al. 2008b), potentially by reducing oxidative stress. Additionally, increased physical exercise which increases both BDNF and antioxidant defense in brain is also protective against LTIH spatial memory impairments (Gozal et al. 2010). An important source of oxidative stress seems to be NADPH oxidase, in that mice deficient in one of the key subunits for NADPH oxidase are resistant to both the LTIH-induced oxidative stress and spatial memory impairments (Nair et al. 2011). Of interest NADPH oxidase activity in the hippocampi of wild-type mice gradually climbs over the first week of life and then plateaus (Nair et al. 2011). Additional sustained sources of oxidative stress in LTIH within the hippocampus include HIF-1α and endoplasmic reticulum oxidoreductin-1 like (ERO-1L) that are both elevated on a sustained basis in the hippocampus (Chou et al. 2013). Angiotensin II inhibition can prevent oxidative stress, lipid peroxidation, and inflammatory responses (Yuan et al. 2015b). Of interest, angiotensin II activation in the carotid sinus also potentiates NADPH oxidase activation, and is therefore responsible in large part for the NADPH oxidase ROS. Overall, the above research supports clinical trials of angiotensin blocker medications and NADPH oxidase inhibitors to reduce both cardiovascular and central nervous system morbidities associated with OSA.

11.5 Molecular Mechanisms by Which LTIH Impairs Wakefulness

Residual sleepiness persists in over 10% of patients in which OSA and other sleep disorders have been treated (Gasa et al. 2013). This finding raises the possibility that OSA through IH or sleep fragmentation might injure neurons essential for alertness and optimal wakefulness. Veasey et al. (2004a) examined the effects of 8 week of severe LTIH (40 events/h to oxyhemoglobin saturation nadirs of 75%) on spontaneous wakefulness in a 24-h period and sleepiness as measured with a mouse version of the multiple sleep latency test (Veasey et al. 2004b). To determine whether sleepiness was affected and whether the effect could persist, wake parameters were assessed for 2 and 24 week into recovery in normoxia after LTIH. Total sleep time was increased for a 24-h period in LTIH mice by 2 and ½ h. Both NREM and REM sleep times increased, and effects were present at least 6 mos into recovery (Veasey et al. 2004a). LTIH also significantly reduced sleep latency (Veasey et al. 2004a). Lipid peroxidation, which signifies both oxidative and nitrative stress, was increased in the lateral hypothalamus and basal forebrain (Veasey et al. 2004a). In a follow-up study, the role of NO in wake impairments was addressed by studying the effects of LTIH on wakefulness in mice with and without inducible NOS (iNOS) (Zhan et al. 2005a). That transgenic absence of iNOS prevented the wake impairments, LTIH oxidative and inflammatory responses strongly support a critical role for ROS and NO in both behavioral and molecular responses to LTIH (Zhan et al. 2005a). Importantly, NADPH oxidase is central to the iNOS activation, as well as the downstream oxidative stress, inflammatory response, and wake impairments, in that all can be prevented in mice with either transgenic absence or pharmacologic inhibition of NADPH oxidase (Zhan et al. 2005b). As with acute IH, female mice conferred some resistance to IH injury to wake impairments (Sanfilippo-Cohn et al. 2006). The most important finding in this series of studies was that catecholaminergic wake-activate neurons, the noradrenergic locus coeruleus and the dopaminergic ventral periacqueductal gray neurons were not only less responsive but lost with LTIH (Zhu et al. 2007). This injury effect as well was an NADPH oxidase-dependent effect.

Residual sleepiness impacts the well-being and safety of patients with OSA and injury to wake-activated neurons may also contribute to depression, cognitive impairments, and in the case of the noradrenergic locus coeruleus neurons, injury can accelerate cognitive decline, and amyloid plaques in Alzheimer's disease (Weinshenker 2008). Thus, identifying therapies that protect wake-activate neurons and wakefulness in persons with OSA should be a high priority in sleep medicine. It is important to note that there have been intermittent hypoxia trials in humans to assess effects on cognition. When limited to one 90-min episode of hypoxia with oxyhemoglobin saturation nadirs of 85% three times 1 week and three times at 80% the next, older humans improved in cognitive performances (executive function) using a within-subject assessment (Schega et al. 2016). Weiss et al. (2009) examined the effects of an IH pattern that modeled moderate OSA with 20 events/h and desaturations into the high to mid-80th %-ile. Exposures were given 9 h/night for 28 days. Using a within-study design the researchers did not observe any differences in cognitive performance. However, the sample size was small ($n = 8$), and all were healthy young adults. Additionally, there was no control group to exclude learning effects with some of the tests over time. Thus, it remains unknown whether humans are resistant to IH effects on cognition and sleepiness; whether LTIH effects are evident only with severe hypoxia and more frequent events, or whether comorbidities influence cognitive and sleepiness effects of LTIH.

11.6 LTIH Injury to Upper Airway Motoneurons

Another group of neurons that may be injured by LTIH are upper airway dilator motoneurons that are critical for pharyngeal patency. Several studies have shown injury to the nerves in upper airway dilator muscles and changes in the muscles consistent with nerve injury (Saboisky et al. 2012; Ramchandren et al. 2010; Boyd et al. 2004). LTIH has been shown to influence upper airway motoneurons activity. Specifically, the effects of LTIH on hypoglossal nerve responses to excitatory neurochemicals serotonin and glutamate have been examined and shown to be markedly reduced in animals after LTIH (Veasey et al. 2004c). This supports the view that severe LTIH leads to major disruption in functional responsiveness of upper airway motoneurons. Endoplasmic reticulum stress has been shown in the LTIH exposed motoneurons (Zhu et al. 2008). The molecular basis of this hypoglossal neuron injury involves endoplasmic reticulum dyshomeostasis as evidenced by increased C/EBP homologous binding protein (CHOP) in these motoneurons that could be prevented by enhancing an adaptive ER stress response (eIF-2a) (Zhu et al. 2008). (For further discussion of the role of CHOP, see Chap. 7) Importantly, CHOP plays a major role in both the NADPH oxidase and inflammatory responses. The transgenic absence of CHOP prevents oxidative, nitrative, and inflammatory injuries in upper airway motoneurons, including hypoglossal neurons. Additionally, CHOP is essential for the HIF1a response to LTIH at motoneurons, and thus may be the most upstream pathway component identified to date (Chou et al. 2013).

11.7 LTIH Effect on Glial Cells

Glial cells within the central nervous system include astrocytes, microglia, and oligodendrocytes. Recent reports suggest that these cells, too, maybe affected by IH. Specifically, very severe LTIH (60 events/h to a fraction of inspired oxygen of 5%) causes a subtle increase in a number of astrocytes in the dorsal hippocampus in adult mice (Sapin et al. 2015). Whether this gliosis contributes to injury or is protective is not known. As with neuronal responses to IH, microglia responses may be beneficial with mild exposures and harmful with more severe exposures (Kiernan et al. 2016). The clearest evidence of glial injury from IH involves oligodendrocytes. Severe LTIH disturbs the ultrastructure of myelin and reduces myelin proteins (Veasey et al. 2013; Kim et al. 2015). Importantly, this is true in developing rats as well upon exposure to LTIH (Cai et al. 2012). Individuals with OSA have increased white matter lesions, and the prevalence increases with OSA severity (Kim et al. 2013).

11.8 Concluding Remarks

IH in humans with OSA occurs across a vast spectrum of severity, defined by the frequency and severity of oxyhemoglobin desaturation. Several mild IH events can augment ventilation and upper airway patency, while the more severe events have lasting effects on neuronal function and survival in selectively vulnerable groups of neurons and may impact glial function. NADPH oxidase plays a vital role in both LTF plasticity and neuronal injury and degradation. Because NADPH oxidase may also contribute to metabolic disturbances in OSA and to cardiovascular pathophysiology, this oxidase should be a major target for pharmacotherapies to prevent the major comorbidities in OSA. As CHOP is upstream to NADPH oxidase, this too may be a promising target for preventative therapies. Collectively, animal studies have successfully provided a translational platform, ripe for implementation science.

Acknowledgment Support from NIH grants R01 HL096037.

References

Alberghina M, Giuffrida AM. Effect of hypoxia on the incorporation of [2-3H] glycerol and [1-14C]-palmitate into lipids of various brain regions. J Neurosci Res. 1981;6(3):403–19.

Altland PD. Recovery rate from some of the effects of chronic intermittent hypoxia in rats. Anat Rec. 1948;101(4):668.

Anderson CA, Dick TE, Orem J. Respiratory responses to tracheobronchial stimulation during sleep and wakefulness in the adult cat. Sleep. 1996;19(6):472–8.

Austin AW, Wissmann T, von Kanel R. Stress and hemostasis: an update. Semin Thromb Hemost. 2013;39(8):902–12.

Baker TL, Mitchell GS. Episodic but not continuous hypoxia elicits long-term facilitation of phrenic motor output in rats. J Physiol. 2000;529(Pt 1):215–9.

Baker-Herman TL, Mitchell GS. Phrenic long-term facilitation requires spinal serotonin receptor activation and protein synthesis. J Neurosci. 2002;22(14):6239–46.

Bao G, Metreveli N, Li R, Taylor A, Fletcher EC. Blood pressure response to chronic episodic hypoxia: role of the sympathetic nervous system. J Appl Physiol (1985). 1997;83(1):95–101.

Behan M, Wenninger JM. Sex steroidal hormones and respiratory control. Respir Physiol Neurobiol. 2008;164(1–2):213–21.

Behan M, Zabka AG, Mitchell GS. Age and gender effects on serotonin-dependent plasticity in respiratory motor control. Respir Physiol Neurobiol. 2002;131(1–2):65–77.

Boyd JH, Petrof BJ, Hamid Q, Fraser R, Kimoff RJ. Upper airway muscle inflammation and denervation changes in obstructive sleep apnea. Am J Respir Crit Care Med. 2004;170(5): 541–6.

Buckler KJ. Effects of exogenous hydrogen sulphide on calcium signalling, background (TASK) K channel activity and mitochondrial function in chemoreceptor cells. Pflugers Arch. 2012;463(5): 743–54.

Cai J, Tuong CM, Zhang Y, Shields CB, Guo G, Fu H, et al. Mouse intermittent hypoxia mimicking apnoea of prematurity: effects on myelinogenesis and axonal maturation. J Pathol. 2012;226(3): 495–508.

Chou YT, Zhan G, Zhu Y, Fenik P, Panossian L, Li Y, et al. C/EBP homologous binding protein (CHOP) underlies neural injury in sleep apnea model. Sleep. 2013;36(4):481–92.

Decker MJ, Hue GE, Caudle WM, Miller GW, Keating GL, Rye DB. Episodic neonatal hypoxia evokes executive dysfunction and regionally specific alterations in markers of dopamine signaling. Neuroscience. 2003;117(2):417–25.

Dempsey JA, Veasey SC, Morgan BJ, O'Donnell CP. Pathophysiology of sleep apnea. Physiol Rev. 2010;90(1):47–112.

Dougherty BJ, Fields DP, Mitchell GS. Mammalian target of rapamycin is required for phrenic long-term facilitation following severe but not moderate acute intermittent hypoxia. J Neurophysiol. 2015;114(3):1784–91.

Douglas NJ, White DP, Pickett CK, Weil JV, Zwillich CW. Respiration during sleep in normal man. Thorax. 1982;37(11):840–4.

Douglas RM, Miyasaka N, Takahashi K, Latuszek-Barrantes A, Haddad GG, Hetherington HP. Chronic intermittent but not constant hypoxia decreases NAA/Cr ratios in neonatal mouse hippocampus and thalamus. Am J Physiol Regul Integr Comp Physiol. 2007;292(3): R1254–9.

Dwinell MR, Janssen PL, Bisgard GE. Lack of long-term facilitation of ventilation after exposure to hypoxia in goats. Respir Physiol. 1997;108(1):1–9.

Fletcher EC. An animal model of the relationship between systemic hypertension and repetitive episodic hypoxia as seen in sleep apnoea. J Sleep Res. 1995;4(S1):71–7.

Fletcher EC, Lesske J, Qian W, Miller CC 3rd, Unger T. Repetitive, episodic hypoxia causes diurnal elevation of blood pressure in rats. Hypertension. 1992;19(6 Pt 1):555–61.

Fletcher EC, Bao G, Miller CC 3rd. Effect of recurrent episodic hypocapnic, eucapnic, and hypercapnic hypoxia on systemic blood pressure. J Appl Physiol (1985). 1995;78(4):1516–21.

Fuller DD, Baker TL, Behan M, Mitchell GS. Expression of hypoglossal long-term facilitation differs between substrains of Sprague-Dawley rat. Physiol Genomics. 2001;4(3):175–81.

Gasa M, Tamisier R, Launois SH, Sapene M, Martin F, Stach B, et al. Residual sleepiness in sleep apnea patients treated by continuous positive airway pressure. J Sleep Res. 2013;22(4):389–97.

Gilmartin GS, Lynch M, Tamisier R, Weiss JW. Chronic intermittent hypoxia in humans during 28 nights results in blood pressure elevation and increased muscle sympathetic nerve activity. Am J Physiol Heart Circ Physiol. 2010;299(3):H925–31.

Goldbart A, Cheng ZJ, Brittian KR, Gozal D. Intermittent hypoxia induces time-dependent changes in the protein kinase B signaling pathway in the hippocampal CA1 region of the rat. Neurobiol Dis. 2003a;14(3):440–6.

Goldbart A, Row BW, Kheirandish L, Schurr A, Gozal E, Guo SZ, et al. Intermittent hypoxic exposure during light phase induces changes in cAMP response element binding protein activity in the rat CA1 hippocampal region: water maze performance correlates. Neuroscience. 2003b;122(3):585–90.

Gozal D, Daniel JM, Dohanich GP. Behavioral and anatomical correlates of chronic episodic hypoxia during sleep in the rat. J Neurosci. 2001;21(7):2442–50.

Gozal E, Gozal D, Pierce WM, Thongboonkerd V, Scherzer JA, Sachleben LR Jr, et al. Proteomic analysis of CA1 and CA3 regions of rat hippocampus and differential susceptibility to intermittent hypoxia. J Neurochem. 2002;83(2):331–45.

Gozal D, Nair D, Goldbart AD. Physical activity attenuates intermittent hypoxia-induced spatial learning deficits and oxidative stress. Am J Respir Crit Care Med. 2010;182(1):104–12.

Greenberg HE, Sica AL, Scharf SM, Ruggiero DA. Expression of c-fos in the rat brainstem after chronic intermittent hypoxia. Brain Res. 1999;816(2):638–45.

Hayashi F, Coles SK, Bach KB, Mitchell GS, McCrimmon DR. Time-dependent phrenic nerve responses to carotid afferent activation: intact vs. decerebellate rats. Am J Phys. 1993;265(4 Pt 2):R811–9.

Heinicke K, Prommer N, Cajigal J, Viola T, Behn C, Schmidt W. Long-term exposure to intermittent hypoxia results in increased hemoglobin mass, reduced plasma volume, and elevated erythropoietin plasma levels in man. Eur J Appl Physiol. 2003;88(6):535–43.

Hermans RH, Hunter DE, McGivern RF, Cain CD, Longo LD. Behavioral sequelae in young rats of acute intermittent antenatal hypoxia. Neurotoxicol Teratol. 1992;14(2):119–29.

Janssen PL, Fregosi RF. No evidence for long-term facilitation after episodic hypoxia in spontaneously breathing, anesthetized rats. J Appl Physiol (1985). 2000;89(4):1345–51.

Jelkmann W. Erythropoietin after a century of research: younger than ever. Eur J Haematol. 2007;78(3):183–205.

Katragadda S, Xie A, Puleo D, Skatrud JB, Morgan BJ. Neural mechanism of the pressor response to obstructive and nonobstructive apnea. J Appl Physiol (1985). 1997;83(6):2048–54.

Kiernan EA, Smith SM, Mitchell GS, Watters JJ. Mechanisms of microglial activation in models of inflammation and hypoxia: implications for chronic intermittent hypoxia. J Physiol. 2016;594(6):1563–77.

Kim H, Yun CH, Thomas RJ, Lee SH, Seo HS, Cho ER, et al. Obstructive sleep apnea as a risk factor for cerebral white matter change in a middle-aged and older general population. Sleep. 2013;36(5):709–15B.

Kim LJ, Martinez D, Fiori CZ, Baronio D, Kretzmann NA, Barros HM. Hypomyelination, memory impairment, and blood-brain barrier permeability in a model of sleep apnea. Brain Res. 2015;1597:28–36.

Kirino T, Sano K. Selective vulnerability in the gerbil hippocampus following transient ischemia. Acta Neuropathol. 1984;62(3):201–8.

Kreisman NR, Soliman S, Gozal D. Regional differences in hypoxic depolarization and swelling in hippocampal slices. J Neurophysiol. 2000;83(2):1031–8.

Kumar P, Prabhakar NR. Peripheral chemoreceptors: function and plasticity of the carotid body. Compr Physiol. 2012;2(1):141–219.

Kumar GK, Nanduri J, Peng YJ, Prabhakar NR. Neuromolecular mechanisms mediating the effects of chronic intermittent hypoxia on adrenal medulla. Respir Physiol Neurobiol. 2015;209:115–9.

Leal G, Comprido D, Duarte CB. BDNF-induced local protein synthesis and synaptic plasticity. Neuropharmacology. 2014;76(Pt C):639–56.

Li Q, Sun B, Wang X, Jin Z, Zhou Y, Dong L, et al. A crucial role for hydrogen sulfide in oxygen sensing via modulating large conductance calcium-activated potassium channels. Antioxid Redox Signal. 2010;12(10):1179–89.

Ling L, Fuller DD, Bach KB, Kinkead R, Olson EB Jr, Mitchell GS. Chronic intermittent hypoxia elicits serotonin-dependent plasticity in the central neural control of breathing. J Neurosci. 2001;21(14):5381–8.

Liu Y, Ji ES, Xiang S, Tamisier R, Tong J, Huang J, et al. Exposure to cyclic intermittent hypoxia increases expression of functional NMDA receptors in the rat carotid body. J Appl Physiol (1985). 2009;106(1):259–67.

Makarenko VV, Nanduri J, Raghuraman G, Fox AP, Gadalla MM, Kumar GK, et al. Endogenous H2S is required for hypoxic sensing by carotid body glomus cells. Am J Physiol Cell Physiol. 2012;303(9):C916–23.

Meyer U, Doelle B. Long-lasting shifts in ribosomal systems of hippocampal granular neurons due to early postnatal hypoxia. J Hirnforsch. 1988;29(3):237–42.

Millhorn DE, Eldridge FL, Waldrop TG. Prolonged stimulation of respiration by a new central neural mechanism. Respir Physiol. 1980;41(1):87–103.

Nagata N, Saji M, Ito T, Ikeno S, Takahashi H, Terakawa N. Repetitive intermittent hypoxia-ischemia and brain damage in neonatal rats. Brain Dev. 2000;22(5):315–20.

Nair D, Dayyat EA, Zhang SX, Wang Y, Gozal D. Intermittent hypoxia-induced cognitive deficits are mediated by NADPH oxidase activity in a murine model of sleep apnea. PLoS One. 2011;6 (5):e19847.

Nanduri J, Wang N, Yuan G, Khan SA, Souvannakitti D, Peng YJ, et al. Intermittent hypoxia degrades HIF-2alpha via calpains resulting in oxidative stress: implications for recurrent apnea-induced morbidities. Proc Natl Acad Sci U S A. 2009;106(4):1199–204.

Nichols NL, Dale EA, Mitchell GS. Severe acute intermittent hypoxia elicits phrenic long-term facilitation by a novel adenosine-dependent mechanism. J Appl Physiol (1985). 2012;112(10): 1678–88.

Nieto FJ, Young TB, Lind BK, Shahar E, Samet JM, Redline S, et al. Association of sleep-disordered breathing, sleep apnea, and hypertension in a large community-based study. Sleep Heart Health Study. JAMA. 2000;283(14):1829–36.

Payne RS, Goldbart A, Gozal D, Schurr A. Effect of intermittent hypoxia on long-term potentiation in rat hippocampal slices. Brain Res. 2004;1029(2):195–9.

Peng YJ, Prabhakar NR. Reactive oxygen species in the plasticity of respiratory behavior elicited by chronic intermittent hypoxia. J Appl Physiol (1985). 2003;94(6):2342–9.

Peng YJ, Yuan G, Ramakrishnan D, Sharma SD, Bosch-Marce M, Kumar GK, et al. Heterozygous HIF-1alpha deficiency impairs carotid body-mediated systemic responses and reactive oxygen species generation in mice exposed to intermittent hypoxia. J Physiol. 2006;577(Pt 2):705–16.

Peng YJ, Yuan G, Khan S, Nanduri J, Makarenko VV, Reddy VD, et al. Regulation of hypoxia-inducible factor-alpha isoforms and redox state by carotid body neural activity in rats. J Physiol. 2014;592(17):3841–58.

Piehl Aulin K, Svedenhag J, Wide L, Berglund B, Saltin B. Short-term intermittent normobaric hypoxia—haematological, physiological and mental effects. Scand J Med Sci Sports. 1998;8(3): 132–7.

Pokala P, Llanera M, Sherwood J, Scharf S, Steinberg H. Erythropoietin response in subjects with obstructive sleep apnea. Am J Respir Crit Care Med. 1995;151(6):1862–5.

Prabhakar NR, Semenza GL. Oxygen sensing and homeostasis. Physiology (Bethesda). 2015;30(5): 340–8.

Ramchandren S, Gruis KL, Chervin RD, Lisabeth LD, Concannon M, Wolfe J, et al. Hypoglossal nerve conduction findings in obstructive sleep apnea. Muscle Nerve. 2010;42(2):257–61.

Remmers JE, deGroot WJ, Sauerland EK, Anch AM. Pathogenesis of upper airway occlusion during sleep. J Appl Physiol Respir Environ Exerc Physiol. 1978;44(6):931–8.

Row BW, Kheirandish L, Neville JJ, Gozal D. Impaired spatial learning and hyperactivity in developing rats exposed to intermittent hypoxia. Pediatr Res. 2002;52(3):449–53.

Saboisky JP, Stashuk DW, Hamilton-Wright A, Carusona AL, Campana LM, Trinder J, et al. Neurogenic changes in the upper airway of patients with obstructive sleep apnea. Am J Respir Crit Care Med. 2012;185(3):322–9.

Sanfilippo-Cohn B, Lai S, Zhan G, Fenik P, Pratico D, Mazza E, et al. Sex differences in susceptibility to oxidative injury and sleepiness from intermittent hypoxia. Sleep. 2006;29(2):152–9.

Sapin E, Peyron C, Roche F, Gay N, Carcenac C, Savasta M, et al. Chronic intermittent hypoxia induces chronic low-grade neuroinflammation in the dorsal hippocampus of mice. Sleep. 2015;38(10):1537–46.

Schega L, Peter B, Brigadski T, Lessmann V, Isermann B, Hamacher D, et al. Effect of intermittent normobaric hypoxia on aerobic capacity and cognitive function in older people. J Sci Med Sport/Sports Med Aust. 2016;19(11):941–5.

Schmidt-Kastner R, Freund TF. Selective vulnerability of the hippocampus in brain ischemia. Neuroscience. 1991;40(3):599–636.

Semenza GL, Prabhakar NR. The role of hypoxia-inducible factors in carotid body (patho) physiology. J Physiol. 2018;596(15):2977–83.

Serra I, Alberghina M, Viola M, Giuffrida AM. Effect of hypoxia on nucleic acid and protein synthesis in different brain regions. Neurochem Res. 1981;6(5):595–605.

Shahar E, Whitney CW, Redline S, Lee ET, Newman AB, Nieto FJ, et al. Sleep-disordered breathing and cardiovascular disease: cross-sectional results of the Sleep Heart Health Study. Am J Respir Crit Care Med. 2001;163(1):19–25.

Shiomi T, Guilleminault C, Stoohs R, Schnittger I. Leftward shift of the interventricular septum and pulsus paradoxus in obstructive sleep apnea syndrome. Chest. 1991;100(4):894–902.

Sica AL, Greenberg HE, Scharf SM, Ruggiero DA. Immediate-early gene expression in cerebral cortex following exposure to chronic-intermittent hypoxia. Brain Res. 2000;870(1–2):204–10.

Somers VK, Mark AL, Abboud FM. Potentiation of sympathetic nerve responses to hypoxia in borderline hypertensive subjects. Hypertension. 1988;11(6 Pt 2):608–12.

Stone KL, Blackwell TL, Ancoli-Israel S, Barrett-Connor E, Bauer DC, Cauley JA, et al. Sleep disordered breathing and risk of stroke in older community-dwelling men. Sleep. 2016;39(3):531–40.

Takemoto O, Tomimoto H, Yanagihara T. Induction of c-fos and c-Jun gene products and heat shock protein after brief and prolonged cerebral ischemia in gerbils. Stroke. 1995;26(9):1639–48.

Telezhkin V, Brazier SP, Cayzac SH, Wilkinson WJ, Riccardi D, Kemp PJ. Mechanism of inhibition by hydrogen sulfide of native and recombinant BKCa channels. Respir Physiol Neurobiol. 2010;172(3):169–78.

Terada J, Mitchell GS. Diaphragm long-term facilitation following acute intermittent hypoxia during wakefulness and sleep. J Appl Physiol (1985). 2011;110(5):1299–310.

Tjong YW, Li M, Hung MW, Wang K, Fung ML. Nitric oxide deficit in chronic intermittent hypoxia impairs large conductance calcium-activated potassium channel activity in rat hippocampal neurons. Free Radic Biol Med. 2008a;44(4):547–57.

Tjong YW, Li MF, Hung MW, Fung ML. Melatonin ameliorates hippocampal nitric oxide production and large conductance calcium-activated potassium channel activity in chronic intermittent hypoxia. J Pineal Res. 2008b;44(3):234–43.

Tolle FA, Judy WV, Yu PL, Markand ON. Reduced stroke volume related to pleural pressure in obstructive sleep apnea. J Appl Physiol Respir Environ Exerc Physiol. 1983;55(6):1718–24.

Veasey SC, Davis CW, Fenik P, Zhan G, Hsu YJ, Pratico D, et al. Long-term intermittent hypoxia in mice: protracted hypersomnolence with oxidative injury to sleep-wake brain regions. Sleep. 2004a;27(2):194–201.

Veasey SC, Yeou-Jey H, Thayer P, Fenik P. Murine multiple sleep latency test: phenotyping sleep propensity in mice. Sleep. 2004b;27(3):388–93.

Veasey SC, Zhan G, Fenik P, Pratico D. Long-term intermittent hypoxia: reduced excitatory hypoglossal nerve output. Am J Respir Crit Care Med. 2004c;170(6):665–72.

Veasey SC, Lear J, Zhu Y, Grinspan JB, Hare DJ, Wang S, et al. Long-term intermittent hypoxia elevates cobalt levels in the brain and injures white matter in adult mice. Sleep. 2013;36(10):1471–81.

Wang GL, Semenza GL. General involvement of hypoxia-inducible factor 1 in transcriptional response to hypoxia. Proc Natl Acad Sci U S A. 1993;90(9):4304–8.

Wang ZY, Baker TL, Keith IM, Mitchell GS, Bisgard GE. Continuous, but not episodic hypoxia, induces CREB phosphorylation in rat carotid body type I cells. Adv Exp Med Biol. 2000;475: 631–5.

Weinshenker D. Functional consequences of locus coeruleus degeneration in Alzheimer's disease. Curr Alzheimer Res. 2008;5(3):342–5.

Weiss MD, Tamisier R, Boucher J, Lynch M, Gilmartin G, Weiss JW, et al. A pilot study of sleep, cognition, and respiration under 4 weeks of intermittent nocturnal hypoxia in adult humans. Sleep Med. 2009;10(7):739–45.

Wilkerson JE, Mitchell GS. Daily intermittent hypoxia augments spinal BDNF levels, ERK phosphorylation and respiratory long-term facilitation. Exp Neurol. 2009;217(1):116–23.

Young T, Peppard P. Sleep-disordered breathing and cardiovascular disease: epidemiologic evidence for a relationship. Sleep. 2000;23(Suppl 4):S122–6.

Yuan G, Adhikary G, McCormick AA, Holcroft JJ, Kumar GK, Prabhakar NR. Role of oxidative stress in intermittent hypoxia-induced immediate early gene activation in rat PC12 cells. J Physiol. 2004;557(Pt 3):773–83.

Yuan G, Vasavda C, Peng YJ, Makarenko VV, Raghuraman G, Nanduri J, et al. Protein kinase G-regulated production of H2S governs oxygen sensing. Sci Signal. 2015a;8(373):ra37.

Yuan X, Guo X, Deng Y, Zhu D, Shang J, Liu H. Chronic intermittent hypoxia-induced neuronal apoptosis in the hippocampus is attenuated by telmisartan through suppression of iNOS/NO and inhibition of lipid peroxidation and inflammatory responses. Brain Res. 2015b;1596:48–57.

Yuan G, Peng YJ, Khan SA, Nanduri J, Singh A, Vasavda C, et al. H2S production by reactive oxygen species in the carotid body triggers hypertension in a rodent model of sleep apnea. Sci Signal. 2016;9(441):ra80.

Zabka AG, Behan M, Mitchell GS. Long term facilitation of respiratory motor output decreases with age in male rats. J Physiol. 2001;531(Pt 2):509–14.

Zhan G, Fenik P, Pratico D, Veasey SC. Inducible nitric oxide synthase in long-term intermittent hypoxia: hypersomnolence and brain injury. Am J Respir Crit Care Med. 2005a;171(12): 1414–20.

Zhan G, Serrano F, Fenik P, Hsu R, Kong L, Pratico D, et al. NADPH oxidase mediates hypersomnolence and brain oxidative injury in a murine model of sleep apnea. Am J Respir Crit Care Med. 2005b;172(7):921–9.

Zhu Y, Fenik P, Zhan G, Mazza E, Kelz M, Aston-Jones G, et al. Selective loss of catecholaminergic wake active neurons in a murine sleep apnea model. J Neurosci. 2007;27(37):10060–71.

Zhu Y, Fenik P, Zhan G, Sanfillipo-Cohn B, Naidoo N, Veasey SC. Eif-2a protects brainstem motoneurons in a murine model of sleep apnea. J Neurosci. 2008;28(9):2168–78.

Part IV
Narcolepsy

Chapter 12
Narcolepsy and Orexin/Hypocretin

Fu Long Xiao, Jun Zhang, and Fang Han

Abstract Narcolepsy is characterized by excessive daytime sleepiness, cataplexy, sleep paralysis, hypnagogic and hypnopompic hallucination, and disturbed nocturnal sleep. A deficient endogenous orexin system due to neuronal loss of orexin neurons in the hypothalamus is the main pathophysiological mechanism for narcolepsy in humans. Recent advances have shown the value of finding decreased cerebrospinal fluid orexin in the diagnosis of human narcolepsy, and the role of the human leucocyte antigen (HLA) gene in the pathogenesis of narcolepsy. Also, there is information on the association between respiratory regulation and the orexin system. Animal models have been used in the pharmacologic study of narcolepsy. Knowledge of how therapeutic agents used to treat narcolepsy act and the underlying neuronal mechanisms come from studies in animal models. Orexin replacement is likely to be a future treatment option for orexin-deficient narcolepsy patients. In this chapter, we will discuss the biology of the orexin system, the clinical aspects of narcolepsy, and examples of translation from basic science research into clinical practice in the field of narcolepsy.

Keywords Narcolepsy · Orexin/Hypocretin

Abbreviations

BST	Bed nucleus of the stria terminalis
CSF	Cerebrospinal fluid
DAT	Dopaminergic transporter
DMN	Dorsal medial hypothalamic nucleus
DR	Dorsal raphe
EDS	Excessive daytime sleepiness

F. L. Xiao · F. Han (✉)
Department of Respiratory Medicine, Peking University People's Hospital, Beijing, China

J. Zhang
Department of Neurology, Peking University People's Hospital, Beijing, China

A. I. Pack, Q. Y. Li (eds.), *Sleep and its Disorders*, Translational Medicine Research,
https://doi.org/10.1007/978-94-024-2168-2_12

GHB	Gamma-hydroxybutyrate
HLA	Human leukocyte antigen
LC	Locus coeruleus
LDT	Laterodorsal tegmental nucleus
MAOI	Monoamine oxidase inhibitor
Orx1	Orexin-1
Orx2	Orexin-2
OSAHS	Obstructive sleep apnea-hypopnea syndrome
PPT	Pedunculopontine nucleus
SNRI	Serotonin norepinephrine reuptake inhibitor
SSRI	Selective serotonin reuptake inhibitor
TCA	Tricyclic antidepressant
TMN	Tuberomammillary nucleus
VLPO	Ventrolateral preoptic nucleus
VTA	Ventral tegmental area

12.1 Biology of Orexin System

The orexin system is conserved across many mammalian species. The orexin system consists of two neuropeptides, orexin-A (or orexin-1) and orexin-B (or orexin-2), and two G-protein-coupled receptors, orexin-1 (Orx1) and orexin-2 (Orx2) receptor. In 1996, a set of neuropeptides associated with the secretin of hormones were isolated from the rat lateral hypothalamus by the process of directional tag PCR subtraction cloning (Gautvik et al. 1996). The cloning of the neuropeptides gene from rat and mouse, the location of the peptide-generating cell bodies and a description of their neuro-connections were first presented in 1997 (Ebrahim et al. 2002). In 1998, the discovery of hypocretin/orexin was reported independently by two groups using different techniques from rat brain: de Lecea et al. (1998) identified the pro-hormone pre-prohypocretin and its peptide products hypocretin-1 and -2 by nucleotide sequencing (de Lecea et al. 1998); at the same time, Sakurai et al. (1998) also reported orexin-1 and -2 by orphan receptor cloning. However, hypocretin and orexin are proven to be synonymous. In this chapter we will use the term orexin.

12.1.1 Orexin and Orexin Receptors

Orexins constitute a novel peptide family with no significant structural similarities to known families of regulatory peptides. Orx1 and Orx2 are generated from a common precursor polypeptide, pre-pro-orexin, with usual proteolytic processing presumably by pro-hormone convertases (Fig. 12.1). Orx1 is a 33-amino acid peptide of 3562 Daltons (Da) with two sets of intrachain disulfide bonds. It has an N-terminal

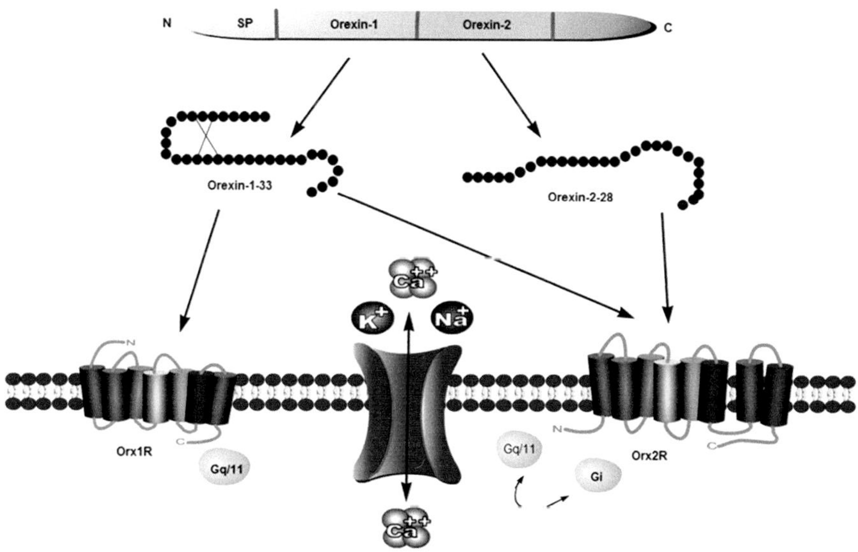

Fig. 12.1 Molecular basis of the orexin system

pyroglutamyl residue and C-terminal amidation (Sakurai et al. 1998). The primary structure of Orx1 predicted from the cDNA sequences is completely conserved among different mammalian species (rat, cow, dog, pig, and human). Orx2 from rat is a 28-amino acid, C-terminally amidated linear peptide of 2937 Da, which is 46% (13/28) same to the sequence of Orx1. The C-terminal half of Orx2 is very similar to that of Orx1 (73%; 11/15), whereas the N-terminal half is variable. Orx2 also has a high degree of sequence conservation among species.

The two orexin receptors, Orx1 receptor (Orx1R) and Orx2 receptor (Orx2R) from human brain, have an identical amino acid sequence of 64% (Tsujino and Sakurai 2009). Amino acid identities between human and rat counterparts of each of these receptors are 94% for Orx1R and 95% for Orx2R, suggesting that both receptor genes are highly conserved among species (Sakurai et al. 1998). Orx1R has a greater affinity for Orx1 than Orx2, whereas Orx2R has a similar affinity for both kinds of Orexins (Sakurai et al. 1998) (Fig. 12.1). Studies in animal brain tissues indicate a complexity in the signal transduction of Orexins (Kukkonen et al. 2002) including the following: direct coupling to nonselective cationic channels (Brown et al. 2002; Yang and Ferguson 2003); transient receptor potential channels (Sergeeva et al. 2003); electrogenic sodium–calcium exchangers (Eriksson et al. 2001; Wu et al. 2002); inhibition of GIRK channels that have previously been activated by somatostatin; nociception or the mu-opioid agonist DAMGO (Hoang et al. 2003); and unusual Ca^{2+}-dependent signaling pathways associated with activation of mitogen-activated protein kinase (Kukkonen et al. 2002; Lund et al. 2000), and/or thapsigargin- and cAMP-PKA-sensitive pathways (Korotkova et al. 2002, 2003; Yamanaka et al. 2003a). Furthermore, Orx1R is coupled to the $G_{q/11}$ class of G protein, which lead to activation of phospholipase C with subsequent triggering of the phosphatidylinositol cascade. Orx2R is shown to be connected with both $G_{q/11}$ and inhibitory G_i proteins when expressed in cell lines (Zhu et al. 2003) (Fig. 12.1).

The characteristic distribution of the Orexin receptors has led some researchers to hypothesize a more sleep-specific role for the Orx1R than Orx2R (Ebrahim et al. 2002). Both orexin receptors are expressed in brain regions, which receive dense orexin innervations (Tsujino and Sakurai 2009). Orx1R and Orx2R show partially overlapping but mainly unique and supplementary distribution patterns, indicating that they play distinct physiological roles (Tsujino and Sakurai 2009). Orx1R is expressed in many brain regions, such as the prefrontal and infralimbic cortex, hippocampus, amygdala, and bed nucleus of the stria terminalis (BST), paraventricular thalamic nucleus, anterior hypothalamus, dorsal raphe (DR), ventral tegmental area (VTA), locus coeruleus (LC), and laterodorsal tegmental nucleus (LDT)/pedunculopontine nucleus (PPT) (Trivedi et al. 1998). Orx2R is also expressed in the amygdala and BST, paraventricular thalamic nucleus, DR, VTA, and LDT/PPT (Lu et al. 2000). Orx2R is also abundantly expressed in the arcuate nucleus, tuberomammillary nucleus (TMN), dorsal medial hypothalamic nucleus (DMN), paraventricular nucleus, lateral hypothalamic area, cornu ammonis 3 in the hippocampus, and medial septal nucleus (Lu et al. 2000). These histological findings suggest that orexin receptors are likely to play a broad regulatory role in the central nervous system and could regulate feeding, autonomic control, sleep, and memory, and play a role in the reward system.

12.1.2 Orexin-Producing Neuron and Its Neuronal Innervation

In both human and rat brains, orexin-producing neurons are exclusively localized in the perifornical area and the lateral and posterior hypothalamic area (Date et al. 1999). These cells diffusely project to the supra-tentorium structure (Fig. 12.2), excluding the cerebellum (Peyron et al. 1998), which suggests that brain areas are widely influenced by orexin neuronal activity. Moreover, the heaviest staining of orexin-immunoreactive neuronal innervation was detected in the paraventricular thalamus nucleus, arcuate nucleus of the hypothalamus, raphe nuclei, TMN, and LC (Tsujino and Sakurai 2009).

In rat, the orexin-producing neurons are specific to the hypothalamus and have widespread neuronal projections with the densest extra-hypothalamic projection to the noradrenergic LC and lesser projections to the basal ganglia, thalamic regions, the medullary reticular formation, and the nucleus of the solitary tract within the central nervous system. Whereas, there are minor projections to cortical regions, central and anterior amygdaloid nuclei, and the olfactory bulb (Gautvik et al. 1996; Mignot 2000; Peyron et al. 1998). In humans, the distribution of orexin-producing neurons is restricted to the dorsolateral hypothalamus with extensive dense projections to the LC, dorsal raphe nuclei, amygdala, suprachiasmatic nucleus, basal

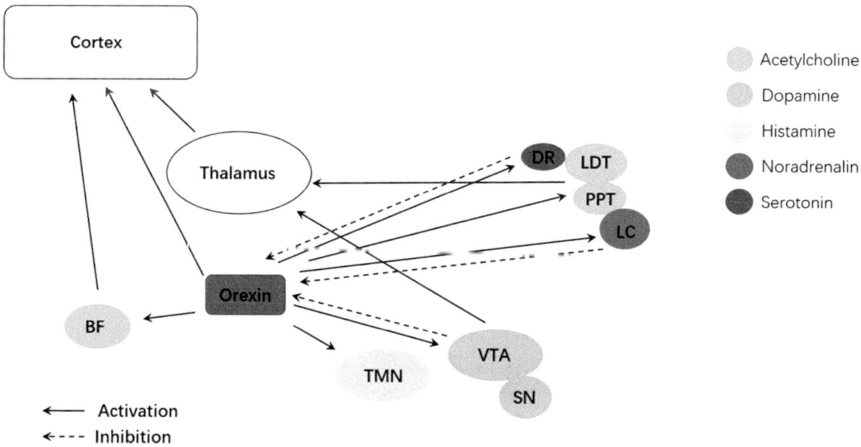

Fig. 12.2 Projections of orexin-producing neurons in the brain, including the main monoaminergic and cholinergic regions where orexin receptors are enriched. *BF* Basal forebrain, *DR* Dorsal raphe, *LC* Locus coeruleus; *LDT* Laterodorsal tegmental nucleus, *PPT* Pedunculopontine tegmental nucleus, *SN* Substantia nigra, *TMN* Tuberomamillary nucleus, *VTA* Ventral tegmental area

forebrain, brainstem, and spinal cord (Peyron et al. 2000; Thannickal et al. 2000; van den Pol 1999). Orexin neurons are innervated by many neurons, including from the lateral parabrachial nucleus, amygdala, BST, lateral septum, ventrolateral preoptic nucleus (VLPO), medial and lateral preoptic areas, basal forebrain, posterior/dorsomedial hypothalamus, VTA, and median raphe nuclei (Tsujino and Sakurai 2009). These neurons that project to orexin neurons are located in regions associated with emotion (Tsujino and Sakurai 2009). Also, the orexin neurons are innervated from the arcuate nucleus associated with energy homeostasis, namely by agouti-related peptide and α-melanin-stimulating hormone-immunoreactive fibers (Broberger et al. 1998).

12.1.3 Neurochemical Interactions of the Orexin

Orexin is thought to act primarily as an excitatory neurotransmitter (de Lecea et al. 1998; Kilduff and Peyron 2000; Sutcliffe and de Lecea 2000). Intracerebroventricular administration of orexin directly stimulates cells in the LC noradrenergic system in rats and monkeys, indicating involvement of orexin in various central functions associated with the noradrenergic system, including vigilance, attention, learning, and memory (Horvath et al. 1999). It also suggested that orexin has an excitatory action on serotonin, histamine, acetylcholine, and dopamine neurons, with a facilitatory role on gamma-aminobutyric acid (GABA) and glutamate-mediated neurotransmission (Ida et al. 2000; van den Pol et al. 1998).

Several neurotransmitters and neuromodulators which activate or inhibit the action of orexin neurons have been identified by electrophysiological studies using transgenic mice (Tsujino and Sakurai 2009). Both noradrenaline and serotonin (5-HT) hyperpolarize and inhibit the activity of orexin neurons by α_2-adrenergic receptors and 5-HT_{1A}-receptors, respectively (Yamanaka et al. 2002). Cholinergic neurons result in both activated and inhibitory actions on orexin neurons through M3-muscarinic receptors (Yamanaka et al. 2003b). However, histamine seems to have no impact on orexin neurons. Furthermore, although orexin neurons do not modify the activity of dopamine receptors, dopamine can inhibit orexin neurons through α_2-adrenergic receptors (Yamanaka et al. 2006). Administration of ionotropic glutamate receptor agonists excites orexin neurons, whereas glutamate antagonists reduce their activity (Li et al. 2002). Glutamatergic neurons can excite orexin neurons (Li et al. 2002). But GABAergic neurons also have a strong effect on orexin neuronal activity (Xie et al. 2006).

Other physiological mechanisms also affect the activity of orexin neurons. Cholecystokinin, as well as neurotensin, oxytocin, and vasopressin excite orexin neurons (Tsujino et al. 2005). Adenosine has been demonstrated to inhibit orexin neurons through A_1 receptors, which might be part of the sleep-facilitating effect of adenosine (Liu and Gao 2007). Fluctuations in CO_2 and pH level also play an important role in the activity of orexin neurons, with increased excitability following acidification and depressed excitability following alkalinization (Williams et al. 2007). This mechanism could explain the role of orexin neurons in the regulation of respiration (Nakamura et al. 2007) (see further below).

12.1.4 Physiological Functions of Orexin

Regulation of the sleep–wake cycle is a primary role of orexin but orexin also has been identified as playing a role in various other functions including feeding and energy homeostasis, neuroendocrine regulation, gastrointestinal and cardiovascular system management, respiratory control, water equilibrium, and autonomic regulation (Edwards et al. 1999; Haynes et al. 1999; Ida et al. 2000; Kirchgessner and Liu 1999; Kuru et al. 2000; Moriguchi et al. 1999; Sakurai et al. 1998; van den Pol et al. 1998). Orexin is involved in the control of other behaviors, such as reward-associated behaviors and emotional processing (de Lecea and Huerta 2014; Ida et al. 1999; Li et al. 2014). Metabolic rate can be increased by administration of orexin in rats and hypoglycemia as a result of administration of insulin can excite up to one-third of orexin-containing neurons. This infers that there is a participation of orexin neurons in regulation of metabolism (Moriguchi et al. 1999; Samson and Resch 2000; Sutcliffe and de Lecea 2000). With respect to neuroendocrine mechanisms, orexin results in a decreased level of prolactin and growth hormone in plasma, combined with an increased level of corticotropin, cortisol, insulin, and luteinizing hormone (Ida et al. 2000; Sutcliffe and de Lecea 2000; van den Pol et al. 1998). Administration of orexin in the central nervous system can improve water consumption, stimulate gastric acid secretion, and increase intestinal movement (Kirchgessner and Liu 1999; Sutcliffe and de Lecea 2000). Mean arterial blood pressure and heart rate can also be increased by orexin (Kilduff and Peyron 2000). Dense distribution of orexin neurons ending in the caudal region of the sacral cord supports the role of orexin in the control of the autonomic nervous system (van den Pol 1999).

In vivo single-unit brain recordings in rats indicate that orexin neuronal firing activity is not only dependent on the behavioral state, but is also associated with specific waking activities, with a maximum firing rate in goal-oriented behaviors such as food seeking and a low firing rate during quiet wakefulness, with a minimum firing rate in slow-wave sleep and tonic REM sleep (Grivel et al. 2005; Kiyashchenko et al. 2002; Mileykovskiy et al. 2005). Orexin is involved in emotional processing. This is a topic of translational research that has a high potential for new pharmaceutical approaches (Johnson et al. 2010; Lutter et al. 2008; Scott et al. 2011). Orexin and its receptor are also being studied as therapeutic targets for mood disorders (Liblau et al. 2015).

12.2 Clinical Aspects of Narcolepsy

Gélineáu first described the term "narcolepsy" in 1880 in a patient with excessive daytime sleepiness, sleep attacks, and episodes of muscle weakness induced by emotions (see Nishino 2007a). Narcolepsy is a chronic neurological condition but is not a progressive disorder (Nishino 2007a). It affects approximately 1 in 2000 individuals in the United States (Mignot 1998). Males and females are both affected. The onset of the disease usually occurs during adolescence. Most cases of human narcolepsy are sporadic; while genetic and environmental factors are also significant for the pathogenesis of narcolepsy, with a few familial cases of human narcolepsy reported (Guilleminault et al. 1989).

12.2.1 Epidemiology

Narcolepsy affects 0.03–0.16% of the general population in various ethnic groups (Hublin et al. 1994; Ohayon et al. 2002; Silber et al. 2002; Wing et al. 2002). There is a spectrum of narcolepsy phenotypes, including narcolepsy with cataplexy (narcolepsy Type 1), narcolepsy without catalepsy and secondary narcolepsy (2014). The prevalence of narcolepsy with catalepsy is between 25 and 50 per 100,000 (de Lecea et al. 1998). Data about incidence is limited. Narcolepsy with cataplexy has an incidence of 0.74 per 100,000 person-years (Silber et al. 2002). The symptoms begin to manifest in the second decade of life among the majority of patients, and the distribution is bimodal, with a large peak around puberty and a smaller peak between 35 and 45 years of age (Dauvilliers et al. 2001). An earlier onset age of narcolepsy has been reported among Chinese cases (Dauvilliers et al. 2001). Although it was thought originally that there was no obvious gender disparity in the prevalence of narcolepsy, newer information indicate that men are more commonly affected, with narcolepsy occurring 1.6 times more frequently than in women (Han et al. 2011; Longstreth et al. 2007). Most cases of narcolepsy in humans are sporadic. Up to 5% are familial cases, and the risk of a first-degree relative suffering narcolepsy-cataplexy is 1–2%, which is 10–40 times higher than that for the general population (Mignot 1998).

12.2.2 *Clinical Manifestation of Narcolepsy*

The classic tetrad of core symptoms for narcolepsy are excessive daytime sleepiness (EDS), cataplexy, hypnagogic, and/or hypnopompic hallucination and sleep paralysis, with disturbed nocturnal sleep. Not all symptoms may be present in an individual patient, and the symptoms may vary in frequency and intensity over time. EDS and cataplexy are the main symptoms of narcolepsy, with the main complaint being EDS.

12.2.2.1 Excessive Daytime Sleepiness and Related Symptoms

After disease onset, EDS persists throughout the patient's life. It results in unwanted episodes of sleep during monotonous sedentary activities and also under circumstances when the patients are involved in a task, such as eating, walking, talking, cycling, or driving. As a result, patients with narcolepsy have a threefold increased risk of motor vehicle accidents due to lapses in attention and lack of alertness (Sakurai 2013). The EDS can be relieved by short naps (from a few seconds to several minutes), but in most situations the sensation of waking up refreshed only lasts from 1 h to several hours before the next feeling of sleepiness. That short naps are refreshing is considered to be diagnostic (Nishino 2007a) and can be helpful in differentiating narcolepsy from other causes of EDS. Sleepiness also happens in irresistible waves in patients with narcolepsy, which is best called "sleep attacks." Sleep attacks may occur in very common situations, such as in the middle of a meal, a conversation, or a bicycle ride. Patients may continue their activities in a semi-conscious status with blurred writing or speaking, which is also described as "automatic behavior" (Nishino 2007a). Abnormalities in learning and impaired attention are frequently associated with narcolepsy, but objective psychophysiological testing is generally normal (Rogers and Rosenberg 1990).

EDS is usually the first symptom of narcolepsy to appear, followed by the other three symptoms (Nishino 2007a). The onset of cataplexy typically happens within 5 years following the presentation of EDS in about two-thirds of patients (Ohayon et al. 2002). The mean duration of onset of hypnagogic and/or hypnopompic hallucination and sleep paralysis is also 2–7 years after that of EDS (Kales et al. 1982).

12.2.2.2 Cataplexy

Cataplexy occurs in 60–70% of narcolepsy patients (Nishino 2007a). It is a diagnostic and unique manifestation of narcolepsy. It is characterized by sudden episodes of bilateral muscle weakness induced by strong emotions, especially positive emotions such as joking, laughing, or a pleasant surprise, and less frequently by negative emotions such as anger. In most circumstances, the loss of muscle tone is mild and happens as a simple buckling of the knees, dropping of the head, flickering of facial muscles, sagging of the jaw, or weakness in the arms. Blurred speech or mutism can also be considered manifestations of cataplexy. Loss of muscle tone can, however, be more severe with individuals falling to the ground. Episodes of cataplexy usually last for a few seconds to several minutes. For children with recent-onset narcolepsy or those cases after sudden withdrawal of anti-cataplexy drugs, cataplexy episodes can occasionally continue for several hours. This is described as "status cataplecticus" (Han et al. 2011; Poryazova et al. 2005). The frequency of cataplexy varies widely between different patients, from rare events over long periods in some cases to numerous attacks per day in others. Poor sleep can worsen cataplexy. It often improves with advancing age. In rare cases, cataplexy can disappear completely, and in most cases it can, with time, be better controlled, particularly after the patients have learned to control their emotions (Hublin et al. 1994).

Awareness of their surroundings is conserved throughout the cataplexy attack, unless the patient suddenly falls asleep or has hypnagogic hallucinations. Falls and injuries occur rarely because patients are often aware of these attacks and take actions to protect themselves by finding support or sitting down as they perceive that the cataplexy is starting. Tone of antigravity muscles can be affected in cataplexy, leading to a progressive collapse of the subject. Respiration may become irregular during an attack, but activity of the diaphragm is not affected. Neurological examination performed at the time of cataplexy shows a suppression of the patellar reflex and sometimes a positive Babinski's sign (Nishino 2007a).

12.2.2.3 Sleep Paralysis

Sleep paralysis presents in 20–50% of all narcolepsy patients (Hublin et al. 1994), and it is often associated with hypnagogic hallucination. Sleep paralysis is described as an inability to carry out voluntary movements at the onset of sleep, or upon awakening from sleep. The patients are unable to perform any movement, even a simple action such as lifting a finger or breathing deeply. The patient is aware of this condition and can recall it completely later. Sleep paralysis may continue for a few minutes and is often interrupted by noise or other external stimulation. The symptom is often troublesome in narcolepsy cases, particularly when accompanied by terrifying hallucinations (Dahlitz and Parkes 1993). Patients may experience extreme anxiety related to fear of dying as a result of sleep paralysis.

Sleep paralysis is not specific to narcolepsy. Sleep paralysis occurs as an isolated symptom among 5–40% of the general population who do not have narcolepsy (Dahlitz and Parkes 1993; Fukuda et al. 1987; Goode 1962). The occurrence of isolated sleep paralysis is amplified by sleep deprivation.

12.2.2.4 Hypnagogic and Hypnopompic Hallucinations

Abnormal visual or auditory perceptions which happen at the time of falling asleep (hypnagogic) or on waking up (hypnopompic) are often reported in cases with narcolepsy (Goode 1962). These hallucinations are often unpleasant and are related to an emotion of fear or threat (Dahlitz and Parkes 1993). Polysomnography studies suggest that these hallucinations most often occur during REM sleep (Chetrit et al. 1994). The episodes are often difficult to distinguish from nightmares or unpleasant dreams, which can also occur in narcolepsy.

Hypnagogic hallucinations are often related to sleep attacks, and the patients can recall the content of the hallucinations. The hallucinations are usually complex, vivid, and dream-mimic experiences, and may be followed by an attack of cataplexy or sleep paralysis. Other common hallucinations observed at sleep onset include primary feelings (i.e., light touching and rubbing), changes in location of body parts (e.g., arm or leg). The hallucinations described in narcolepsy should be distinguished from hallucinations reported in schizophrenia or other psychotic disorders. Patients with narcolepsy reporting these hallucinations may be misdiagnosed.

12.2.2.5 Other Important Symptoms

One of the most common symptoms of narcolepsy is disturbed nocturnal sleep, namely insomnia, which is characterized as difficulty in maintaining nighttime sleep. Narcolepsy patients fall asleep easily, but wake up after a short sleep and are unable to fall asleep again for an hour or so. As for total sleep time, narcolepsy patients typically spend the same time in bed as normal individuals over the 24-h cycle (Broughton et al. 1988; Hishikawa et al. 1976; Montplaisir et al. 1978). But narcolepsy patients usually suffer from insomnia. Other sleep-related problems are periodic leg movements (Mosko et al. 1984), REM behavior disorder, parasomnias (Schenck and Mahowald 1992), and obstructive sleep apnea (Chokroverty 1986; Mosko et al. 1984).

Metabolic disorders were also reported in narcolepsy patients several decades ago. Obesity (Honda et al. 1986; Schuld et al. 2000), insulin-resistant diabetes (Honda et al. 1986), reduced food intake (Lammers et al. 1996), and lower blood pressure and temperature (Mayer et al. 1997) have all been described in patients with narcolepsy. However, these findings are not considered to be specific since they may be secondary to sleepiness or inactivity during the daytime. It has also been shown, however, that these metabolic disorders could be the result of orexin deficiency (Nishino et al. 2001).

Narcolepsy interferes with every aspect of daily life. The negative social impact, working disability, depression in mood have also been extensively described (Aldrich 1989).

12.2.3 *Diagnosis*

12.2.3.1 Polysomnography, Symptoms, and Sleep Evaluations

The diagnosis of narcolepsy is based on clinical symptomatology, with EDS daily for at least 3 months, combined with a clear history of cataplexy (2014). Objective tests to assist diagnosis include nocturnal polysomnography followed by a daytime multiple sleep latency test (MSLT) and measurement of orexin-1 concentrations in CSF. According to ICSD-3 (2014), the diagnosis of narcolepsy requires a clinical history of EDS and a positive MSLT result, with a mean sleep-onset latency of 8 min or less and two or more sleep-onset REM periods (SOREMPs). Sleep prior to the MSLT must be at least 6 h to allow proper interpretation of results (Nishino 2007a). The standard MSLT consists of five naps, scheduled at 2 h intervals starting between 9 and 10 am (Carskadon et al. 1986; Chervin et al. 1995; Richardson et al. 1978). The test is terminated after a sleep period lasting 15 min or after 20 min if the patients did not fall asleep. SOREMs are defined as the occurrence of REM sleep within 15 min after sleep onset. In addition, hypersomnia should not result from other sleep disorders or substance abuse. In the ICSD-2 guideline, an MSLT is not required for the diagnosis of narcolepsy with definite cataplexy. Although neither the MSLT results nor the orexin-1 levels in CSF measurements will affect the treatment strategy, obtaining objective data is still recommended before the beginning of life-long therapy even in patients with cataplexy (2014). The MSLT is also the accepted standard for evaluating the severity of EDS and the appearance of SOREMs. However, the diagnostic value of a single MSLT for narcolepsy is limited since around 15% of patients with narcolepsy-cataplexy have normal or more frequently, borderline MSLT results. On the other hand, typical narcolepsy-like MSLT results have been reported in a small number of patients with sleep breathing disorders and even normal individuals. A nocturnal polysomnography is also useful for the diagnosis of other sleep disorders related to EDS, such as periodic limb movement disorder and sleep breathing disorders.

Other objective methods have been developed to assess EDS in narcolepsy, such as the sleep latency on the maintenance of wakefulness test (MWT) (Mitler et al. 1998). In the MWT, the subject is told to attempt to remain awake. Generally, this method is not used for the diagnosis, but it is useful to evaluate the impact of treatment with psychostimulant drugs (Mitler et al. 1998).

12.2.3.2 Biological Markers

In addition to the role of clinical factors and polysomnography in diagnosis, it has been shown that HLA typing, i.e., DQB1*0602, is supportive of the diagnosis, but the specificity of DQB1*0602 positive is very low (Mignot 1998). Quantification of CSF orexin-1 has also become a positive criterion for the diagnosis of narcolepsy (Mignot et al. 2002; Ripley et al. 2001). A concentration of CSF orexin-1 below 110 pg/mL is highly specific (99%) and sensitive (87%) for narcolepsy, and is more specific than the MSLT (Han 2012b). Low CSF orexin-1 levels in DQB1*0602 negative patients without cataplexy occurs in less than 1% of all patients with narcolepsy. Low CSF orexin-1 concentration is typically positive for patients with narcolepsy with DQB1*0602. Evaluation of CSF orexin-1 is currently advocated in a situation when there is a borderline MSLT result, such as in children who are unable to follow the instructions for MSLT, patients with psychiatric, neurological or medical disorders, and those with drugs or substances usage, which can change the sleep latency and the latency to REM sleep (Bourgin et al. 2008; Dauvilliers et al. 2007).

12.2.3.3 Diagnosis of Narcolepsy

Narcolepsy is categorized as type 1 (narcolepsy with catalepsy) and type 2 (narcolepsy without catalepsy). Type-1 narcolepsy is a distinct phenomenon with definitive diagnostic criteria. However, type-2 narcolepsy remains a "developing diagnosis," and it is controversial whether type-2 narcolepsy is a specific condition or part of the spectrum of narcolepsy and idiopathic hypersomnia.

According to ICSD-3 (2014), type-1 narcolepsy requires the following (see Table 12.1): (A) excessive daytime sleepiness lasting at least 3 months; (B) definite history of cataplexy; (C) abnormal MSLT (mean sleep latency ≤8 min and 2 or more SOREMPs); (D) CSF orexin-1 concentrations ≤110 pg/mL, or

Table 12.1 Diagnostic criteria for narcolepsy from ICSD-3 (2014)

Type-1 narcolepsy	Type-2 narcolepsy
1. Excessive daytime sleepiness lasting at least 3 months	1. Excessive daytime sleepiness lasting at least 3 months
2. Definite history of cataplexy	2. Definite no history of cataplexy
3. Abnormal MSLT (mean sleep latency ≤8 min and 2 or more SOREMPs)	3. Abnormal MSLT (mean sleep latency ≤8 min and 2 or more SOREMPs)
4. CSF orexin-1 concentrations ≤110 pg/mL, or one-third of mean normal values	4. CSF orexin-1 concentrations >110 pg/mL, or one-third of mean normal values
	5. Excluding hypersomnia due to other disorders and/or diseases resulted in abnormal MSLT

Once the definitive cataplexy is reported or the CSF orexin-1 levels are decreased to concentrations ≤110 pg/mL or one-third of mean normal values, then the patients would be considered to have type-1 narcolepsy

one-third of mean normal values. Definite type-1 narcolepsy requires meeting the items of A+B+C or A+B+D. Low levels of CSF orexin-1 are specific for type-1 narcolepsy and can confirm the diagnosis. Nocturnal polysomnography SOREMPs can also be included in the total for SOREMPs.

Type-2 narcolepsy requires the followings: (A) excessive daytime sleepiness lasting at least 3 months; (B) no history of cataplexy; (C) abnormal MSLT (mean sleep latency $\leq$8 min and 2 or more SOREMPs); (D) CSF orexin-1 concentrations $>$110 pg/mL, or greater than one-third of mean normal values; (E) excluding hypersomnia due to other disorders and/or diseases resulting in abnormal MSLT. The diagnosis of type-2 narcolepsy is controversial and requires meeting all of the items discussed above (see Table 12.1).

12.2.3.4 Differential Diagnosis

Narcolepsy needs to be distinguished from other forms of hypersomnia, such as sleep breathing disorders, idiopathic hypersomnia, and chronic insufficient sleep (Dauvilliers 2006). The occurrence of cataplexy is an obvious feature in distinguishing narcolepsy from other forms of hypersomnia. Also becoming refreshed after a short nap is considered to be of diagnostic value, as this may distinguish narcolepsy from idiopathic hypersomnia. Cataplexy should be differentiated from other events, such as those that occur in psychiatric disorders or epilepsy. Narcolepsy also needs to be distinguished from neurological conditions such as syncope, drop attack, or attacks of a histrionic nature. Symptomatic or secondary narcolepsy due to other medical disorders may occur with cataplexy, and neurological examinations and brain imaging scans can be helpful for diagnosis of these conditions.

12.3 Narcolepsy and Orexin: From Basic Science Research into Clinical Practice

12.3.1 Deficient Orexin in Narcolepsy and Diagnostic Value of CSF Orexin Measurement

12.3.1.1 Dog and Rodent Models of Narcolepsy

Animal models first demonstrated the involvement of orexin deficiency in narcolepsy (Sakurai 2013). Mice lacking either the *orexin* gene (*prepro-orexin* knockout mice) or orexin-producing neurons (*orexin/ataxin-3* transgenic mice), or dogs and mice with mutations in the orexin-2 receptor that rendered it ineffective, show a narcoleptic phenotype, including disrupted sleep–wake regulation and sudden atonia of muscles (Beuckmann et al. 2004; Chemelli et al. 1999; Hara et al. 2001; Lin et al. 1999; Willie et al. 2003).

Mignot and colleagues described that dogs with a mutation in the orexin-2 receptor are similar to humans with narcolepsy (Lin et al. 1999). As in human narcolepsy, canine narcolepsy shows cataplexy, sleepiness (such as decreased sleep latency) and SOREMPs (Nishino and Mignot 1997). The narcoleptic dogs have fragmented sleep/wake patterns and they do not maintain long bouts of wakefulness or sleep (Kaitin et al. 1986a, b; Nishino et al. 2000a). Narcoleptic Dobermans showed decreased sleep latency and reduced latency to REM sleep (Nishino et al. 2000a). Canine cataplexy is typically induced by playing with other dogs or with human caretakers; presentation of food (especially favored food) is a powerful precipitant. This has led to the use of food elicited cataplexy as a test for narcolepsy in canine models. Sexual activity will often elicit cataplexy in male narcoleptic canines (Boehmer et al. 2004; Nishino and Mignot 1997). Canines with narcolepsy usually have about two episodes of cataplexy/hour during the day, but in the Food Elicited Cataplexy Test, a narcoleptic dog can have five or more events of cataplexy in just 1 or 2 min (Nishino et al. 1989, 2000a). Canine cataplexy is not triggered by startling loud noises.

Cataplexy in dogs typically shows a progressive inhibition of muscle tone, with the hindlimbs involved first (Fujiki et al. 2002). Hindlimb weakness often resolves in a few seconds in the case of partial cataplexy, or it may spread to the forelimbs and somatic muscles, resulting in generalized weakness (Scammell et al. 2009). In narcoleptic dogs, all the limbs may collapse at the same time (Fujiki et al. 2002). Even though the dog collapses to the ground, it may continue to eat, suggesting the tone of the cranial muscles can be preserved. But, these cranial muscles might also be fully atonic in cataplexy (Scammell et al. 2009). The eyes are open during the cataplectic attacks, with eyes following objects of interest, indicating the preservation of consciousness during cataplexy in both human and dogs (Nishino et al. 1995). The duration of cataplexy can range from a few seconds to several minutes in dogs (Nishino et al. 1989, 2000a). Longer durations may be reported in a situation like REM sleep with closure of the eyes, rapid eye movements and distal muscle twitching (Siegel et al. 1991).

Typical murine models of narcolepsy with cataplexy have been produced with removal of the *prepro-orexin* gene or transgenic expression of a toxic protein which selectively kills orexin-producing neurons (Chemelli et al. 1999; Hara et al. 2001). As in human narcolepsy, murine narcolepsy shows cataplexy, impaired maintenance of wakefulness and fragmented sleep (Chemelli et al. 1999; Hara et al. 2001). As a mouse changes from normal activity into cataplexy, the EEG shifts from a waking pattern to that for REM sleep or pre-REM sleep (Chemelli et al. 1999; Hara et al. 2001; Willie et al. 2003). Cataplexy in rodent is similar to human cataplexy (Chemelli et al. 1999; Hara et al. 2001; Willie et al. 2003). Cataplexy is more frequent with emotional stimulation, such as social interaction, enriched environment (novel toys, fresh bedding, etc.) and in the open field (Chemelli et al. 1999; Espana et al. 2007). Mild fasting, restricted feeding programs, and presentation of favored food can make the cataplectic attacks more frequent, but these situations are not as effective as the Food Elicited Cataplexy Test, which is employed in identification of canine cataplexy (Nishino and Mignot 1997; Scammell et al. 2009). Also, cataplexy associated with sexual activity is not common in narcoleptic rodents (Scammell et al. 2009). At the onset of cataplexy, the mouse suddenly ceases motor activity, combined with an ataxic gait due to loss of tone in muscles (Willie et al. 2003). Then the mouse collapses prone, falling to one side for 30 s to 2 min, which is similar to what occurs in human and canine cataplexy (Chemelli et al. 1999; Hara et al. 2001; Mochizuki et al. 2004; Willie et al. 2003). At the end of an attack, the mouse rapidly recovers from cataplexy and often restarts its ongoing activity (Espana et al. 2007). Consciousness is still maintained during the cataplectic episode, with eyes open and weak vigilance (Willie et al. 2003).

12.3.1.2 Orexin Deficiency in Human Narcolepsy

In contrast to animal models, most human cases of narcolepsy are not due to mutations in the orexin or orexin receptor genes (Han 2012b). The first link between orexin dysfunction and narcolepsy in humans came from a clinical report of nine human narcolepsy patients who were found to have very low levels of orexin-1 in the cerebrospinal fluid (CSF) as compared with healthy subjects (Nishino et al. 2000b). Seven of these narcoleptic subjects were reported to have undetectable orexin-1 levels, while two narcoleptic patients had normal levels of orexin-1. All the eight healthy control subjects had normal levels of orexin-1. This result indicated that human narcolepsy may be caused by a deficiency in orexin (Nishino et al. 2000b). Subsequently, autopsy studies of human narcolepsy patients indicated a loss of orexin peptides in the cortex and pons, with an 80–100% reduction in the number of orexin-producing neurons in the hypothalamus (Peyron et al. 2000; Thannickal et al. 2000). A possible explanation is that the orexin-producing neurons may be destroyed by an autoimmune mechanism associated with the specific HLA genotype in narcolepsy patients (Mignot 2014). There are just a hundred thousand orexin-producing neurons located in the hypothalamus and a specific lesion in these cells has not been reported in most other neurological disorders (Mignot 2014).

More studies have supported the concept of human narcolepsy is the direct result of loss of orexin-producing neurons (Han 2012b). Peyron et al. reported a total loss of orexin in the brains of six narcoleptic cases using in situ hybridization and radioimmunoassay of the perifornical hypothalamus (Peyron et al. 2000). There was no evidence of inflammatory pathology in all the six brains, albeit many years after the initial presentation (Peyron et al. 2000). Another study demonstrated an 85–95% decline in the number of orexin-producing neurons in four narcoleptic brains by using immunocytochemistry (Thannickal et al. 2000). Moreover, in both studies, it was suggested that the melanin-concentrating hormone neurons, which are situated close to the orexin-producing neurons in hypothalamus, were intact in the narcoleptic brains. This suggested that the putative autoimmune process was relatively specific for orexin-producing neurons (Peyron et al. 2000; Thannickal et al. 2000). Additional studies also found that loss of orexin cells in the hypothalamus, rather than failure of orexin expression, was the main pathological mechanism (Blouin et al. 2005; Crocker et al. 2005). Some studies also found an increased number of histaminergic cells in the tuberomammillary nucleus of the hypothalamus in narcoleptic brains. This may be a compensatory mechanism of the wake-promoting system following the loss of orexin-producing neurons (John et al. 2013; Valko et al. 2013).

12.3.1.3 Similar Phenotype of Narcolepsy-Cataplexy in Humans and Mice

Orexin−/− mice showed a phenotype similar to human narcolepsy-cataplexy (Chemelli et al. 1999). However, these mice can be divided into two different phenotypes according to the behavioral characterization, pharmacological, and electrophysiological features (Sakurai 2013). One is "abrupt attack," which presents as a sudden loss of muscle tone during obvious emotional stimulation (Willie et al. 2003). EEG recording indicate that abrupt attacks in *Orexin−/−* mice are the result of abnormal transitions from wakefulness directly to REM sleep. The other type is "gradual attack," in which the attack begins during quiet wakefulness, with a transition over a period of several seconds to a collapsed posture. EEG recording shows that a gradual attack in *Orexin−/−* mice is the result of a switch from wakefulness to NREM sleep, which may correspond to "sleep attacks" in human narcolepsy patients (Sakurai 2013). It is proposed that the abrupt and gradual attacks are similar to cataplexy and sleep attacks in human narcolepsy-cataplexy, respectively (Sakurai 2013).

Similar to *Orexin−/−* mice, human narcolepsy-cataplexy can also be divided into two phenotypes caused by two different pathological mechanisms (Sakurai 2013). One is characterized by difficulty in maintaining long periods of wakefulness, with abrupt transitions from waking to NREM sleep. This phenotype manifests as excessive daytime sleepiness, resulting in sleep attacks. Animal studies indicate that sleep attacks result from deficiency in Orx2 (Mignot 1998). The other phenotype is cataplexy attacks, with pathological REM sleep intrusions into wakefulness. Administration of tricyclic antidepressants, serotonin-specific reuptake inhibitors (SSRIs), and serotonin/noradrenaline reuptake inhibitors (SNRI) can suppress the cataplexy attack, indicating a role for dysfunctional monoaminergic neurotransmission in the pathophysiology of cataplexy (Poryazova et al. 2005). Animal studies indicate that a cataplexy attack might result from abnormal function of both orexin receptors (Poryazova et al. 2005; Willie et al. 2003), although more studies are required to establish the mechanism of cataplexy.

12.3.1.4 Measurement of CSF Orexin in the Diagnosis of Narcolepsy

A low CSF level of orexin-1 is now one of the diagnostic criteria for narcolepsy-cataplexy according to the 3rd edition of the International Classification of Sleep Disorders (ICSD-3) (2014). Narcolepsy-cataplexy is considered to be more closely associated with orexin deficiency as compared with narcolepsy without cataplexy.

Interestingly, there was previously no available diagnostic biomarker for narcolepsy, and the definite diagnosis was often delayed for several years after the onset of symptoms (Nishino and Kanbayashi 2005). Basic science research in animal models of narcolepsy has led to the identification of the role of orexin-1 deficiency in the pathogenesis of narcolepsy. As a result, measurement of decreased CSF orexin-1 has proven to be a more specific test than the MSLT (Han 2012b; Nishino 2007a).

Decreased levels of CSF orexin-1 are also seen in a few other neurological diseases, specifically Guillain-Barre syndrome and Ma2 positive paraneoplastic syndrome (Nishino et al. 2003; Overeem et al. 2004). However, these neurological diseases are easily distinguished from narcolepsy clinically. About 10% of narcolepsy-cataplexy cases have, however, normal CSF orexin-1 (Krahn et al. 2002; Mignot et al. 2002; Nishino et al. 2001). It is controversial whether the orexin system is abnormal or not in these rare patients. Deficiency in orexin receptors and dysfunction in its downstream pathway might be the pathological mechanism in these patients (Nishino 2007a). But this cannot be currently verified.

12.3.2 HLA Genetic Marker in Narcolepsy

The HLA genes, also called major histocompatibility (MHC) genes, are located on human chromosome 6. The HLA locus encompasses genes encoding for HLA class I molecules (HLA-A, HLA-B, and HLA-C), which present antigenic peptides to the T-cell receptors (TCR) at the surface of $CD8^{+}$T cells. HLA class II molecules (HLA-DR, HLA-DQ, and HLA-DP) present antigenic peptides to TCR on $CD4^{+}$T cells. HLA polymorphisms contribute to genetic variations in the immune response (McDevitt and Tyan 1968). HLA polymorphisms regulate immune responses to infections, but they are also associated with autoimmune disorders (Dausset 1972). Over the past 30 years, a better understanding of the genetic basis of narcolepsy has shown that narcolepsy is strongly associated with a specific HLA allele, DQB1*0602. This polymorphism is consistently present in 90–100% of patients across different ethnic groups (Mignot et al. 2001). As a result, it has long been speculated that the pathogenesis of narcolepsy results from an autoimmune-mediated mechanism (Kadotani et al. 1998). The identification of the Tribbles homolog 2 (Trib2, an antigen abundantly expressed on orexin-producing neurons) reactive antibodies (Cvetkovic-Lopes et al. 2010); the association of polymorphisms in the T-cell receptor alpha locus and the purinergic receptor subtype 2Y11 (P2RY11) loci found in genome-wide association studies (Hallmayer et al. 2009; Han et al. 2012a; Kornum et al. 2011b) all add further support for the proposed autoimmune mechanism.

The first report about HLA relationship with narcolepsy was from Juli and Honda, they reported that all Japanese narcolepsy-cataplexy cases (22 male and 18 female patients) included in the study carried HLA-DR2 gene, while only 49.1% control subjects carried HLA-DR2 gene, indicating an absolute association with HLA-DR2 in the Japanese narcolepsy patients (Juji et al. 1984). Guilleminault and his colleagues, however, found that very rare DR2-negative narcolepsy patients were found in American (Guilleminault and Grumet 1986). This is in conflict with Japanese research described above (Juji et al. 1984). The possible explanation for this conflict may be the ethnic difference in linkage disequilibrium between DR2 and other narcolepsy-associated genes. On the other hand, diagnostic criteria also affected the findings of association between HLA-DR2 and narcolepsy (Matsuki et al. 1987). In German Caucasoids narcolepsy patients, Gertrud et al. found that 57 out of 58 unrelated patients (98.3%) carried HLA-DR2 and DQw1 (Mueller-Eckhardt et al. 1986), which was demonstrated as the subtype of HLADQ0602 by high resolution analysis. While the HLA-DR and HLA-DQ region is compact, containing in sequence the DRA gene (practically monomorphic), accessory DRB genes (DRB3,4,5 genes present in some but not all haplotypes), the DRB1 gene (a very polymorphic gene), and finally the polymorphic DQA1 and DQB1 loci. In Caucasians and Japanese, linkage disequilibrium between DQ and DR is remarkable such that almost all DQB1*06:02 alleles are linked with DQA1*01:02 and DRB1*15:01 (DR2), making it difficult to distinguish whether the effect is caused by DR or DQ (Mignot 2014). In the early 1990s, studies in African Americans showed additional diversity in DR-DQ haplotypes, such that DQB1*06:02 was detected not only in linkage with DRB1*15:01, but also in linkage with DRB1*11:01 and more rarely DRB1*12:02 (Behar et al. 1995; Fernandez-Vina et al. 1991; Mignot et al. 1997). There are less DR2 carriers in African American narcoleptic cases (Neely et al. 1986), and the detection of HLA-DR and HLA-DQ associations in this ethnic group seem to be significant (Neely et al. 1986).

Mignot and his colleagues reported that all African American patients with narcolepsy carried both DQA1*01:02 and DQB1*06:02 (Matsuki et al. 1992; Mignot et al. 1994); while in many instances, DRB1*15 (DR2) was not detected. This demonstrates that the primary association is with HLA-DQ, not DR, and more particularly with the DQ heterodimer DQ0602 that encodes DQA1*01:02 and DQB1*06:02. This was replicated in Chinese patients with narcolepsy, we found that DRB1*15:01 alone does not predispose to narcolepsy in the context of the DRB1*15:01, DQA1*01:02, and DQB1*06:01 in South China (Han et al. 2012b). The data illustrated the extraordinary conservation of HLA class II effects in narcolepsy across populations and show that DRB1*15:01 has no effect on narcolepsy susceptibility in the absence of DQB1*06:02 (Han et al. 2012b). In follow-up studies, Mignot and his colleagues found a number of very rare cases of DQB1*06:02-positive cases that carried various DRB1 alleles by screening hundreds of patients. Alleles such as DRB1*03:01, DRB1*08:01, DRB1*08:06, and DRB1*16:01 are only exceptionally detected in control subjects (Mignot et al. 1993, 1997), confirming the abundance of these rare DQ0602 haplotypes in narcolepsy. Other HLA alleles genes encoding MHC I molecules can also predispose individuals to narcolepsy, including HLA-A*11:01, HLA-B*35:01, HLA-B*51:01, and HLA-C*04:01 (Tafti et al. 2016). Current findings suggest antigen presentation by the heterodimer DQ0602 (MHC II molecule) to T cells may be central to the pathogenesis of narcolepsy (Latorre et al. 2018; Luo et al. 2018; Irukayama-Tomobe et al. 2017).

As described above, studies have demonstrated that the best genetic marker for narcolepsy is the closely linked HLA-DQB1*06:01 and DQA1*01:02 loci (encoding the DQ0602 heterodimer) rather than HLA-DR2.

12.3.3 *Narcolepsy and Sleep Apnea*

A 9–19% prevalence of obstructive sleep apnea-hypopnea syndrome (OSAHS) has been detected in narcoleptic patients based on polysomnography studies (Han et al. 2010; Pataka et al. 2012). Recent research based on studies on a large number of narcolepsy patients demonstrated a 26% incidence of OSAHS among narcolepsy-cataplexy cases with a mean age of 45 years. There is a higher apnea-hypopnea index and lower minimal oxygen saturation for the nonobese young narcoleptic patients during nocturnal sleep compared with the age- and gender-matched control subjects (Han et al. 2010). The exact mechanisms linking narcolepsy and OSAHS are still unknown. It is suggested that a deficiency in orexin inclines narcoleptic patients to obesity, and the risk of further weight gain is still high even after the initiation of treatment, which means OSAHS is more likely to appear over time (Schuld et al. 2000). In addition to concurrent obesity, it has been proposed that abnormalities in respiratory regulation occur in narcoleptic patients, since the impaired central control of breathing during sleep has been implicated in these populations (Han 2012a).

12.3.3.1 Respiratory Regulation and Orexin/Hypocretin in Narcoleptic Animal Models

The hypothalamus, in which orexin-producing neurons are located, has long been considered as being involved in respiratory regulation (Kuwaki 2010). Recent studies indicate that this effect is partially mediated by the orexin system. Orexin-producing neurons may participate in breathing control with the changing of consciousness. Neuronal projections from orexin-producing neurons include ascending pathways to arousal regulation regions such as the thalamus and cortex, and descending pathways to brainstem regulating nuclei, such as the raphe nuclei, nucleus tractus solitarius, the rostral ventrolateral medulla as well as to phrenic and hypoglossal nuclei (Kuwaki 2010; Williams and Burdakov 2008). Both the Orx2 receptor and the Orx1 receptor are expressed in brainstem respiratory centers, and the orexin-producing neurons also serve as acid and CO_2 sensors, as well as receiving afferent signals from amygdala and the bed nucleus of the stria terminals (Williams and Burdakov 2008). Activation of orexin receptors at different locations in the brainstem and spinal cord can influence the ventilatory rate and depth, as well as the coordination between upper airway and thoracic pump muscles. Microperfusion of orexin either to sites in the pre-Bötzinger region in the medulla or phrenic nucleus leads to a dose-dependent, a significant increase in diaphragm electromyographic activity (Nattie and Li 2010). Injection of orexin into the hypoglossal motor nucleus increases genioglossus muscle activity. Moreover, administration of orexin-2 to the pontine respiratory center can increase the pre-inspiratory activity of the hypoglossal nerve, which is necessary for the maintenance of upper airway patency (Kuwaki et al. 2010).

From studies in knockout mice, Kuwaki and his colleagues proposed that orexin plays a role in central chemoreception (Nattie and Li 2010). Increased respiratory activity due to excitation of the hypothalamus is absent in the knockout mice lacking the orexin gene (Kuwaki et al. 2010). Orexin-producing neurons have been demonstrated to be the most CO_2/H^+-sensitive neurons in brain based on in vitro studies (Williams et al. 2007). These neurons can be excited by CO_2 in vivo (Sunanaga et al. 2009). In the orexin genetic knockout mice, administration of exogenous orexin can partially recover the attenuated respiratory response to hypercapnia (Han 2012b). The respiratory response to hypoxia is, however, not different in orexin knockout mice compared to wild-type mice (Han 2012b). Antagonists to Orx1 and Orx2 receptors may lead to a decrease in the CO_2 ventilatory response in wild-type mice, especially in the waking state (Han 2012b). The excitatory effect of Orx2 on ventilation is more obvious than Orx1, whereas Orx1 has a more profound impact on sleep. This suggests that the respiratory effect of orexin is independent of its effect on sleep at least to some degree. Orexin may also be involved in the stabilization of ventilation (Han 2012b). Long-term respiratory facilitation, which is considered necessary to stabilize breathing and prevent sleep apnea, was absent in orexin genetic knockout mice. Orexin knockout mice have also more frequent apneas during sleep (Han 2012b).

12.3.3.2 Respiratory Regulation and Orexin/Hypocretin in Human Narcolepsy

In narcolepsy, nocturnal sleep may be disturbed by coexistent OSAHS, which can result from a dysfunction of respiratory control (Strohl et al. 1986). Orexin plays a role in suppression of central sleep apnea (Kuwaki 2008, 2010; Nakamura et al. 2007). Deficiency in orexin might therefore lead to a higher incidence of central sleep apnea in patients with narcolepsy. Long-term nocturnal sleep disturbance in narcoleptic patients may also contribute to alterations in the chemo-responsiveness and mimic the alterations produced by sleep deprivation (White et al. 1983). Fragmented sleep and hypoxia resulting from coexistent OSAHS may further impair the ventilatory responsiveness of narcoleptic patients (Han et al. 2001). An altered hypoxic responsiveness, but not hypercapnic response, was detected in human narcolepsy. This contrasts with the findings in orexin knockout mice (Han et al. 2010; Williams et al. 2007). Further analysis reveals that the disordered hypoxic response in human narcolepsy was independent of body mass index, age, gender, and the severity of narcolepsy symptoms such as sleepiness and cataplexy. It also had no relationship with orexin deficiency. An unexpected finding was that the mechanism for abnormal hypoxic response in human narcolepsy may result from HLADQB1*06:02 rather than the disease itself (Han 2012b). For normal subjects who carry the HLADQB1*06:02, the same abnormal hypoxic response could also be found as in narcoleptic patients with HLADQB1*06:02 (Han 2012b). However, since the pathogenesis of narcolepsy is an autoimmune disorder, it has been reported that HLADQB1*06:02 associated immune-mediated destruction of type I glomus cells in the carotid bodies (the peripheral chemoreceptor for detection of hypoxia) might contribute to the abnormal hypoxic response in human narcolepsy (Kornum et al. 2011a).

12.3.4 Treatment of Narcolepsy

Animal models, especially canine models, have been used to understand the neuronal mechanisms that underlie the pharmacological control of narcolepsy (Nishino 2007a). The cholinergic system, which plays a significant role in triggering REM sleep and REM sleep atonia, was identified as an investigatory target (Nishino 2007b). Although cholinergic blockade with muscarinic antagonists could significantly reduce cataplexy in canine models, this class of compounds has not been used in human narcolepsy due to their obvious peripheral side effects (Nishino 2007a). Treatment of narcolepsy is focused on control of the two core symptoms, excessive daytime sleepiness, and cataplexy. Recently, disturbed nocturnal sleep is increasingly recognized as an important symptom of narcolepsy. Generally speaking, all therapeutic agents used to treat cataplexy are aimed to act on the monoaminergic system (Nishino 2007a). Wakefulness-stimulant drugs such as modafinil and amphetamine are used to treat excessive daytime sleepiness (Sakurai 2013). Modulation of γ-aminobutyric acid B ($GABA_B$) receptors or histamine H_3 receptors (H_3R) has effects on both EDS and cataplexy (Thorpy 2020). Pitolisant, an H_3R antagonist, and solriamfetol, a dopamine and norepinephrine reuptake inhibitor, are the most recently approved treatments for narcolepsy EDS in the European Union (pitolisant) and the United States (pitolisant and solriamfetol) (Thorpy 2020). Several new agents are being developed and tested as potential treatments for EDS and cataplexy in narcolepsy (Thorpy 2020), including novel oxybate formulations (once-nightly [FT218]; low sodium [JZP-258]), a selective norepinephrine reuptake inhibitor (AXS-12), and a product combining modafinil and an astroglial connexin inhibitor (THN102). Continuous deep brain stimulation to lateral hypothalamus and zona incerta dose-responsively reversed sleep and cataplexy episodes in narcolepsy mouse model without negative sequelae (Rogers et al. 2020). Since the finding of association between Orexin/hypocretin and narcolepsy, this system has been a target for therapy. Previous studies showed that central administration of orexin can ameliorate cataplexy and improve the wakefulness in narcolepsy animals (Zeitzer et al. 2006), which demonstrated that deficiency of orexin does not induce a permanent inability in orexin system. Thus, pharmacological modulation aims to the orexin system and sets an example for the ideal approach to narcolepsy treatment. Promising orexin-based narcolepsy treatment includes orexin administration via different pathways (intravenous, intranasal, intra-cerebral ventricle), gene therapy, orexin cell transplantation, and orexin-receptor agonists. The blood–brain barrier is the most common limitation in delivery of therapeutics to the brain.

Orexin Administration
Hagan et al. (1999) revealed that intracerebroventricular administration of orexin-A improved arousal and locomotor activity in rats and increased locus coeruleus neuronal firing in vitro. Dube et al. (1999) administered orexin-A and -B into rats' brain via microinjection and observed that orexin-A enhanced the food intake after application to the lateral hypothalamus, paraventricular nucleus, whereas orexin-B was not effective at any of these sites, which concluded the hypothesis that the responsiveness of both orexins in different brain sites are not identical.

Intravenous administering of a therapeutic amount of orexin resulted in a decrease or even completed elimination of cataplexy in narcolepsy animal models. Conversely, high doses of orexin-A led to a significant worsening in cataplexy (John et al. 2000; Kiyashchenko et al. 2001). Microinjection of orexin-A into the locus coeruleus in rats improved their muscle tone and prevented cataplexy, whereas microinjection of the same amount of orexin-A into areas ventral to the locus coeruleus caused an acute loss of muscle tone (John et al. 2000). It indicates that lower doses of orexin-A stimulate the brain monoaminergic system and the muscle tone facilitatory system (Wu et al. 1999), whereas higher doses of orexin-A inversely activate the muscle tone inhibitory system (John et al. 2000; Lai and Siegel 1988). Moreover, no effect on cataplexy or wakefulness was observed after intravenous or intracerebroventricular administration of orexin-A at a similar dose to narcolepsy animals with orexin-receptor 2 mutation (Fujiki et al. 2003).

Intranasal delivery of drugs is an optimal option for the treatment of neurodegenerative diseases due to the noninvasive administration mode. Dhuria et al. (2009) compared the intranasal and intravenous infusion of orexin-A to the central and peripheral nervous systems in rats, respectively and concluded that intranasal delivery is preferable over intravenous administration after detecting the pharmacokinetics of orexin-A. Intranasal delivery of orexin-A resulted in a ten-fold lower concentration in the blood and lower concentrations in the kidneys, liver, and muscle compared with those observed on an equivalent intravenous administration, but similar concentrations were observed in multiple brain regions (hippocampus, hypothalamus, cerebellum, medulla, olfactory bulbs, and anterior olfactory nucleus) in both intranasal and intravenous administrations. Thus, the intranasal route seems to be optimal for the delivery of orexins to the brain and might be a potential treatment strategy (Dhuria et al. 2009). The intranasal administration for orexin provides a more effective method for future in vivo research in the field of orexin peptides and their effects (Deadwyler et al. 2007).

Gene Therapy
Canines with orexin-receptor mutations (Gulyani et al. 2002; Lin et al. 1999) and mice with knockdown of orexin and orexin-receptor genes (Chemelli et al. 1999; Kalogiannis et al. 2011), or orexin-producing neurons deletion in the lateral hypothalamus (Hara et al. 2001; Kantor et al. 2013; Tabuchi et al. 2014) can be served as narcolepsy animal models.

In narcolepsy mice with orexin gene knockout, orexin gene transfer to neurons in the lateral hypothalamus using replication-defective herpes simplex virus 1 (HSV-1) reduces cataplexy and restores normal sleep–wake cycle during the 4-day lifetime of the vector (Liu et al. 2008). However, unlike those in orexin gene knockout mice, orexin neurons are missing in human narcolepsy patients as well as in another animal model, orexin-ataxin-3 mice (Hara et al. 2001). Orexin neurons project to wide areas of the brain (Peyron et al. 1998), including the dorsal pons, which involve in the maintenance of muscle tone during waking. Indeed, transfer of the orexin gene to surrogate neurons in the dorsal pons using an adeno-associated virus (AAV) vector decreased cataplexy and restored normal sleep–wake cycle 3 weeks after injection in orexin gene knockout mice (Blanco-Centurion et al. 2013). More specifically, restoration of orexin receptor expression in the serotonergic neurons in dorsal raphe nuclei decreased cataplexy and orexin receptor expression in noradrenergic neurons in the locus coeruleus consolidated sleep fragmentation in orexin receptor knockout mice (Hasegawa et al. 2014).

Cell Transplantation

It is not known in which brain regions the loss of orexin signaling contributes most significantly to narcolepsy. Some studies suggest that orexin innervation deficiency in pontine reticular formation plays a crucial role in the development of narcolepsy (Blanco-Centurion et al. 2004). Orexin neurons grafted onto the pons can survive most likely because the pons is mainly innervated by orexin neurons and secretes factors stimulating axonal growth in orexin neurons (Peyron et al. 1998). The main interest is now focused on the derivation of orexin neuroblasts for transplantation from stem cells. This concept can promote higher rates of graft survival and functional integration into host brain tissue.

Once the orexin neuron survival rate problem is resolved, the question of whether transplanted orexin neurons indeed restore sleep–wake cycle in narcolepsy animal models will remain. Arias-Carrion and Murillo-Rodriguez reported the first evidence that transplantation of orexin neurons into the lateral hypothalamus diminishes narcolepsy-like behaviors in narcolepsy rats (Arias-Carrion and Murillo-Rodriguez 2014).

Orexin Receptor Agonists

Nonpeptide orexin receptor agonists, currently under development, may be promising candidates for treating narcolepsy. Peripheral administration of YNT-185, a nonpeptide orexin-2 receptor agonist, significantly ameliorates the narcolepsy symptoms in narcolepsy model mice (Irukayama-Tomobe et al. 2017). YNT-185 also improves wakefulness in wild-type mice, suggesting that orexin receptor agonists may be useful for treating sleepiness due to other disorders (Irukayama-Tomobe et al. 2017). However, YNT-185 was limited in vivo efficacy and appears not suitable for further clinical development. A second orexin 2 receptor-selective agonist, TAK-925, when injected intravenously showed robust wake-promoting effects in wild-type mice and nonhuman primates (marmosets and cynomolgus monkeys), and increased wakefulness time and completely removed daytime sleepiness and cataplexy in orexin deficiency narcolepsy mice (Yukitake et al. 2019).

Preliminary data also showed that TAK-925 attenuated the body weight gain in orexin/ataxin-3 mice (another narcolepsy animal model) without changing the daily food intake (Yukitake et al. 2019). These results persisted after 14 days of systemic administration, favoring that, TAK-925 may treat a broad range of narcolepsy symptoms without causing orexin receptor desensitization. New promising nonpeptide orexin receptor agonists are also currently under development. In the future, the use of orexin 2 receptor agonists as efficient stimulants could also be of interest in decreasing daytime sleepiness in patients with type 2 narcolepsy and idiopathic hypersomnia, conditions with normal CSF orexin levels.

Immune-Based Therapy

Current treatment for narcolepsy is only symptomatic based on our understanding of the neuro-pathophysiology of narcolepsy. However, deficiency in orexin resulting from a possible autoimmune mechanism is the core pathophysiology of narcolepsy. So far, in animal models, orexin peptides or orexin-producing neuronal transplantation are orexin-based therapies for a new approach to treatment of narcolepsy.

Immune-based therapy, such as intravenous immunoglobulins (IVIgs), corticosteroids, and plasmapheresis, have been tested in several cases given the role of autoimmune mechanisms (Dauvilliers et al. 2004; Lecendreux et al. 2003). If applied at disease onset, immune-based therapy might modify the course of narcolepsy but delays in recognition of the disease limit this approach. Attempts to use immune-based therapy in narcolepsy patients have been reported and summarized (Barateau and Dauvilliers 2019), but they are all uncontrolled case studies, with very small numbers of involved patients. IVIgs were usually evaluated, possibly due to the good efficacy and tolerability in other autoimmune disorders. One adult patient received IVIg treatment 15 days after narcolepsy onset and completely reversed EDS and cataplexy, with normalized orexin levels in CSF (Dauvilliers et al. 2009). But the difficulty is to administer the treatment at very early narcolepsy onset and the destruction of orexin neurons may still be reversed at that period. So, there is no current evidence to guide these immunomodulatory treatments in narcolepsy. Other innovative immune-based treatments in narcolepsy were proposed: natalizumab, fingolimod, abatacept, monoclonal antibodies targeting T or B cells, tumor necrosis factor alpha blockers, anakinra, antigen-specific therapies, or cyclophosphamide (Barateau et al. 2017). But these medications may also have the risk of serious side effects. In future clinical trials, immune-based drugs should be given to highly selected narcolepsy patients: these patients should have an ongoing autoimmune response (Barateau and Dauvilliers 2019). More randomized controlled trials and animal model studies are being conducted to study the benefits of immune-based therapy in narcolepsy.

12.4 Conclusion

This is an exciting time for narcolepsy research. Over the last two decades, we have learned much about the pathogenesis of the condition and the key role that orexin plays. Animals models—both in dogs and mice—have played a major role in new discoveries. While we have not yet reached the goal of orexin replacement in humans, there have been extensive clinical trials with respect to medications to combat excessive sleepiness and cataplexy. Thus, the current treatment of narcolepsy has a much more solid scientific base. We can anticipate more progress in the future that should avoid the problem of cases of the disorder going for years unrecognized and untreated.

References

Aldrich MS. Automobile accidents in patients with sleep disorders. Sleep. 1989;12:487–94.

American Academy of Sleep Medicine. The international classification of sleep disorders. Westchester: American Academy of Sleep Medicine; 2014.

Arias-Carrion O, Murillo-Rodriguez E. Effects of hypocretin/orexin cell transplantation on narcoleptic-like sleep behavior in rats. PLoS One. 2014;9:e95342.

Barateau L, Dauvilliers Y. Recent advances in treatment for narcolepsy. Ther Adv Neurol Disord. 2019;12:1756286419875622.

Barateau L, Liblau R, Peyron C, Dauvilliers Y. Narcolepsy type 1 as an autoimmune disorder: evidence, and implications for pharmacological treatment. CNS Drugs. 2017;31:821–34.

Behar E, Lin X, Grumet FC, Mignot E. A new DRB1*1202 allele (DRB1*12022) found in association with DQA1*0102 and DQB1*0602 in two black narcoleptic subjects. Immunogenetics. 1995;41:52.

Beuckmann CT, Sinton CM, Williams SC, Richardson JA, Hammer RE, Sakurai T, Yanagisawa M. Expression of a poly-glutamine-ataxin-3 transgene in orexin neurons induces narcolepsy-cataplexy in the rat. J Neurosci. 2004;24:4469–77.

Blanco-Centurion C, Gerashchenko D, Salin-Pascual RJ, Shiromani PJ. Effects of hypocretin2-saporin and antidopamine-beta-hydroxylase-saporin neurotoxic lesions of the dorsolateral pons on sleep and muscle tone. Eur J Neurosci. 2004;19:2741–52.

Blanco-Centurion C, Liu M, Konadhode R, Pelluru D, Shiromani PJ. Effects of orexin gene transfer in the dorsolateral pons in orexin knockout mice. Sleep. 2013;36:31–40.

Blouin AM, Thannickal TC, Worley PF, Baraban JM, Reti IM, Siegel JM. Narp immunostaining of human hypocretin (orexin) neurons: loss in narcolepsy. Neurology. 2005;65:1189–92.

Boehmer LN, Wu MF, John J, Siegel JM. Treatment with immunosuppressive and anti-inflammatory agents delays onset of canine genetic narcolepsy and reduces symptom severity. Exp Neurol. 2004;188:292–9.

Bourgin P, Zeitzer JM, Mignot E. CSF hypocretin-1 assessment in sleep and neurological disorders. Lancet Neurol. 2008;7:649–62.

Broberger C, De Lecea L, Sutcliffe JG, Hokfelt T. Hypocretin/orexin- and melanin-concentrating hormone-expressing cells form distinct populations in the rodent lateral hypothalamus: relationship to the neuropeptide Y and agouti gene-related protein systems. J Comp Neurol. 1998;402:460–74.

Broughton R, Dunham W, Newman J, Lutley K, Duschesne P, Rivers M. Ambulatory 24 hour sleep-wake monitoring in narcolepsy-cataplexy compared to matched controls. Electroencephalogr Clin Neurophysiol. 1988;70:473–81.

Brown RE, Sergeeva OA, Eriksson KS, Haas HL. Convergent excitation of dorsal raphe serotonin neurons by multiple arousal systems (orexin/hypocretin, histamine and noradrenaline). J Neurosci. 2002;22:8850–9.

Carskadon MA, Dement WC, Mitler MM, Roth T, Westbrook PR, Keenan S. Guidelines for the multiple sleep latency test (MSLT): a standard measure of sleepiness. Sleep. 1986;9:519–24.

Chemelli RM, Willie JT, Sinton CM, Elmquist JK, Scammell T, Lee C, Richardson JA, Williams SC, Xiong Y, Kisanuki Y, Fitch TE, Nakazato M, Hammer RE, Saper CB, Yanagisawa M. Narcolepsy in orexin knockout mice: molecular genetics of sleep regulation. Cell. 1999;98:437–51.

Chervin RD, Kraemer HC, Guilleminault C. Correlates of sleep latency on the multiple sleep latency test in a clinical population. Electroencephalogr Clin Neurophysiol. 1995;95:147–53.

Chetrit M, Besset A, Damci D, Lelarge C, Billiard M. Hypnogogic hallucinations associated with sleep onset REM period in narcolepsy-cataplexy. J Sleep Res. 1994;3:43.

Chokroverty S. Sleep apnea in narcolepsy. Sleep. 1986;9:250–3.

Crocker A, Espana RA, Papadopoulou M, Saper CB, Faraco J, Sakurai T, Honda M, Mignot E, Scammell TE. Concomitant loss of dynorphin, NARP, and orexin in narcolepsy. Neurology. 2005;65:1184–8.

Cvetkovic-Lopes V, Bayer L, Dorsaz S, Maret S, Pradervand S, Dauvilliers Y, Lecendreux M, Lammers GJ, Donjacour CE, Du Pasquier RA, Pfister C, Petit B, Hor H, Muhlethaler M, Tafti M. Elevated Tribbles homolog 2-specific antibody levels in narcolepsy patients. J Clin Invest. 2010;120:713–9.

Dahlitz M, Parkes JD. Sleep paralysis. Lancet. 1993;341:406–7.

Date Y, Ueta Y, Yamashita H, Yamaguchi H, Matsukura S, Kangawa K, Sakurai T, Yanagisawa M, Nakazato M. Orexins, orexigenic hypothalamic peptides, interact with autonomic, neuroendocrine and neuroregulatory systems. Proc Natl Acad Sci U S A. 1999;96:748–53.

Dausset J. Correlation between histocompatibility antigens and susceptibility to illness. Prog Clin Immunol. 1972;1:183–210.

Dauvilliers Y. Differential diagnosis in hypersomnia. Curr Neurol Neurosci Rep. 2006;6:156–62.

Dauvilliers Y, Montplaisir J, Molinari N, Carlander B, Ondze B, Besset A, Billiard M. Age at onset of narcolepsy in two large populations of patients in France and Quebec. Neurology. 2001;57: 2029–33.

Dauvilliers Y, Carlander B, Rivier F, Touchon J, Tafti M. Successful management of cataplexy with intravenous immunoglobulins at narcolepsy onset. Ann Neurol. 2004;56:905–8.

Dauvilliers Y, Arnulf I, Mignot E. Narcolepsy with cataplexy. Lancet. 2007;369:499–511.

Dauvilliers Y, Abril B, Mas E, Michel F, Tafti M. Normalization of hypocretin-1 in narcolepsy after intravenous immunoglobulin treatment. Neurology. 2009;73:1333–4.

de Lecea L, Huerta R. Hypocretin (orexin) regulation of sleep-to-wake transitions. Front Pharmacol. 2014;5:16.

de Lecea L, Kilduff TS, Peyron C, Gao X, Foye PE, Danielson PE, Fukuhara C, Battenberg EL, Gautvik VT, Bartlett FS 2nd, Frankel WN, van den Pol AN, Bloom FE, Gautvik KM, Sutcliffe JG. The hypocretins: hypothalamus-specific peptides with neuroexcitatory activity. Proc Natl Acad Sci U S A. 1998;95:322–7.

Deadwyler SA, Porrino L, Siegel JM, Hampson RE. Systemic and nasal delivery of orexin-A (Hypocretin-1) reduces the effects of sleep deprivation on cognitive performance in nonhuman primates. J Neurosci. 2007;27:14239–47.

Dhuria SV, Hanson LR, Frey WH 2nd. Intranasal drug targeting of hypocretin-1 (orexin-A) to the central nervous system. J Pharm Sci. 2009;98:2501–15.

Dube MG, Kalra SP, Kalra PS. Food intake elicited by central administration of orexins/ hypocretins: identification of hypothalamic sites of action. Brain Res. 1999;842:473–7.

Ebrahim IO, Howard RS, Kopelman MD, Sharief MK, Williams AJ. The hypocretin/orexin system. J R Soc Med. 2002;95:227–30.

Edwards CM, Abusnana S, Sunter D, Murphy KG, Ghatei MA, Bloom SR. The effect of the orexins on food intake: comparison with neuropeptide Y, melanin-concentrating hormone and galanin. J Endocrinol. 1999;160:R7–12.

Eriksson KS, Sergeeva O, Brown RE, Haas HL. Orexin/hypocretin excites the histaminergic neurons of the tuberomammillary nucleus. J Neurosci. 2001;21:9273–9.

Espana RA, McCormack SL, Mochizuki T, Scammell TE. Running promotes wakefulness and increases cataplexy in orexin knockout mice. Sleep. 2007;30:1417–25.

Fernandez-Vina M, Moraes JR, Moraes ME, Miller S, Stastny P. HLA class II haplotypes in Amerindians and in black North and South Americans. Tissue Antigens. 1991;38:235–7.

Fujiki N, Morris L, Mignot E, Nishino S. Analysis of onset location, laterality and propagation of cataplexy in canine narcolepsy. Psychiatry Clin Neurosci. 2002;56:275–6.

Fujiki N, Yoshida Y, Ripley B, Mignot E, Nishino S. Effects of IV and ICV hypocretin-1 (orexin A) in hypocretin receptor-2 gene mutated narcoleptic dogs and IV hypocretin-1 replacement therapy in a hypocretin-ligand-deficient narcoleptic dog. Sleep. 2003;26:953–9.

Fukuda K, Miyasita A, Inugami M, Ishihara K. High prevalence of isolated sleep paralysis: kanashibari phenomenon in Japan. Sleep. 1987;10:279–86.

Gautvik KM, de Lecea L, Gautvik VT, Danielson PE, Tranque P, Dopazo A, Bloom FE, Sutcliffe JG. Overview of the most prevalent hypothalamus-specific mRNAs, as identified by directional tag PCR subtraction. Proc Natl Acad Sci U S A. 1996;93:8733–8.

Goode GB. Sleep paralysis. Arch Neurol. 1962;6:228–34.

Grivel J, Cvetkovic V, Bayer L, Machard D, Tobler I, Muhlethaler M, Serafin M. The wake-promoting hypocretin/orexin neurons change their response to noradrenaline after sleep deprivation. J Neurosci. 2005;25:4127–30.

Guilleminault C, Grumet C. HLA-DR2 and narcolepsy: not all narcoleptic-cataplectic patients are DR2. Hum Immunol. 1986;17:1–2.

Guilleminault C, Mignot E, Grumet FC. Familial patterns of narcolepsy. Lancet. 1989;2:1376–9.

Gulyani S, Wu MF, Nienhuis R, John J, Siegel JM. Cataplexy-related neurons in the amygdala of the narcoleptic dog. Neuroscience. 2002;112:355–65.

Hagan JJ, Leslie RA, Patel S, Evans ML, Wattam TA, Holmes S, Benham CD, Taylor SG, Routledge C, Hemmati P, Munton RP, Ashmeade TE, Shah AS, Hatcher JP, Hatcher PD, Jones DN, Smith MI, Piper DC, Hunter AJ, Porter RA, Upton N. Orexin A activates locus coeruleus cell firing and increases arousal in the rat. Proc Natl Acad Sci U S A. 1999;96:10911–6.

Hallmayer J, Faraco J, Lin L, Hesselson S, Winkelmann J, Kawashima M, Mayer G, Plazzi G, Nevsimalova S, Bourgin P, Hong SC, Honda Y, Honda M, Hogl B, Longstreth WT Jr, Montplaisir J, Kemlink D, Einen M, Chen J, Musone SL, Akana M, Miyagawa T, Duan J, Desautels A, Erhardt C, Hesla PE, Poli F, Frauscher B, Jeong JH, Lee SP, Ton TG, Kvale M, Kolesar L, Dobrovolna M, Nepom GT, Salomon D, Wichmann HE, Rouleau GA, Gieger C, Levinson DF, Gejman PV, Meitinger T, Young T, Peppard P, Tokunaga K, Kwok PY, Risch N, Mignot E. Narcolepsy is strongly associated with the T-cell receptor alpha locus. Nat Genet. 2009;41:708–11.

Han F. Respiratory regulation in narcolepsy. Sleep Breath. 2012a;16:241–5.

Han F. Sleepiness that cannot be overcome: narcolepsy and cataplexy. Respirology. 2012b;17: 1157–65.

Han F, Chen E, Wei H, He Q, Ding D, Strohl KP. Treatment effects on carbon dioxide retention in patients with obstructive sleep apnea-hypopnea syndrome. Chest. 2001;119:1814–9.

Han F, Mignot E, Wei YC, Dong SX, Li J, Lin L, An P, Wang LH, Wang JS, He MZ, Gao HY, Li M, Gao ZC, Strohl KP. Ventilatory chemoresponsiveness, narcolepsy-cataplexy and human leukocyte antigen DQB1*0602 status. Eur Respir J. 2010;36:577–83.

Han F, Lin L, Li J, Aran A, Dong SX, An P, Zhao L, Li M, Li QY, Yan H, Wang JS, Gao HY, Li M, Gao ZC, Strohl KP, Mignot E. Presentations of primary hypersomnia in Chinese children. Sleep. 2011;34:627–32.

Han F, Lin L, Li J, Aran A, Dong SX, An P, Zhao L, Li QY, Yan H, Wang JS, Gao HY, Li M, Gao ZC, Strohl KP, Mignot E. TCRA, P2RY11, and CPT1B/CHKB associations in Chinese narcolepsy. Sleep Med. 2012a;13:269–72.

Han F, Lin L, Li J, Dong SX, An P, Zhao L, Liu NY, Li QY, Yan H, Gao ZC, Faraco J, Strohl KP, Liu X, Miyadera H, Mignot E. HLA-DQ association and allele competition in Chinese narcolepsy. Tissue Antigens. 2012b;80:328–35.

Hara J, Beuckmann CT, Nambu T, Willie JT, Chemelli RM, Sinton CM, Sugiyama F, Yagami K, Goto K, Yanagisawa M, Sakurai T. Genetic ablation of orexin neurons in mice results in narcolepsy, hypophagia, and obesity. Neuron. 2001;30:345–54.

Hasegawa E, Yanagisawa M, Sakurai T, Mieda M. Orexin neurons suppress narcolepsy via 2 distinct efferent pathways. J Clin Invest. 2014;124:604–16.

Haynes AC, Jackson B, Overend P, Buckingham RE, Wilson S, Tadayyon M, Arch JR. Effects of single and chronic intracerebroventricular administration of the orexins on feeding in the rat. Peptides. 1999;20:1099–105.

Hishikawa Y, Wakamatsu H, Furuya E, Sugita Y, Masaoka S. Sleep satiation in narcoleptic patients. Electroencephalogr Clin Neurophysiol. 1976;41:1–18.

Hoang QV, Bajic D, Yanagisawa M, Nakajima S, Nakajima Y. Effects of orexin (hypocretin) on GIRK channels. J Neurophysiol. 2003;90:693–702.

Honda Y, Doi Y, Ninomiya R, Ninomiya C. Increased frequency of non-insulin-dependent diabetes mellitus among narcoleptic patients. Sleep. 1986;9:254–9.

Horvath TL, Peyron C, Diano S, Ivanov A, Aston-Jones G, Kilduff TS, van Den Pol AN. Hypocretin (orexin) activation and synaptic innervation of the locus coeruleus noradrenergic system. J Comp Neurol. 1999;415:145–59.

Hublin C, Kaprio J, Partinen M, Koskenvuo M, Heikkila K, Koskimies S, Guilleminault C. The prevalence of narcolepsy: an epidemiological study of the Finnish Twin Cohort. Ann Neurol. 1994;35:709–16.

Ida T, Nakahara K, Katayama T, Murakami N, Nakazato M. Effect of lateral cerebroventricular injection of the appetite-stimulating neuropeptide, orexin and neuropeptide Y, on the various behavioral activities of rats. Brain Res. 1999;821:526–9.

Ida T, Nakahara K, Kuroiwa T, Fukui K, Nakazato M, Murakami T, Murakami N. Both corticotropin releasing factor and neuropeptide Y are involved in the effect of orexin (hypocretin) on the food intake in rats. Neurosci Lett. 2000;293:119–22.

Irukayama-Tomobe Y, Ogawa Y, Tominaga H, Ishikawa Y, Hosokawa N, Ambai S, Kawabe Y, Uchida S, Nakajima R, Saitoh T, Kanda T, Vogt K, Sakurai T, Nagase H, Yanagisawa M. Nonpeptide orexin type-2 receptor agonist ameliorates narcolepsy-cataplexy symptoms in mouse models. Proc Natl Acad Sci U S A. 2017;114:5731–6.

John J, Wu MF, Siegel JM. Systemic administration of hypocretin-1 reduces cataplexy and normalizes sleep and waking durations in narcoleptic dogs. Sleep Res Online. 2000;3:23–8.

John J, Thannickal TC, McGregor R, Ramanathan L, Ohtsu H, Nishino S, Sakai N, Yamanaka A, Stone C, Cornford M, Siegel JM. Greatly increased numbers of histamine cells in human narcolepsy with cataplexy. Ann Neurol. 2013;74:786–93.

Johnson PL, Truitt W, Fitz SD, Minick PE, Dietrich A, Sanghani S, Traskman-Bendz L, Goddard AW, Brundin L, Shekhar A. A key role for orexin in panic anxiety. Nat Med. 2010;16:111–5.

Juji T, Satake M, Honda Y, Doi Y. HLA antigens in Japanese patients with narcolepsy. All the patients were DR2 positive. Tissue Antigens. 1984;24:316–9.

Kadotani H, Faraco J, Mignot E. Genetic studies in the sleep disorder narcolepsy. Genome Res. 1998;8:427–34.

Kaitin KI, Kilduff TS, Dement WC. Evidence for excessive sleepiness in canine narcoleptics. Electroencephalogr Clin Neurophysiol. 1986a;64:447–54.

Kaitin KI, Kilduff TS, Dement WC. Sleep fragmentation in canine narcolepsy. Sleep. 1986b;9:116–9.

Kales A, Soldatos CR, Bixler EO, Caldwell A, Cadieux RJ, Verrechio JM, Kales JD. Narcolepsy-cataplexy. II. Psychosocial consequences and associated psychopathology. Arch Neurol. 1982;39:169–71.

Kalogiannis M, Hsu E, Willie JT, Chemelli RM, Kisanuki YY, Yanagisawa M, Leonard CS. Cholinergic modulation of narcoleptic attacks in double orexin receptor knockout mice. PLoS One. 2011;6:e18697.

Kantor S, Mochizuki T, Lops SN, Ko B, Clain E, Clark E, Yamamoto M, Scammell TE. Orexin gene therapy restores the timing and maintenance of wakefulness in narcoleptic mice. Sleep. 2013;36:1129–38.

Kilduff TS, Peyron C. The hypocretin/orexin ligand-receptor system: implications for sleep and sleep disorders. Trends Neurosci. 2000;23:359–65.

Kirchgessner AL, Liu M. Orexin synthesis and response in the gut. Neuron. 1999;24:941–51.

Kiyashchenko LI, Mileykovskiy BY, Lai YY, Siegel JM. Increased and decreased muscle tone with orexin (hypocretin) microinjections in the locus coeruleus and pontine inhibitory area. J Neurophysiol. 2001;85:2008–16.

Kiyashchenko LI, Mileykovskiy BY, Maidment N, Lam HA, Wu MF, John J, Peever J, Siegel JM. Release of hypocretin (orexin) during waking and sleep states. J Neurosci. 2002;22:5282–6.

Kornum BR, Faraco J, Mignot E. Narcolepsy with hypocretin/orexin deficiency, infections and autoimmunity of the brain. Curr Opin Neurobiol. 2011a;21:897–903.

Kornum BR, Kawashima M, Faraco J, Lin L, Rico TJ, Hesselson S, Axtell RC, Kuipers H, Weiner K, Hamacher A, Kassack MU, Han F, Knudsen S, Li J, Dong X, Winkelmann J, Plazzi G, Nevsimalova S, Hong SC, Honda Y, Honda M, Hogl B, Ton TG, Montplaisir J, Bourgin P, Kemlink D, Huang YS, Warby S, Einen M, Eshragh JL, Miyagawa T, Desautels A, Ruppert E, Hesla PE, Poli F, Pizza F, Frauscher B, Jeong JH, Lee SP, Strohl KP, Longstreth WT Jr, Kvale M, Dobrovolna M, Ohayon MM, Nepom GT, Wichmann HE, Rouleau GA, Gieger C, Levinson DF, Gejman PV, Meitinger T, Peppard P, Young T, Jennum P, Steinman L, Tokunaga K, Kwok PY, Risch N, Hallmayer J, Mignot E. Common variants in P2RY11 are associated with narcolepsy. Nat Genet. 2011b;43:66–71.

Korotkova TM, Eriksson KS, Haas HL, Brown RE. Selective excitation of GABAergic neurons in the substantia nigra of the rat by orexin/hypocretin in vitro. Regul Pept. 2002;104:83–9.

Korotkova TM, Sergeeva OA, Eriksson KS, Haas HL, Brown RE. Excitation of ventral tegmental area dopaminergic and nondopaminergic neurons by orexins/hypocretins. J Neurosci. 2003;23:7–11.

Krahn LE, Pankratz VS, Oliver L, Boeve BF, Silber MH. Hypocretin (orexin) levels in cerebrospinal fluid of patients with narcolepsy: relationship to cataplexy and HLA DQB1*0602 status. Sleep. 2002;25:733–6.

Kukkonen JP, Holmqvist T, Ammoun S, Akerman KE. Functions of the orexinergic/hypocretinergic system. Am J Physiol Cell Physiol. 2002;283:C1567–91.

Kuru M, Ueta Y, Serino R, Nakazato M, Yamamoto Y, Shibuya I, Yamashita H. Centrally administered orexin/hypocretin activates HPA axis in rats. Neuroreport. 2000;11:1977–80.

Kuwaki T. Orexinergic modulation of breathing across vigilance states. Respir Physiol Neurobiol. 2008;164:204–12.

Kuwaki T. Hypothalamic modulation of breathing. Adv Exp Med Biol. 2010;669:243–7.

Kuwaki T, Li A, Nattie E. State-dependent central chemoreception: a role of orexin. Respir Physiol Neurobiol. 2010;173:223–9.

Lai YY, Siegel JM. Medullary regions mediating atonia. J Neurosci. 1988;8:4790–6.

Lammers GJ, Pijl H, Iestra J, Langius JA, Buunk G, Meinders AE. Spontaneous food choice in narcolepsy. Sleep. 1996;19:75–6.

Latorre D, Kallweit U, Armentani E, Foglierini M, Mele F, Cassotta A, Jovic S, Jarrossay D, Mathis J, Zellini F, Becher B, Lanzavecchia A, Khatami R, Manconi M, Tafti M, Bassetti CL, Sallusto F. T cells in patients with narcolepsy target self-antigens of hypocretin neurons. Nature. 2018;562:63–8.

Lecendreux M, Maret S, Bassetti C, Mouren MC, Tafti M. Clinical efficacy of high-dose intravenous immunoglobulins near the onset of narcolepsy in a 10-year-old boy. J Sleep Res. 2003;12:347–8.

Li Y, Gao XB, Sakurai T, van den Pol AN. Hypocretin/Orexin excites hypocretin neurons via a local glutamate neuron-A potential mechanism for orchestrating the hypothalamic arousal system. Neuron. 2002;36:1169–81.

Li J, Hu Z, de Lecea L. The hypocretins/orexins: integrators of multiple physiological functions. Br J Pharmacol. 2014;171:332–50.

Liblau RS, Vassalli A, Seifinejad A, Tafti M. Hypocretin (orexin) biology and the pathophysiology of narcolepsy with cataplexy. Lancet Neurol. 2015;14:318–28.

Lin L, Faraco J, Li R, Kadotani H, Rogers W, Lin X, Qiu X, de Jong PJ, Nishino S, Mignot E. The sleep disorder canine narcolepsy is caused by a mutation in the hypocretin (orexin) receptor 2 gene. Cell. 1999;98:365–76.

Liu ZW, Gao XB. Adenosine inhibits activity of hypocretin/orexin neurons by the A1 receptor in the lateral hypothalamus: a possible sleep-promoting effect. J Neurophysiol. 2007;97:837–48.

Liu M, Thankachan S, Kaur S, Begum S, Blanco-Centurion C, Sakurai T, Yanagisawa M, Neve R, Shiromani PJ. Orexin (hypocretin) gene transfer diminishes narcoleptic sleep behavior in mice. Eur J Neurosci. 2008;28:1382–93.

Longstreth WT Jr, Koepsell TD, Ton TG, Hendrickson AF, van Belle G. The epidemiology of narcolepsy. Sleep. 2007;30:13–26.

Lu XY, Bagnol D, Burke S, Akil H, Watson SJ. Differential distribution and regulation of OX1 and OX2 orexin/hypocretin receptor messenger RNA in the brain upon fasting. Horm Behav. 2000;37:335–44.

Lund PE, Shariatmadari R, Uustare A, Detheux M, Parmentier M, Kukkonen JP, Akerman KE. The orexin OX1 receptor activates a novel Ca2+ influx pathway necessary for coupling to phospholipase C. J Biol Chem. 2000;275:30806–12.

Luo G, Ambati A, Lin L, Bonvalet M, Partinen M, Ji X, Maecker HT, Mignot EJ. Autoimmunity to hypocretin and molecular mimicry to flu in type 1 narcolepsy. Proc Natl Acad Sci U S A. 2018;115:E12323–32.

Lutter M, Krishnan V, Russo SJ, Jung S, McClung CA, Nestler EJ. Orexin signaling mediates the antidepressant-like effect of calorie restriction. J Neurosci. 2008;28:3071–5.

Matsuki K, Honda Y, Juji T. Diagnostic criteria for narcolepsy and HLA-DR2 frequencies. Tissue Antigens. 1987;30:155–60.

Matsuki K, Grumet FC, Lin X, Gelb M, Guilleminault C, Dement WC, Mignot E. DQ (rather than DR) gene marks susceptibility to narcolepsy. Lancet. 1992;339:1052.

Mayer G, Hellmann F, Leonhard E, Meier-Ewert K. Circadian temperature and activity rhythms in unmedicated narcoleptic patients. Pharmacol Biochem Behav. 1997;58:395–402.

McDevitt HO, Tyan ML. Genetic control of the antibody response in inbred mice. Transfer of response by spleen cells and linkage to the major histocompatibility (H-2) locus. J Exp Med. 1968;128:1–11.

Mignot E. Genetic and familial aspects of narcolepsy. Neurology. 1998;50:S16–22.

Mignot E. Perspectives in narcolepsy and hypocretin (orexin) research. Sleep Med. 2000;1:87–90.

Mignot EJ. History of narcolepsy at Stanford University. Immunol Res. 2014;58:315–39.

Mignot E, Lin X, Hesla PE, Dement WC, Guilleminault C, Grumet FC. A novel HLA DR17, DQ1 (DQA1-0102/DQB1-0602 positive) haplotype predisposing to narcolepsy in Caucasians. Sleep. 1993;16:764–5.

Mignot E, Lin X, Arrigoni J, Macaubas C, Olive F, Hallmayer J, Underhill P, Guilleminault C, Dement WC, Grumet FC. DQB1*0602 and DQA1*0102 (DQ1) are better markers than DR2 for narcolepsy in Caucasian and black Americans. Sleep. 1994;17:S60–7.

Mignot E, Kimura A, Lattermann A, Lin X, Yasunaga S, Mueller-Eckhardt G, Rattazzi C, Lin L, Guilleminault C, Grumet FC, Mayer G, Dement WC, Underhill P. Extensive HLA class II studies in 58 non-DRB1*15 (DR2) narcoleptic patients with cataplexy. Tissue Antigens. 1997;49:329–41.

Mignot E, Lin L, Rogers W, Honda Y, Qiu X, Lin X, Okun M, Hohjoh H, Miki T, Hsu S, Leffell M, Grumet F, Fernandez-Vina M, Honda M, Risch N. Complex HLA-DR and -DQ interactions confer risk of narcolepsy-cataplexy in three ethnic groups. Am J Hum Genet. 2001;68:686–99.

Mignot E, Lammers GJ, Ripley B, Okun M, Nevsimalova S, Overeem S, Vankova J, Black J, Harsh J, Bassetti C, Schrader H, Nishino S. The role of cerebrospinal fluid hypocretin measurement in the diagnosis of narcolepsy and other hypersomnias. Arch Neurol. 2002;59:1553–62.

Mileykovskiy BY, Kiyashchenko LI, Siegel JM. Behavioral correlates of activity in identified hypocretin/orexin neurons. Neuron. 2005;46:787–98.

Mitler MM, Walsleben J, Sangal RB, Hirshkowitz M. Sleep latency on the maintenance of wakefulness test (MWT) for 530 patients with narcolepsy while free of psychoactive drugs Electroencephalogr Clin Neurophysiol. 1998;107:33–8.

Mochizuki T, Crocker A, McCormack S, Yanagisawa M, Sakurai T, Scammell TE. Behavioral state instability in orexin knock-out mice. J Neurosci. 2004;24:6291–300.

Montplaisir J, Billiard M, Takahashi S, Bell IR, Guilleminault C, Dement WC. Twenty-four-hour recording in REM-narcoleptics with special reference to nocturnal sleep disruption. Biol Psychiatry. 1978;13:73–89.

Moriguchi T, Sakurai T, Nambu T, Yanagisawa M, Goto K. Neurons containing orexin in the lateral hypothalamic area of the adult rat brain are activated by insulin-induced acute hypoglycemia. Neurosci Lett. 1999;264:101–4.

Mosko SS, Shampain DS, Sassin JF. Nocturnal REM latency and sleep disturbance in narcolepsy. Sleep. 1984;7:115–25.

Mueller-Eckhardt G, Meier-Ewert K, Schendel DJ, Reinecker FB, Multhoff G, Mueller-Eckhardt C. HLA and narcolepsy in a German population. Tissue Antigens. 1986;28:163–9.

Nakamura A, Zhang W, Yanagisawa M, Fukuda Y, Kuwaki T. Vigilance state-dependent attenuation of hypercapnic chemoreflex and exaggerated sleep apnea in orexin knockout mice. J Appl Physiol (1985). 2007;102:241–8.

Nattie E, Li A. Central chemoreception in wakefulness and sleep: evidence for a distributed network and a role for orexin. J Appl Physiol (1985). 2010;108:1417–24.

Neely SE, Rosenberg RS, Spire JP, Antel J, Arnason BGW. Familial Narcolepsy and Hla Antigens. Ann Neurol. 1986;20:168.

Nishino S. Clinical and neurobiological aspects of narcolepsy. Sleep Med. 2007a;8:373–99.

Nishino S. Narcolepsy: pathophysiology and pharmacology. J Clin Psychiatry. 2007b;68(Suppl 13):9–15.

Nishino S, Kanbayashi T. Symptomatic narcolepsy, cataplexy and hypersomnia, and their implications in the hypothalamic hypocretin/orexin system. Sleep Med Rev. 2005;9:269–310.

Nishino S, Mignot E. Pharmacological aspects of human and canine narcolepsy. Prog Neurobiol. 1997;52:27–78.

Nishino S, Mignot E, Fruhstorfer B, Dement WC, Hayaishi O. Prostaglandin E2 and its methyl ester reduce cataplexy in canine narcolepsy. Proc Natl Acad Sci U S A. 1989;86:2483–7.

Nishino S, Tafti M, Reid MS, Shelton J, Siegel JM, Dement WC, Mignot E. Muscle atonia is triggered by cholinergic stimulation of the basal forebrain: implication for the pathophysiology of canine narcolepsy. J Neurosci. 1995;15:4806–14.

Nishino S, Riehl J, Hong J, Kwan M, Reid M, Mignot E. Is narcolepsy a REM sleep disorder? Analysis of sleep abnormalities in narcoleptic Dobermans. Neurosci Res. 2000a;38:437–46.

Nishino S, Ripley B, Overeem S, Lammers GJ, Mignot E. Hypocretin (orexin) deficiency in human narcolepsy. Lancet. 2000b;355:39–40.

Nishino S, Ripley B, Overeem S, Nevsimalova S, Lammers GJ, Vankova J, Okun M, Rogers W, Brooks S, Mignot E. Low cerebrospinal fluid hypocretin (Orexin) and altered energy homeostasis in human narcolepsy. Ann Neurol. 2001;50:381–8.

Nishino S, Kanbayashi T, Fujiki N, Uchino M, Ripley B, Watanabe M, Lammers GJ, Ishiguro H, Shoji S, Nishida Y, Overeem S, Toyoshima I, Yoshida Y, Shimizu T, Taheri S, Mignot E. CSF hypocretin levels in Guillain-Barre syndrome and other inflammatory neuropathies. Neurology. 2003;61:823–5.

Ohayon MM, Priest RG, Zulley J, Smirne S, Paiva T. Prevalence of narcolepsy symptomatology and diagnosis in the European general population. Neurology. 2002;58:1826–33.

Overeem S, Dalmau J, Bataller L, Nishino S, Mignot E, Verschuuren J, Lammers GJ. Hypocretin-1 CSF levels in anti-Ma2 associated encephalitis. Neurology. 2004;62:138–40.

Pataka AD, Frangulyan RR, Mackay TW, Douglas NJ, Riha RL. Narcolepsy and sleep-disordered breathing. Eur J Neurol. 2012;19:696–702.

Peyron C, Tighe DK, van den Pol AN, de Lecea L, Heller HC, Sutcliffe JG, Kilduff TS. Neurons containing hypocretin (orexin) project to multiple neuronal systems. J Neurosci. 1998;18:9996–10015.

Peyron C, Faraco J, Rogers W, Ripley B, Overeem S, Charnay Y, Nevsimalova S, Aldrich M, Reynolds D, Albin R, Li R, Hungs M, Pedrazzoli M, Padigaru M, Kucherlapati M, Fan J, Maki R, Lammers GJ, Bouras C, Kucherlapati R, Nishino S, Mignot E. A mutation in a case of early onset narcolepsy and a generalized absence of hypocretin peptides in human narcoleptic brains. Nat Med. 2000;6:991–7.

Poryazova R, Siccoli M, Werth E, Bassetti CL. Unusually prolonged rebound cataplexy after withdrawal of fluoxetine. Neurology. 2005;65:967–8.

Richardson GS, Carskadon MA, Flagg W, Van den Hoed J, Dement WC, Mitler MM. Excessive daytime sleepiness in man: multiple sleep latency measurement in narcoleptic and control subjects. Electroencephalogr Clin Neurophysiol. 1978;45:621–7.

Ripley B, Overeem S, Fujiki N, Nevsimalova S, Uchino M, Yesavage J, Di Monte D, Dohi K, Melberg A, Lammers GJ, Nishida Y, Roelandse FW, Hungs M, Mignot E, Nishino S. CSF hypocretin/orexin levels in narcolepsy and other neurological conditions. Neurology. 2001;57: 2253–8.

Rogers AE, Rosenberg RS. Tests of memory in narcoleptics. Sleep. 1990;13:42–52.

Rogers AA, Aiani LM, Blanpain LT, Yuxian S, Moore R, Willie JT. Deep brain stimulation of hypothalamus for narcolepsy-cataplexy in mice. Brain Stimul. 2020;13:1305–16.

Sakurai T. Orexin deficiency and narcolepsy. Curr Opin Neurobiol. 2013;23:760–6.

Sakurai T, Amemiya A, Ishii M, Matsuzaki I, Chemelli RM, Tanaka H, Williams SC, Richarson JA, Kozlowski GP, Wilson S, Arch JR, Buckingham RE, Haynes AC, Carr SA, Annan RS, McNulty DE, Liu WS, Terrett JA, Elshourbagy NA, Bergsma DJ, Yanagisawa M. Orexins and orexin receptors: a family of hypothalamic neuropeptides and G protein-coupled receptors that regulate feeding behavior. Cell. 1998;92:1. page following 696

Samson WK, Resch ZT. The hypocretin/orexin story. Trends Endocrinol Metab. 2000;11:257–62.

Scammell TE, Willie JT, Guilleminault C, Siegel JM, International Working Group on Rodent Models of Narcolepsy. A consensus definition of cataplexy in mouse models of narcolepsy. Sleep. 2009;32:111–6.

Schenck CH, Mahowald MW. Motor dyscontrol in narcolepsy: rapid-eye-movement (REM) sleep without atonia and REM sleep behavior disorder. Ann Neurol. 1992;32:3–10.

Schuld A, Hebebrand J, Geller F, Pollmacher T. Increased body-mass index in patients with narcolepsy. Lancet. 2000;355:1274–5.

Scott MM, Marcus JN, Pettersen A, Birnbaum SG, Mochizuki T, Scammell TE, Nestler EJ, Elmquist JK, Lutter M. Hcrtr1 and 2 signaling differentially regulates depression-like behaviors. Behav Brain Res. 2011;222:289–94.

Sergeeva OA, Korotkova TM, Scherer A, Brown RE, Haas HL. Co-expression of non-selective cation channels of the transient receptor potential canonical family in central aminergic neurones. J Neurochem. 2003;85:1547–52.

Siegel JM, Nienhuis R, Fahringer HM, Paul R, Shiromani P, Dement WC, Mignot E, Chiu C. Neuronal activity in narcolepsy: identification of cataplexy-related cells in the medial medulla. Science. 1991;252:1315–8.

Silber MH, Krahn LE, Olson EJ, Pankratz VS. The epidemiology of narcolepsy in Olmsted County, Minnesota: a population-based study. Sleep. 2002;25:197–202.

Strohl KP, Cherniack NS, Gothe B. Physiologic basis of therapy for sleep apnea. Am Rev Respir Dis. 1986;134:791–802.

Sunanaga J, Deng BS, Zhang W, Kanmura Y, Kuwaki T. CO2 activates orexin-containing neurons in mice. Respir Physiol Neurobiol. 2009;166:184–6.

Sutcliffe JG, de Lecea L. The hypocretins: excitatory neuromodulatory peptides for multiple homeostatic systems, including sleep and feeding. J Neurosci Res. 2000;62:161–8.

Tabuchi S, Tsunematsu T, Black SW, Tominaga M, Maruyama M, Takagi K, Minokoshi Y, Sakurai T, Kilduff TS, Yamanaka A. Conditional ablation of orexin/hypocretin neurons: a new mouse model for the study of narcolepsy and orexin system function. J Neurosci. 2014;34:6495–509.

Tafti M, Lammers GJ, Dauvilliers Y, Overeem S, Mayer G, Nowak J, Pfister C, Dubois V, Eliaou JF, Eberhard HP, Liblau R, Wierzbicka A, Geisler P, Bassetti CL, Mathis J, Lecendreux M, Khatami R, Heinzer R, Haba-Rubio J, Feketeova E, Baumann CR, Kutalik Z, Tiercy JM. Narcolepsy-associated HLA class I alleles implicate cell-mediated cytotoxicity. Sleep. 2016;39:581–7.

Thannickal TC, Moore RY, Nienhuis R, Ramanathan L, Gulyani S, Aldrich M, Cornford M, Siegel JM. Reduced number of hypocretin neurons in human narcolepsy. Neuron. 2000;27:469–74.

Thorpy MJ. Recently approved and upcoming treatments for narcolepsy. CNS Drugs. 2020;34:9–27.

Trivedi P, Yu H, MacNeil DJ, Van der Ploeg LH, Guan XM. Distribution of orexin receptor mRNA in the rat brain. FEBS Lett. 1998;438:71–5.

Tsujino N, Sakurai T. Orexin/hypocretin: a neuropeptide at the interface of sleep, energy homeostasis, and reward system. Pharmacol Rev. 2009;61:162–76.

Tsujino N, Yamanaka A, Ichiki K, Muraki Y, Kilduff TS, Yagami K, Takahashi S, Goto K, Sakurai T. Cholecystokinin activates orexin/hypocretin neurons through the cholecystokinin A receptor. J Neurosci. 2005;25:7459–69.

Valko PO, Gavrilov YV, Yamamoto M, Reddy H, Haybaeck J, Mignot E, Baumann CR, Scammell TE. Increase of histaminergic tuberomammillary neurons in narcolepsy. Ann Neurol. 2013;74: 794–804.

van den Pol AN. Hypothalamic hypocretin (orexin): robust innervation of the spinal cord. J Neurosci. 1999;19:3171–82.

van den Pol AN, Gao XB, Obrietan K, Kilduff TS, Belousov AB. Presynaptic and postsynaptic actions and modulation of neuroendocrine neurons by a new hypothalamic peptide, hypocretin/orexin. J Neurosci. 1998;18:7962–71.

White DP, Douglas NJ, Pickett CK, Zwillich CW, Weil JV. Sleep deprivation and the control of ventilation. Am Rev Respir Dis. 1983;128:984–6.

Williams RH, Burdakov D. Hypothalamic orexins/hypocretins as regulators of breathing. Expert Rev Mol Med. 2008;10:e28.

Williams RH, Jensen LT, Verkhratsky A, Fugger L, Burdakov D. Control of hypothalamic orexin neurons by acid and CO2. Proc Natl Acad Sci U S A. 2007;104:10685–90.

Willie JT, Chemelli RM, Sinton CM, Tokita S, Williams SC, Kisanuki YY, Marcus JN, Lee C, Elmquist JK, Kohlmeier KA, Leonard CS, Richardson JA, Hammer RE, Yanagisawa M. Distinct narcolepsy syndromes in Orexin receptor-2 and Orexin null mice: molecular genetic dissection of Non-REM and REM sleep regulatory processes. Neuron. 2003;38:715–30.

Wing YK, Li RH, Lam CW, Ho CK, Fong SY, Leung T. The prevalence of narcolepsy among Chinese in Hong Kong. Ann Neurol. 2002;51:578–84.

Wu MF, Gulyani SA, Yau E, Mignot E, Phan B, Siegel JM. Locus coeruleus neurons: cessation of activity during cataplexy. Neuroscience. 1999;91:1389–99.

Wu M, Zhang Z, Leranth C, Xu C, van den Pol AN, Alreja M. Hypocretin increases impulse flow in the septohippocampal GABAergic pathway: implications for arousal via a mechanism of hippocampal disinhibition. J Neurosci. 2002;22:7754–65.

Xie X, Crowder TL, Yamanaka A, Morairty SR, Lewinter RD, Sakurai T, Kilduff TS. GABA (B) receptor-mediated modulation of hypocretin/orexin neurones in mouse hypothalamus. J Physiol. 2006;574:399–414.

Yamanaka A, Tsujino N, Funahashi H, Honda K, Guan JL, Wang QP, Tominaga M, Goto K, Shioda S, Sakurai T. Orexins activate histaminergic neurons via the orexin 2 receptor. Biochem Biophys Res Commun. 2002;290:1237–45.

Yamanaka A, Beuckmann CT, Willie JT, Hara J, Tsujino N, Mieda M, Tominaga M, Yagami K, Sugiyama F, Goto K, Yanagisawa M, Sakurai T. Hypothalamic orexin neurons regulate arousal according to energy balance in mice. Neuron. 2003a;38:701–13.

Yamanaka A, Muraki Y, Tsujino N, Goto K, Sakurai T. Regulation of orexin neurons by the monoaminergic and cholinergic systems. Biochem Biophys Res Commun. 2003b;303:120–9.

Yamanaka A, Muraki Y, Ichiki K, Tsujino N, Kilduff TS, Goto K, Sakurai T. Orexin neurons are directly and indirectly regulated by catecholamines in a complex manner. J Neurophysiol. 2006;96:284–98.

Yang B, Ferguson AV. Orexin-A depolarizes nucleus tractus solitarius neurons through effects on nonselective cationic and K+ conductances. J Neurophysiol. 2003;89:2167–75.

Yukitake H, Fujimoto T, Ishikawa T, Suzuki A, Shimizu Y, Rikimaru K, Ito M, Suzuki M, Kimura H. TAK-925, an orexin 2 receptor-selective agonist, shows robust wake-promoting effects in mice. Pharmacol Biochem Behav. 2019;187:172794.

Zeitzer JM, Nishino S, Mignot E. The neurobiology of hypocretins (orexins), narcolepsy and related therapeutic interventions. Trends Pharmacol Sci. 2006;27:368–74.

Zhu Y, Miwa Y, Yamanaka A, Yada T, Shibahara M, Abe Y, Sakurai T, Goto K. Orexin receptor type-1 couples exclusively to pertussis toxin-insensitive G-proteins, while orexin receptor type-2 couples to both pertussis toxin-sensitive and -insensitive G-proteins. J Pharmacol Sci. 2003;92:259–66.

Part V
Circadian Rhythm Disorders

Chapter 13 Circadian Rhythm Sleep–Wake Disorders: Mechanisms and Treatment

Sabra M. Abbott and Phyllis C. Zee

Abstract Nearly all biological processes exhibit circadian rhythms that are generated by circadian clocks in central and peripheral tissues. In mammals a central circadian clock, the suprachiasmatic nucleus helps to align behaviors and physiological processes, including the sleep–wake cycle with the 24-h environment. Disruption of the proper alignment of circadian clocks with the required sleep–wake time leads to development of circadian rhythm sleep–wake disorders. These disorders can develop as a result of pathology at the level of the internal clock, disruption of the ability to receive or process environmental synchronizing signals, or changes to the external environmental time. Treatment of circadian rhythm sleep–wake disorders depends on behavioral adjustments, often in conjunction with specific timing of light and/or melatonin. This chapter will highlight the six primary circadian rhythm sleep–wake disorders, focusing on what is known about their underlying pathogenic mechanisms and the currently recommended treatment strategies.

Keywords Circadian · Suprachiasmatic nucleus · Melatonin · Light · Actigraphy

13.1 Introduction

Circadian rhythms are the near 24-oscillations observed in nearly all physiological processes and behaviors. They serve to align, or entrain, these behaviors with the external environment. While the most apparent of these rhythms is the daily pattern of the sleep–wake cycle, these rhythms can also be observed in everything from feeding behaviors to daily patterns of body temperature and hormone release. In mammals, these rhythms are regulated by the suprachiasmatic nucleus (SCN), a set of paired nuclei, located in the hypothalamus, directly above the optic chiasm (Stephan and Zucker 1972). The SCN sends direct projections to the paraventricular

S. M. Abbott (✉) · P. C. Zee
Center for Circadian and Sleep Medicine, Northwestern University Feinberg School of Medicine, Chicago, IL, USA
e-mail: sabra.abbott@northwestern.edu; p-zee@northwestern.edu

A. I. Pack, Q. Y. Li (eds.), *Sleep and its Disorders*, Translational Medicine Research,
https://doi.org/10.1007/978-94-024-2168-2_13

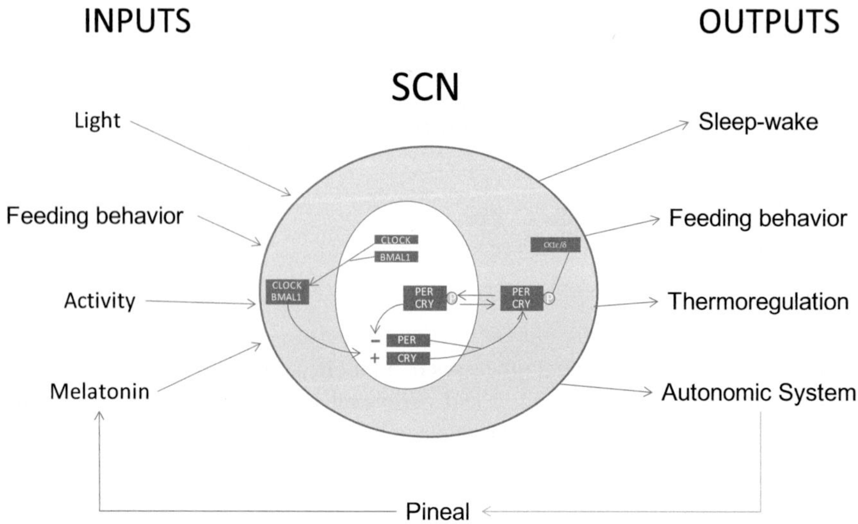

Fig. 13.1 Illustration of the circadian system. Cells within the suprachiasmatic nucleus (SCN) contain a set of core clock genes. The transcription–translation feedback loop completed by these genes maintains the 24-h clock. Peripheral inputs to the SCN can reset or adjust circadian timing, while the SCN in turn provides outputs that regulate the timing of many of these behaviors

nucleus (PVN) of the hypothalamus along with indirect projections to the dorsomedial, ventromedial and lateral hypothalamus, and the superior cervical ganglion (Dai et al. 1998), whereby it influences feeding behavior, metabolism, sleep–wake behaviors and autonomic function (Fig. 13.1).

The SCN is able to maintain a near 24 rhythmicity through a set of core clock genes, which undergo a transcription–translation feedback loop that takes ~24 h to complete. In a simplified version, the mammalian circadian clock, the proteins CLOCK and BMAL1 dimerize, and induce the expression of three Period genes (*hPer1*, *2*, and *3*) and two Cryptochrome genes (*hCry 1* and *2*). PER and CRY dimerize, and are translocated back into the nucleus, where they inhibit their own transcription. The rate of translocation is regulated by the phosphorylation of this dimer by casein kinase Iδ, Iε, and glycogen synthase kinase (GSK). This entire cycle takes ~24 h to complete, and alterations to these clock genes can result in lengthening or shortening of the endogenous period to more or less than 24 h (Lamont et al. 2007). Not only does the SCN contain these core clock genes, they are also found in multiple organ systems throughout the body (Nagoshi et al. 2004), and coordination of these peripheral clocks is important for overall health.

Along with being able to maintain a 24-h rhythm, the SCN is also capable of resetting in response to environmental inputs, in a dose and time-of-day dependent manner. By far the strongest of these resetting signals is light. Light reaches the SCN primarily through melanopsin-containing retinal ganglion cells, which project through the retinohypothalamic tract to the SCN. The pigment melanopsin is maximally sensitive to blue light. However, the traditional rod and cone

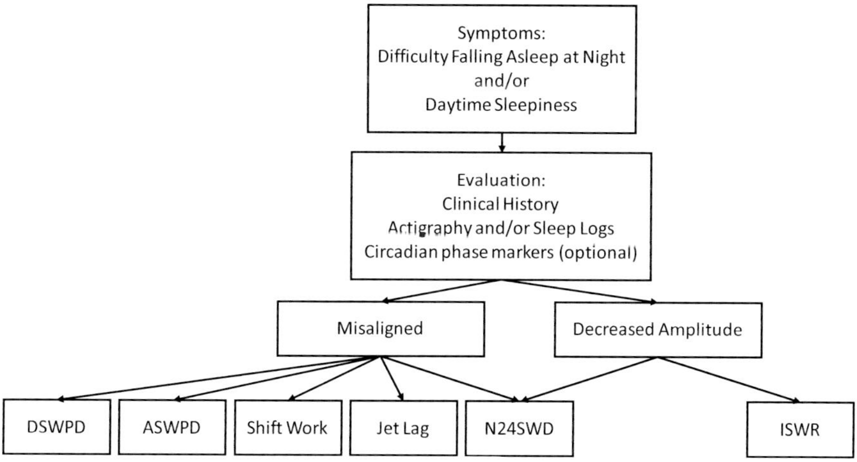

Fig. 13.2 Algorithm for the evaluation of a patient with a circadian rhythm sleep–wake disorder. Treatment strategies are based on targeting the primary underlying problem, either using phase shifting strategies to adjust misalignment, or using strong time cues to improve amplitude

photoreceptors also appear to play a role in irradiance detection (Gooley et al. 2001; van Diepen et al. 2013). Light in the evening, prior to the core body temperature nadir causes delays in the circadian rhythm, while light in the morning, after the core body temperature nadir causes circadian advances (St Hilaire et al. 2012).

Melatonin is one of the other key resetting signals for the mammalian circadian clock. Melatonin is secreted by the pineal gland, and levels normally increase shortly before sleep onset, peaking in the middle of the night, and dropping off the following morning (Lewy and Sack 1989). Opposite to the effects seen with light, melatonin in the evening can cause circadian advances, while melatonin in the morning causes circadian delays (Burgess et al. 2010). The circadian resetting properties of light and melatonin play a key role in the treatment of circadian rhythms sleep–wake disorders.

The circadian rhythm sleep–wake disorders result when there is a mismatch between the internal circadian time and the external environment. Symptoms should be present for at least 3 months. Figure 13.2 outlines a schematic for evaluating a patient suspected to have a circadian rhythm sleep–wake disorder. Delayed sleep–wake phase disorder, advanced sleep–wake phase disorder irregular sleep–wake rhythm disorder and non-24-h sleep–wake rhythm disorder are thought to be primarily due to abnormalities at the level of biological clock, though behavioral factors can often contribute to the development of these disorders. Conversely, shift work disorder and jet lag disorder develop when an individual is behaviorally active during the time period they would normally be sleeping, either because of work requirements or as a result of crossing multiple time zones. However, there are likely biological factors contributing to these disorders as well, as some individuals exposed to these environmental conditions appear to be able to adapt to these symptoms, and do not develop a chronic circadian disorder (ICSD-3 2014). In the

Table 13.1 Summary of the strength of evidence for current treatment strategies for circadian rhythm sleep–wake disorders (Auger et al. 2015)

Diagnosis	Treatment	Evidence
DSWPD	Timed evening melatonin	Weak for
	Post-awakening light	Weak for
ASWPD	Evening light	Weak for
ISWRD	Light therapy	Weak for
	Melatonin in elderly with dementia	Weak against
	Hypnotics for elderly patients	Strong against
N24SWD	Timed melatonin (in blind adults)	Weak for

following sections, we will detail what is currently known about the underlying pathophysiology and treatment options for each of these disorders (Table 13.1).

13.2 Delayed Sleep–Wake Phase Disorder

Patients with delayed sleep–wake phase disorder (DSWPD) have chronic or recurrent habitual sleep times that are significantly later than average, often not going to bed until at least 2 am, or sometimes much later, and are unable to wake until late morning/early afternoon. These individuals are often diagnosed with insomnia due to their difficulty falling asleep, however, if allowed to sleep during their preferred times, sleep duration and quality are normal for their age (ICSD-3 2014). The prevalence of DSWPD varies depending on the population being studied, but can be as high as 7–16% in adolescents and decreases with age (ICSD-3 2014; Paine et al. 2014). In addition, it has been estimated that ~10% of patients presenting to a sleep clinic with a chief complaint of insomnia actually have DSWPD (Flynn-Evans et al. 2017).

The diagnosis of DSWPD is confirmed through the use of sleep logs, preferably with the addition of actigraphy, collected for at least 7 days, but ideally 14 days to confirm a delayed sleep–wake pattern (Fig. 13.3). Standard chronotype questionnaires such as the Munich which measures the actual timing of daily sleep–wake patterns, or the Horne-Ostberg which measures sleep–wake preferences (Zavada et al. 2005) can be used to confirm a later sleep midpoint and evening chronotype, though these are not required for diagnosis. In addition, the pattern of secretion of melatonin can also be measured in the saliva to confirm a delay in the daily onset of melatonin secretion (ICSD-3 2014). Overnight sleep studies are generally not indicated unless there is a concern for another underlying sleep disorder such as obstructive sleep apnea.

The underlying pathophysiology of DSWPD is still not fully understood; however, there are several current theories regarding the underlying mechanism, with varying degrees of supportive evidence: (1) Individuals with DSWPD are either more sensitive to the delaying effects of evening light or less sensitive to the

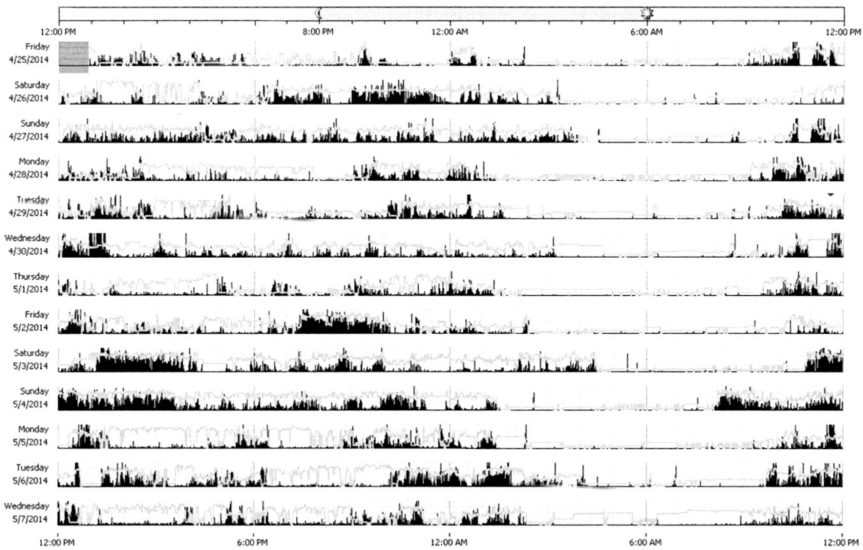

Fig. 13.3 Example actigraphy from a subject with delayed sleep–wake phase disorder. Black bars indicate activity, while the yellow line represents light levels. Each line is 24 h. Sleep onset is typically around 2–3 am, while sleep offset is generally around 10 am

advancing effects of morning light; (2) Due to behavioral changes, individuals with DSWPD are exposed to more light in the evening during times of maximal phase delay, and are exposed to less light in the morning during times of maximal phase advance; or (3) Individuals with DSWPD have a longer intrinsic period, making it more difficult to fully entrain to a 24-h schedule. A very small study of individuals with DSWPD did demonstrate that these individuals exhibit a greater degree of melatonin suppression in response to light, suggesting greater sensitivity to evening light (Aoki et al. 2001). However, similar studies have not been performed evaluating the sensitivity of these individuals to light during the phase advance time. The support for behavioral factors contributing to DSWPD is mixed. Studies in adolescents have demonstrated a greater exposure to evening light, and decreased exposure to morning light in evening type individuals with respect to clock time. However, when corrected for circadian time, there were no significant differences observed suggesting that they are not receiving excess light at circadian times that would promote a delay (Auger et al. 2011). Finally, to evaluate the potential for increased period length as a contributing factor, polymorphisms of core clock genes have been analyzed in individuals with DSWPD. It has been demonstrated that polymorphisms in the gene *hPer3* near the phosphorylation site for CK1ε are associated with DSWPD (Ebisawa et al. 2001). Alterations in phosphorylation presumably affect the degradation rate of hPER3, in turn impacting the overall period.

Treatment of DSWPD focuses on very specific timing of both light exposure and avoidance, along with timed melatonin. In addition, close attention to general principles of sleep hygiene and maintaining a regular sleep–wake schedule are important.

As mentioned previously, phase response curves conducted in healthy controls have demonstrated that light administered prior to the core body temperature minimum induces circadian phase delays, while light administered after the core body temperature nadir induces circadian advances. Based on those principles, it is very important for individuals with DSWPD to both avoid light during their biological evening, and increase light exposure during the biological morning. At least one study has demonstrated that the use of blue light-blocking glasses during the 3 h prior to bedtime results in an increase in total sleep time (Burkhart and Phelps 2009). Combining evening light restriction with 2 h of morning bright light therapy has been demonstrated to successfully advance both the sleep–wake patterns and core body temperature in individuals with DSWPD (Rosenthal et al. 1990; Gradisar et al. 2011). It is always important to time these light interventions based on biological time, rather than clock time, as the biological morning for many individuals with DSWPD often does not occur until early afternoon when based on clock time.

Melatonin has also been successfully used to induce circadian phase advances. Earlier studies demonstrated that administering 5 mg of melatonin 5 h prior to the DLMO resulted in an average phase advance of 1.5 h (Nagtegaal et al. 1998). Later studies compared either 0.3 mg or 3 mg, given anywhere from 1.5 to 6.5 h prior to DLMO. Either dose produced phase advances, in DLMO and sleep offset with greater effects observed the earlier the melatonin was given (Mundey et al. 2005).

Patients may receive additional benefits from the use of a combination of timed light and melatonin along with behavioral interventions. In a placebo controlled trial, subjects took either placebo or melatonin (3 mg) 12 h after awakening, were exposed to either bright or dim light for 30–45 min on awakening, and were instructed to advance their wake time by 1 h each day. Following this protocol, all subjects showed an advance in sleep timing, accompanied by improvement in daytime sleepiness and cognitive function (Saxvig et al. 2014; Wilhelmsen-Langeland et al. 2013). Similar results were found with subjects given 0.5 mg of melatonin 5 h prior to habitual bedtime, accompanied by morning light ranging from 30 min to 2 h. All subjects showed advances in the timing of DLMO, with the largest advances seen following the 2-h light pulse (Crowley and Eastman 2015).

13.3 Advanced Sleep–Wake Phase Disorder

In advanced sleep–wake phase disorder (ASWPD) patients fall asleep and wake up much earlier than desired, with typical bedtimes around 6–9 pm and wake times around 2–5 am. Sleep complaints include difficulty staying awake for evening activities, along with early morning awakenings. If they are able to make themselves stay up later, they develop daytime sleepiness because they are still unable to sleep later. Similar to DSWPD, patients with ASWPD have a normal duration and quality of sleep when allowed to sleep during their preferred times (ICSD-3 2014). The prevalence of ASWPD appears to be lower than that of DSWPD ranging from 1 to 7%, but again depends on age, with the highest prevalence among older males (Paine et al. 2014).

The diagnosis of ASWPD relies on the collection of sleep logs with or without actigraphy to confirm a stable advance in the sleep–wake patterns. Optional chronotype questionnaires will demonstrate a morning chronotype and earlier sleep midpoint. Circadian phase markers such as salivary dim-light melatonin onset can be measured, and will demonstrate a significantly earlier melatonin onset when compared to intermediate individuals. A sleep study is not necessary to confirm the diagnosis unless there is also concern for another underlying sleep disorder (ICSD-3 2014).

There have been several familial cohorts identified with ASWPD (Reid et al. 2001). While a number of different mutations have been identified, the common factor appears to be a mutation either of CKIε or the phosphorylation site for this kinase on the protein hPER2 (Jones et al. 1999; Toh et al. 2001; Xu et al. 2005). The net result of these mutations is that the lack of phosphorylation results in faster translocation of the hPER2/CRY protein dimer back into the nucleus, leading to faster cycling through the transcription/translation feedback loop, resulting in an overall shortened circadian period.

In non-familial cases of ASWPD, theories for potential etiologies are similar to those for DSWPD, ranging from decreased exposure or sensitivity to the delaying effects of light, increased exposure or sensitivity to the advancing effects of light or a shortened circadian period. However, none of these possibilities have been definitively studied in nonfamilial ASWPD to date.

The treatment of ASWPD is primarily dependent on timed light administration. In a pilot study of 9 individuals, 4 h of evening bright light between 2000 and 2400 resulted in a 1–2 h delay in DLMO, a 2–4 h delay in the core body temperature minimum, and an increase in total sleep time of >1 h (Lack and Wright 1993). In another study, 16 patients with ASWPD received a white light pulse (4000 lux) for 2 h at some time between 2000 and 2300, resulting in a delay in core body temperature by ~2 h and an increase in total sleep time by ~1 h (Campbell et al. 1993). A larger cohort of individuals received a 2-h light pulse between 1900 and 2100 and also demonstrated a 2-h phase delay in both DLMO and temperature (Lack et al. 2005). While melatonin theoretically could be used to induce additional phase delays, there are currently no clinical trials investigating the efficacy nor effectiveness of this treatment, and there is some concern that the soporific effects of melatonin may negatively impact daily function, so this is not currently regularly used in clinical practice (Zee 2008).

13.4 Irregular Sleep–Wake Rhythm Disorder

In irregular sleep–wake rhythm disorder (ISWRD) individuals lack a clear 24-h pattern for their sleep–wake schedule. Sleep will occur in at least three distinct bouts throughout the 24-h period, however, the total sleep time is normal for age. The diagnosis of ISWRD is made through a collection of sleep logs and/or actigraphy for at least seven but preferably 14 days (Fig. 13.4). Typically, these individuals will have a longer (<4 h) sleep bout at night, along with several naps throughout the day (ICSD-3 2014).

ISWRD is thought to result from either a dysfunctional SCN that is no longer able to maintain a 24-h rhythm, impaired input to the SCN resulting in an inability to receive normal time cues, or living in an environment that lacks a clear day/night pattern. As a result, ISWRD is generally seen in two main populations, children with neurodevelopmental delays, and adults with neurodegenerative diseases (Zee and Vitiello 2009).

Several pediatric neurodegenerative and developmental disorders have been associated with ISWRD. Children who are congenitally blind with neurodevelopmental delay have been noted to have either a non-24-h sleep–wake pattern (detailed in the next section) or an irregular rest–activity pattern (Okawa et al. 1987) presumably related both to abnormal light input and impairments at the level of the SCN. In children with neuronal ceroid lipofuscinosis (NCL) a neurodegenerative disorder associated with retinal degeneration and optic atrophy, ISWRD is

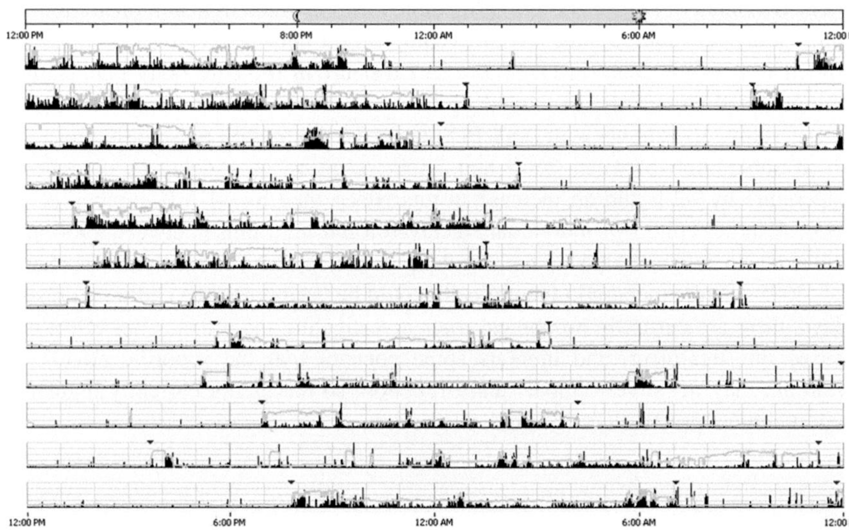

Fig. 13.4 Example actigraphy from a subject with non-24-h sleep–wake rhythm disorder. Black bars indicate activity, while the yellow line represents light levels. Each line is 24 h. The duration of the sleep window remains relatively similar from day to day, however, the onset shifts later by 1–2 h each day. Note the overall amplitude of activity and light

frequently observed. However, interestingly the rest–activity patterns are disrupted early in the illness, while changes in the melatonin and core body temperature rhythms are not observed until much later in the disease course (Heikkila et al. 1995). Angelman syndrome is another neurodevelopmental disorder frequently associated with ISWRD, along with decreases in nocturnal melatonin secretion patterns (Takaesu et al. 2012). In Smith Magenis syndrome, patients have craniofacial abnormalities, and frequently exhibit ISWRD or a complete inversion of the sleep–wake cycle, thought to be related to abnormal patterns of melatonin secretion (Potocki et al. 2000). Finally, ISWRD is frequently observed in children with autism spectrum disorder, thought to be due in part to increased sleep fragmentation as a result of increased sensitivity to external noise (Cortesi et al. 2010).

Multiple studies of elderly individuals with dementia have demonstrated ISWRD either through caretaker assessment of sleep–wake patterns (Okawa et al. 1991) or actigraphy (Witting et al. 1990). The degree of rhythm disruption seems to correlate with the severity of dementia (Witting et al. 1990) and a decreased rest–activity amplitude in healthy controls is actually predictive of development of mild cognitive impairment or dementia over the following 5 years (Tranah et al. 2011). Pathologically, the change in amplitude of rest–activity is also associated with a decrease in the number of cells in the SCN, suggesting impairment at the level of the primary pacemaker (Wang et al. 2015). Autopsy studies have also demonstrated a lack of synchronization of clock gene expression throughout the brain in patients with Alzheimer's disease, suggesting overall circadian desynchrony (Cermakian et al. 2011).

In other populations, ISWRD has also been noted in patients with schizophrenia, more frequently in those with positive symptoms (Afonso et al. 2011), and has been associated with decreased cognitive performance (Bromundt et al. 2011). Finally, direct pathology at the level of the SCN can also be associated with the development of ISWRD. There are case reports of individuals developing ISWRD following traumatic brain injury (Ayalon et al. 2007), gunshot injury to the SCN and optic nerves (DelRosso et al. 2014), or the development of a brain tumor impacting the hypothalamus (Borodkin et al. 2005).

The treatment of ISWRD is aimed to consolidate sleep during the night and promote wakefulness during the day. Thus, multimodal modalities including light, melatonin, and behavioral interventions are recommended. Bright light therapy has primarily been studied in adults with dementia, and has been shown to be beneficial for sleep regardless of the time-of-day administered. Continuous daytime bright light exposure (1000 lux) is associated with increased total sleep time and improved mood (Riemersma-van der Lek et al. 2008). Morning bright light (>2500 lux) increases total sleep time by 20–30 min (Ancoli-Israel et al. 2003), and evening bright light is associated with greater consolidation of the rest–activity rhythm (Ancoli-Israel et al. 2003). In a smaller study of children with neurodevelopmental delay, morning bright light (4500 lux) was associated with normalization of sleep-wake patterns in >50% of children (Guilleminault et al. 1993).

Melatonin has been useful in treating children with ISWRD, however, results are less clear for elderly patients with dementia. In children with severe psychomotor retardation and a decreased amplitude of melatonin secretion, 3 mg of melatonin in the evening resulted in a significant increase in nocturnal sleep and a significant decrease in daytime sleep (Pillar et al. 2000). Similarly, treatment with 1 mg of melatonin in children with Angelman syndrome resulted in more sleep at night and less sleep during the day (Takaesu et al. 2012). In a larger open-label trial, melatonin doses ranging from 2 to 20 mg were shown to normalize sleep–wake patterns in children with developmental delay (Jan et al. 1994). In patients with schizophrenia administering 2 mg of melatonin at bedtime results in improved sleep (Shamir et al. 2000). However, in patients with dementia melatonin alone did not significantly improve actigraphically measured sleep (Serfaty et al. 2002; Singer et al. 2003), and in some cases melatonin alone has been associated with an increased risk for depression in the elderly so it is not recommended as a monotherapy in this age group (Auger et al. 2015).

In elderly patients with ISWRD, a fair amount of success has been found through treatment with mixed modality therapy. This consists of a combination of efforts to keep patients out of bed and alert during the day, using low-level physical activity and at least 30 min of bright (>10,000 lux) light exposure, along with a structured bedtime routine and efforts to minimize light and noise at night. This strategy has been demonstrated to both significantly decrease daytime sleep and improve nighttime sleep (Alessi et al. 2005; McCurry et al. 2005).

13.5 Non-24-Hour Sleep–Wake Rhythm Disorder

In Non-24-hour sleep–wake rhythm disorder (N24SWD), individuals do have a daily pattern to their rest/activity cycle; however, it no longer follows a 24-h pattern, and is instead typically slightly longer than 24 h. As a result, each day individuals go to bed and wake up slightly later with respect to the 24-h clock. Symptoms can range from complaints of insomnia to excessive daytime sleepiness, depending on where their biological clock currently falls with respect to the environment (ICSD-3 2014).

The diagnosis of N24SWD depends on the use of sleep logs and/or actigraphy for at least 14 days, though it is often necessary to observe for longer in order to determine the underlying behavioral pattern. Circadian phase markers such as salivary melatonin can also be obtained. However, in this case, measurements will need to be obtained on two separate occasions to demonstrate the presence of a non-entrained rhythm over time (ICSD-3 2014).

N24SWD is observed in two main populations; blind and sighted individuals, presumably with different underlying pathophysiology. Blind individuals who lack the circadian photic input to the SCN from melanopsin-containing retinal ganglion cells are no longer able to receive environmental light signals to help them entrain to the 24-h environment. However, not all blind individuals develop N24SWD. A recent study of 127 blind individuals demonstrated that 63% of those with no light perception were not entrained, while only 21% of those with light perception were not entrained (Flynn-Evans et al. 2014). It is possible that those individuals without light perception who are unaffected have an internal clock that is closer to 24 h, so it is easier for them to maintain entrainment through non-photic cues, such as social interactions and activity. Sighted individuals with N24SWD are thought to result from a combination of factors. These individuals often initially present as cases of severe DSWPD, and they eventually are unable to maintain entrainment (Hayakawa et al. 2005). There is also evidence that sighted individuals with N24SWD have an internal period that is significantly longer than 24 h, making it more difficult to maintain entrainment through traditional signals (Kitamura et al. 2013). In addition, other potential possibilities include limited exposure to strong entraining signals, or an inability to respond normally to the entraining signals of light.

The treatment of N24SWD is dependent on the underlying etiology. In blind individuals treatment with daily melatonin at a fixed time has been effective. Previous studies have evaluated doses ranging from 10 mg (Sack et al. 2000) to 0.5 mg (Lewy et al. 2001) given 1 h before the desired bedtime. Currently lower doses are preferred. More recently tasimelteon, a melatonin agonist was developed as the first FDA approved medication for the treatment of N24SWD (The Medical Letter 2014). In sighted individuals treatment is more complicated, and there is less data available on effective treatment regimens. Currently, suggestions include a combination of enforcing available entraining signals, including regular timed light exposure, strong social cues and regular sleep–wake cycles. Melatonin may be effective; however, it is not as well studied in sighted N24SWD when compared to blind individuals (Auger et al. 2015).

13.6 Shift Work Disorder

Shift work sleep disorder results when individuals develop sleep complaints as a result of being required to follow a recurrent work schedule that occurs during the time they would normally be sleeping. Symptoms can include both excessive sleepiness while at work, and insomnia when allowed time to sleep. The diagnosis is confirmed with sleep logs and/or actigraphy for at least 14 days, demonstrating a disrupted sleep–wake pattern as a result of this work schedule (ICSD-3 2014).

Of note, not all individuals who are shift workers develop shift work disorder, with some estimates suggesting that only 5–10% of shift workers have shift work sleep disorder (Drake et al. 2004). Factors that may contribute to the development of shift work disorder include age, gender, shift schedule, and circadian preference or chronotype (Harma et al. 1994). Those who are more likely to develop shift work disorder include those with a morning chronotype, older individuals, and individuals with more daytime responsibilities, which may limit their ability to sleep during their time off (Colligan and Rosa 1990). In addition, more recent studies have demonstrated that polymorphisms in the *hPer3* gene have been associated with a greater tendency to develop symptoms of shift work disorder (Gumenyuk et al. 2015; Drake et al. 2015).

In addition to sleep–wake complaints, shift work has been associated with multiple other adverse health outcomes. There appears to be a higher incidence of diabetes (Pan et al. 2011), obesity (Antunes et al. 2010), cardiovascular disease, and stroke (Brown et al. 2009) among shift workers even when controlling for other lifestyle factors. In addition, there is increasing evidence that shift work is associated with an increased risk for cancer, leading to the establishment of shift work as a probable carcinogen (Schernhammer et al. 2001). While there is some evidence that these risks may result from a suppression of the normal nocturnal release of melatonin, underlying circadian misalignment may also be playing a role.

The treatment of shift work disorder can be divided into two main aspects of treatment; improving sleep quality and improving alertness during work hours. To improve sleep quality, it is important to focus on general principles of good sleep hygiene, including maintaining a quiet, cool, and dark environment for sleep. The addition of melatonin can help to both promote sleep, and aid with resetting the circadian clock to the desired sleep time. Melatonin 0.5–3 mg taken 30 min before the desired bedtime has been demonstrated to increase the length of daytime sleep (Sharkey and Eastman 2002). Hypnotics can also be used, with studies demonstrating that zolpidem can increase sleep quality while not significantly impairing next-day performance (Hart et al. 2003).

Multiple strategies can be used to improve daytime alertness. Bright light exposure can help both to improve alertness and help to reset the circadian clock to the new schedule. General recommendations are to obtain 3000–5000 lux of light during the first half of the work schedule (Boivin and James 2002). The re-entraining effects can be further enforced by avoiding bright light by wearing dark glasses for the morning commute home, however, there are some concerns that the loss of the alerting effects of light may increase the risk for fatigue related accidents. Strategic use of napping (as short as 10 min) and caffeine prior to the beginning of the work shift can also be beneficial for improving alertness at work (Schweitzer et al. 2006). Finally, if all of the above are unsuccessful, the stimulants modafinil and armodafinil have been approved for use in the treatment of hypersomnia associated with shift work (Czeisler et al. 2005, 2009). However, of note, while these medications can improve sleepiness at work, a recent study showed that individuals taking these medications still had significant subjective sleepiness in the morning, around the time of the commute home (Drake et al. 2014).

Successful treatment of shift work disorder generally depends on being able to successfully re-entrain the biological clock to the desired schedule. While this can be achieved when living under controlled environments, individuals often have daytime responsibilities on days off that impair their ability to maintain this entrainment continuously. To account for this a shift work simulation study successfully employed a compromise phase strategy, whereby individuals sleep from 8 am to 4 pm on work days, and sleep from 3 am to noon on non-workdays, allowing for daytime activities, without completely losing entrainment to the night shift schedule on days off (Smith et al. 2009).

13.7 Jet Lag Disorder

Jet lag disorder consists of sleep complaints that result from crossing at least two time zones. In addition to complaints of insomnia and/or excessive sleepiness, patients often also develop somatic symptoms such as gastrointestinal distress. Diagnosis is made based on clinical history of experiencing the above symptoms in temporal correlation with jet travel. The potential for and severity of symptoms depends on both the direction of travel and the number of time zones crossed, with eastward travel generally producing more symptoms (ICSD-3 2014).

Treatment of jet lag disorder depends on multiple factors, including the direction of travel, number of time zones crossed, and duration of time spent at the destination. In general, if trips are short (<48 h) it is often easier to try to maintain the home schedule, rather than trying to adapt to the new schedule. For longer trips, targeted use of light and melatonin to reset the clock can be beneficial. In all cases attention to good sleep hygiene is important, making sure that the sleeping environment is cool, dark, and quiet. In addition, adapting behaviors to the new environmental time as soon as possible can be beneficial, including sleeping, and eating meals at the local time. Avoiding excessive alcohol and caffeine can also help to limit the symptoms of jet lag.

When traveling east the goal is to advance, or move the clock earlier. As the human circadian clock naturally is slightly longer than 24 h, most individuals find this transition to be much more challenging than the delays required for traveling west. The required circadian phase shifts are generally accomplished through a combination of timed melatonin, light exposure, and light avoidance. Depending on the commitments prior to travel, attempts can be made to begin to adjust the clock prior to leaving, or can start once arriving at the new destination. If trying to adjust prior to departure, starting 3 days before leaving, patients should take melatonin (1–3 mg) prior to their habitual sleep time, get at least an hour of bright light (5000 lux) in the morning, and move everything 1 h earlier each day (Burgess et al. 2003). At the new time zone, to maximize the ability to re-entrain to the new time zone, general recommendations are to avoid bright light in the morning and maximize bright light exposure in the afternoon (Boulos et al. 1995). In addition, melatonin (2–5 mg) can be taken before bed, both to help advance the clock, and as a mild hypnotic (Suhner et al. 2001). Hypnotics such as zolpidem (10 mg) have also been beneficial for improving sleep in the new location, though were associated with more side effects when compared to melatonin (Suhner et al. 2001).

The goal when traveling west is to delay or move the clock later. As was mentioned previously, it is generally easier for humans to delay than it is to advance. Prior to traveling to the new destination, just one night of bright light exposure prior to bedtime (2 h, ~4000 lux) can effectively delay the clock by ~1.5 h (Canton et al. 2009). After arriving at the new destination, patients should avoid bright light in the morning, and seek bright light in the afternoon/evening to further delay the clock (Boulos et al. 1995). Melatonin (5 mg) right before bedtime may provide additional benefit (Petrie et al. 1993).

13.8 Conclusions

The circadian rhythm sleep–wake disorders encompass a broad range of sleep–wake disruptions. However, the common theme is that individuals develop sleep–wake complaints in relation to their desired or required sleep–wake schedule being out of phase with their biological sleep–wake schedule. Treatment generally focuses on the use of specifically timed light and melatonin to realign the biological time with the desired/required sleep–wake time. In addition to causing significant sleep–wake complaints, the circadian rhythm sleep–wake disorders can be associated with multiple other medical comorbidities, including psychiatric and cardiometabolic disorders, emphasizing the importance of recognizing and treating these disorders. One of the major barriers to diagnosis and treatment of circadian disorders has been the lack of clinically practical biomarkers. Future research to develop circadian sleep biomarkers will allow us to better identify the mechanisms of disease and translate the exciting science of circadian biology to the clinic.

References

Afonso P, Brissos S, Figueira ML, Paiva T. Schizophrenia patients with predominantly positive symptoms have more disturbed sleep-wake cycles measured by actigraphy. Psychiatry Res. 2011;189(1):62–6.

Alessi CA, Martin JL, Webber AP, Cynthia Kim E, Harker JO, Josephson KR. Randomized, controlled trial of a nonpharmacological intervention to improve abnormal sleep/wake patterns in nursing home residents. J Am Geriatr Soc. 2005;53(5):803–10.

Ancoli-Israel S, Gehrman P, Martin JL, Shochat T, Marler M, Corey-Bloom J, et al. Increased light exposure consolidates sleep and strengthens circadian rhythms in severe Alzheimer's disease patients. Behav Sleep Med. 2003;1(1):22–36.

Antunes LC, Levandovski R, Dantas G, Caumo W, Hidalgo MP. Obesity and shift work: chronobiological aspects. Nutr Res Rev. 2010;23(1):155–68.

Aoki H, Ozeki Y, Yamada N. Hypersensitivity of melatonin suppression in response to light in patients with delayed sleep phase syndrome. Chronobiol Int. 2001;18(2):263–71.

Auger RR, Burgess HJ, Dierkhising RA, Sharma RG, Slocumb NL. Light exposure among adolescents with delayed sleep phase disorder: a prospective cohort study. Chronobiol Int. 2011;28(10):911–20.

Auger RR, Burgess HJ, Emens JS, Deriy LV, Thomas SM, Sharkey KM. Clinical Practice Guideline for the Treatment of Intrinsic Circadian Rhythm Sleep-Wake Disorders: Advanced Sleep-Wake Phase Disorder (ASWPD), Delayed Sleep-Wake Phase Disorder (DSWPD), Non-24-Hour Sleep-Wake Rhythm Disorder (N24SWD), and Irregular Sleep-Wake Rhythm Disorder (ISWRD). An update for 2015: an American Academy of Sleep Medicine Clinical Practice Guideline. J Clin Sleep Med. 2015;11(10):1199–236.

Ayalon L, Borodkin K, Dishon L, Kanety H, Dagan Y. Circadian rhythm sleep disorders following mild traumatic brain injury. Neurology. 2007;68(14):1136–40.

Boivin DB, James FO. Circadian adaptation to night-shift work by judicious light and darkness exposure. J Biol Rhythm. 2002;17(6):556–67.

Borodkin K, Ayalon L, Kanety H, Dagan Y. Dysregulation of circadian rhythms following prolactin-secreting pituitary microadenoma. Chronobiol Int. 2005;22(1):145–56.

Boulos Z, Campbell SS, Lewy AJ, Terman M, Dijk DJ, Eastman CI. Light treatment for sleep disorders: consensus report. VII. Jet lag. J Biol Rhythm. 1995;10(2):167–76.

Bromundt V, Koster M, Georgiev-Kill A, Opwis K, Wirz-Justice A, Stoppe G, et al. Sleep-wake cycles and cognitive functioning in schizophrenia. Br J Psychiatry. 2011;198(4):269–76.

Brown DL, Feskanich D, Sanchez BN, Rexrode KM, Schernhammer ES, Lisabeth LD. Rotating night shift work and the risk of ischemic stroke. Am J Epidemiol. 2009;169(11):1370–7.

Burgess HJ, Crowley SJ, Gazda CJ, Fogg LF, Eastman CI. Preflight adjustment to eastward travel: 3 days of advancing sleep with and without morning bright light. J Biol Rhythm. 2003;18(4):318–28.

Burgess HJ, Revell VL, Molina TA, Eastman CI. Human phase response curves to three days of daily melatonin: 0.5 mg versus 3.0 mg. J Clin Endocrinol Metab. 2010;95(7):3325–31.

Burkhart K, Phelps JR. Amber lenses to block blue light and improve sleep: a randomized trial. Chronobiol Int. 2009;26(8):1602–12.

Campbell SS, Dawson D, Anderson MW. Alleviation of sleep maintenance insomnia with timed exposure to bright light. J Am Geriatr Soc. 1993;41(8):829–36.

Canton JL, Smith MR, Choi HS, Eastman CI. Phase delaying the human circadian clock with a single light pulse and moderate delay of the sleep/dark episode: no influence of iris color. J Circadian Rhythms. 2009;7:8.

Cermakian N, Lamont EW, Boudreau P, Boivin DB. Circadian clock gene expression in brain regions of Alzheimer's disease patients and control subjects. J Biol Rhythm. 2011;26(2):160–70.

Colligan MJ, Rosa RR. Shiftwork effects on social and family life. Occup Med. 1990;5(2):315–22.

Cortesi F, Giannotti F, Ivanenko A, Johnson K. Sleep in children with autistic spectrum disorder. Sleep Med. 2010;11(7):659–64.

Crowley SJ, Eastman CI. Phase advancing human circadian rhythms with morning bright light, afternoon melatonin, and gradually shifted sleep: can we reduce morning bright-light duration? Sleep Med. 2015;16(2):288–97.

Czeisler CA, Walsh JK, Roth T, Hughes RJ, Wright KP, Kingsbury L, et al. Modafinil for excessive sleepiness associated with shift-work sleep disorder. N Engl J Med. 2005;353(5):476–86.

Czeisler CA, Walsh JK, Wesnes KA, Arora S, Roth T. Armodafinil for treatment of excessive sleepiness associated with shift work disorder: a randomized controlled study. Mayo Clin Proc. 2009;84(11):958–72.

Dai J, Swaab DF, Van der Vliet J, Buijs RM. Postmortem tracing reveals the organization of hypothalamic projections of the suprachiasmatic nucleus in the human brain. J Comp Neurol. 1998;400(1):87–102.

DelRosso LM, Hoque R, James S, Gonzalez-Toledo E, Chesson AL Jr. Sleep-wake pattern following gunshot suprachiasmatic damage. J Clin Sleep Med. 2014;10(4):443–5.

Drake CL, Roehrs T, Richardson G, Walsh JK, Roth T. Shift work sleep disorder: prevalence and consequences beyond that of symptomatic day workers. Sleep. 2004;27(8):1453–62.

Drake C, Gumenyuk V, Roth T, Howard R. Effects of armodafinil on simulated driving and alertness in shift work disorder. Sleep. 2014;37(12):1987–94.

Drake CL, Belcher R, Howard R, Roth T, Levin AM, Gumenyuk V. Length polymorphism in the period 3 gene is associated with sleepiness and maladaptive circadian phase in night-shift workers. J Sleep Res. 2015;24(3):254–61.

Ebisawa T, Uchiyama M, Kajimura N, Mishima K, Kamei Y, Katoh M, et al. Association of structural polymorphisms in the human period3 gene with delayed sleep phase syndrome. EMBO Rep. 2001;2(4):342–6.

Flynn-Evans EE, Tabandeh H, Skene DJ, Lockley SW. Circadian rhythm disorders and melatonin production in 127 blind women with and without light perception. J Biol Rhythm. 2014;29(3):215–24.

Flynn-Evans EE, Shekleton JA, Miller B, Epstein LJ, Kirsch D, Brogna LA, et al. Circadian phase and phase angle disorders in primary insomnia. Sleep. 2017;40(12) https://doi.org/10.1093/sleep/zsx163.

Gooley JJ, Lu J, Chou TC, Scammell TE, Saper CB. Melanopsin in cells of origin of the retinohypothalamic tract. Nat Neurosci. 2001;4(12):1165.

Gradisar M, Dohnt H, Gardner G, Paine S, Starkey K, Menne A, et al. A randomized controlled trial of cognitive-behavior therapy plus bright light therapy for adolescent delayed sleep phase disorder. Sleep. 2011;34(12):1671–80.

Guilleminault C, McCann CC, Quera-Salva M, Cetel M. Light therapy as treatment of dyschronosis in brain impaired children. Eur J Pediatr. 1993;152(9):754–9.

Gumenyuk V, Belcher R, Drake CL, Roth T. Differential sleep, sleepiness, and neurophysiology in the insomnia phenotypes of shift work disorder. Sleep. 2015;38(1):119–26.

Harma MI, Hakola T, Akerstedt T, Laitinen JT. Age and adjustment to night work. Occup Environ Med. 1994;51(8):568–73.

Hart CL, Ward AS, Haney M, Foltin RW. Zolpidem-related effects on performance and mood during simulated night-shift work. Exp Clin Psychopharmacol. 2003;11(4):259–68.

Hayakawa T, Uchiyama M, Kamei Y, Shibui K, Tagaya H, Asada T, et al. Clinical analyses of sighted patients with non-24-hour sleep-wake syndrome: a study of 57 consecutively diagnosed cases. Sleep. 2005;28(8):945–52.

Heikkila E, Hatonen TH, Telakivi T, Laakso ML, Heiskala H, Salmi T, et al. Circadian rhythm studies in neuronal ceroid-lipofuscinosis (NCL). Am J Med Genet. 1995;57(2):229–34.

ICSD-3. The international classification of sleep disorders: diagnostic and coding manual. 2nd ed. Darien, IL: American Academy of Sleep Medicine; 2014.

Jan JE, Espezel H, Appleton RE. The treatment of sleep disorders with melatonin. Dev Med Child Neurol. 1994;36(2):97–107.

Jones CR, Campbell SS, Zone SE, Cooper F, DeSano A, Murphy PJ, et al. Familial advanced sleep-phase syndrome: a short-period circadian rhythm variant in humans. Nat Med. 1999;5(9): 1062–5.

Kitamura S, Hida A, Enomoto M, Watanabe M, Katayose Y, Nozaki K, et al. Intrinsic circadian period of sighted patients with circadian rhythm sleep disorder, free-running type. Biol Psychiatry. 2013;73(1):63–9.

Lack L, Wright H. The effect of evening bright light in delaying the circadian rhythms and lengthening the sleep of early morning awakening insomniacs. Sleep. 1993;16(5):436–43.

Lack L, Wright H, Kemp K, Gibbon S. The treatment of early-morning awakening insomnia with 2 evenings of bright light. Sleep. 2005;28(5):616–23.

Lamont EW, James FO, Boivin DB, Cermakian N. From circadian clock gene expression to pathologies. Sleep Med. 2007;8(6):547–56.

Lewy AJ, Sack RL. The dim light melatonin onset as a marker for circadian phase position. Chronobiol Int. 1989;6(1):93–102.

Lewy AJ, Bauer VK, Hasler BP, Kendall AR, Pires ML, Sack RL. Capturing the circadian rhythms of free-running blind people with 0.5 mg melatonin. Brain Res. 2001;918(1–2):96–100.

McCurry SM, Gibbons LE, Logsdon RG, Vitiello MV, Teri L. Nighttime insomnia treatment and education for Alzheimer's disease: a randomized, controlled trial. J Am Geriatr Soc. 2005;53(5): 793–802.

Mundey K, Benloucif S, Harsanyi K, Dubocovich ML, Zee PC. Phase-dependent treatment of delayed sleep phase syndrome with melatonin. Sleep. 2005;28(10):1271–8.

Nagoshi E, Saini C, Bauer C, Laroche T, Naef F, Schibler U. Circadian gene expression in individual fibroblasts: cell-autonomous and self-sustained oscillators pass time to daughter cells. Cell. 2004;119(5):693–705.

Nagtegaal JE, Kerkhof GA, Smits MG, Swart AC, Van Der Meer YG. Delayed sleep phase syndrome: a placebo-controlled cross-over study on the effects of melatonin administered five hours before the individual dim light melatonin onset. J Sleep Res. 1998;7(2):135–43.

Okawa M, Nanami T, Wada S, Shimizu T, Hishikawa Y, Sasaki H, et al. Four congenitally blind children with circadian sleep-wake rhythm disorder. Sleep. 1987;10(2):101–10.

Okawa M, Mishima K, Hishikawa Y, Hozumi S, Hori H, Takahashi K. Circadian rhythm disorders in sleep-waking and body temperature in elderly patients with dementia and their treatment. Sleep. 1991;14(6):478–85.

Paine SJ, Fink J, Gander PH, Warman GR. Identifying advanced and delayed sleep phase disorders in the general population: a national survey of New Zealand adults. Chronobiol Int. 2014;31(5): 627–36.

Pan A, Schernhammer ES, Sun Q, Hu FB. Rotating night shift work and risk of type 2 diabetes: two prospective cohort studies in women. PLoS Med. 2011;8(12):e1001141.

Petrie K, Dawson AG, Thompson L, Brook R. A double-blind trial of melatonin as a treatment for jet lag in international cabin crew. Biol Psychiatry. 1993;33(7):526–30.

Pillar G, Shahar E, Peled N, Ravid S, Lavie P, Etzioni A. Melatonin improves sleep-wake patterns in psychomotor retarded children. Pediatr Neurol. 2000;23(3):225–8.

Potocki L, Glaze D, Tan DX, Park SS, Kashork CD, Shaffer LG, et al. Circadian rhythm abnormalities of melatonin in Smith-Magenis syndrome. J Med Genet. 2000;37(6):428–33.

Reid KJ, Chang AM, Dubocovich ML, Turek FW, Takahashi JS, Zee PC. Familial advanced sleep phase syndrome. Arch Neurol. 2001;58(7):1089–94.

Riemersma-van der Lek RF, Swaab DF, Twisk J, Hol EM, Hoogendijk WJ, Van Someren EJ. Effect of bright light and melatonin on cognitive and noncognitive function in elderly residents of group care facilities: a randomized controlled trial. JAMA. 2008;299(22):2642–55.

Rosenthal NE, Joseph-Vanderpool JR, Levendosky AA, Johnston SH, Allen R, Kelly KA, et al. Phase-shifting effects of bright morning light as treatment for delayed sleep phase syndrome. Sleep. 1990;13(4):354–61.

Sack RL, Brandes RW, Kendall AR, Lewy AJ. Entrainment of free-running circadian rhythms by melatonin in blind people. N Engl J Med. 2000;343(15):1070–7.

Saxvig IW, Wilhelmsen-Langeland A, Pallesen S, Vedaa O, Nordhus IH, Bjorvatn B. A randomized controlled trial with bright light and melatonin for delayed sleep phase disorder: effects on subjective and objective sleep. Chronobiol Int. 2014;31(1):72–86.

Schernhammer ES, Laden F, Speizer FE, Willett WC, Hunter DJ, Kawachi I, et al. Rotating night shifts and risk of breast cancer in women participating in the nurses' health study. J Natl Cancer Inst. 2001;93(20):1563–8.

Schweitzer PK, Randazzo AC, Stone K, Erman M, Walsh JK. Laboratory and field studies of naps and caffeine as practical countermeasures for sleep-wake problems associated with night work. Sleep. 2006;29(1):39–50.

Serfaty M, Kennell-Webb S, Warner J, Blizard R, Raven P. Double blind randomised placebo controlled trial of low dose melatonin for sleep disorders in dementia. Int J Geriatr Psychiatry. 2002;17(12):1120–7.

Shamir E, Laudon M, Barak Y, Anis Y, Rotenberg V, Elizur A, et al. Melatonin improves sleep quality of patients with chronic schizophrenia. J Clin Psychiatry. 2000;61(5):373–7.

Sharkey KM, Eastman CI. Melatonin phase shifts human circadian rhythms in a placebo-controlled simulated night-work study. Am J Physiol Regul Integr Comp Physiol. 2002;282(2):R454–63.

Singer C, Tractenberg RE, Kaye J, Schafer K, Gamst A, Grundman M, et al. A multicenter, placebo-controlled trial of melatonin for sleep disturbance in Alzheimer's disease. Sleep. 2003;26(7):893–901.

Smith MR, Fogg LF, Eastman CI. A compromise circadian phase position for permanent night work improves mood, fatigue, and performance. Sleep. 2009;32(11):1481–9.

St Hilaire MA, Gooley JJ, Khalsa SB, Kronauer RE, Czeisler CA, Lockley SW. Human phase response curve to a 1 h pulse of bright white light. J Physiol. 2012;590(13):3035–45.

Stephan FK, Zucker I. Circadian rhythms in drinking behavior and locomotor activity of rats are eliminated by hypothalamic lesions. Proc Natl Acad Sci U S A. 1972;69(6):1583–6.

Suhner A, Schlagenhauf P, Hofer I, Johnson R, Tschopp A, Steffen R. Effectiveness and tolerability of melatonin and zolpidem for the alleviation of jet lag. Aviat Space Environ Med. 2001;72(7): 638–46.

Takaesu Y, Komada Y, Inoue Y. Melatonin profile and its relation to circadian rhythm sleep disorders in Angelman syndrome patients. Sleep Med. 2012;13(9):1164–70.

The Medical Letter. Tasimelteon (Hetlioz) for non-24-hour sleep-wake disorder. Med Lett Drugs Ther. 2014;56(1441):34–5.

Toh KL, Jones CR, He Y, Eide EJ, Hinz WA, Virshup DM, et al. An hPer2 phosphorylation site mutation in familial advanced sleep phase syndrome. Science. 2001;291(5506):1040–3.

Tranah GJ, Blackwell T, Stone KL, Ancoli-Israel S, Paudel ML, Ensrud KE, et al. Circadian activity rhythms and risk of incident dementia and mild cognitive impairment in older women. Ann Neurol. 2011;70(5):722–32.

van Diepen HC, Ramkisoensing A, Peirson SN, Foster RG, Meijer JH. Irradiance encoding in the suprachiasmatic nuclei by rod and cone photoreceptors. FASEB J. 2013;27(10):4204–12.

Wang JL, Lim AS, Chiang WY, Hsieh WH, Lo MT, Schneider JA, et al. Suprachiasmatic neuron numbers and rest-activity circadian rhythms in older humans. Ann Neurol. 2015;78(2):317–22.

Wilhelmsen-Langeland A, Saxvig IW, Pallesen S, Nordhus IH, Vedaa O, Lundervold AJ, et al. A randomized controlled trial with bright light and melatonin for the treatment of delayed sleep phase disorder: effects on subjective and objective sleepiness and cognitive function. J Biol Rhythm. 2013;28(5):306–21.

Witting W, Kwa IH, Eikelenboom P, Mirmiran M, Swaab DF. Alterations in the circadian rest-activity rhythm in aging and Alzheimer's disease. Biol Psychiatry. 1990;27(6):563–72.

Xu Y, Padiath QS, Shapiro RE, Jones CR, Wu SC, Saigoh N, et al. Functional consequences of a CKIdelta mutation causing familial advanced sleep phase syndrome. Nature. 2005;434(7033): 640–4.

Zavada A, Gordijn MC, Beersma DG, Daan S, Roenneberg T. Comparison of the Munich chronotype questionnaire with the Horne-Ostberg's morningness-eveningness score. Chronobiol Int. 2005;22(2):267–78.

Zee PC. Melantonin for the treatment of advanced sleep phase disorder. Sleep. 2008;31(7):923. author reply 5

Zee PC, Vitiello MV. Circadian rhythm sleep disorder: irregular sleep wake rhythm type. Sleep Med Clin. 2009;4(2):213–8.

MIX
Papier aus verantwortungsvollen Quellen
Paper from responsible sources
FSC® C105338

If you have any concerns about our products,
you can contact us on
ProductSafety@springernature.com

In case Publisher is established outside the EU,
the EU authorized representative is:
Springer Nature Customer Service Center GmbH
Europaplatz 3, 69115 Heidelberg, Germany

Printed by Libri Plureos GmbH
in Hamburg, Germany